THE POWER OF BIRTH

STORIES TO EDUCATE, INSPIRE AND EMPOWER

GABRIELLE TARGETT

i

Published by Gabrielle Targett

Fremantle, WA 6162 Australia

Email: alabouroflovecentre@gmail.com

Cover design and photo: Gabrielle Targett

Photo permission Hayley Flemming

National Library of Australia
Cataloguing-in-publication data

ISBN: 9 780975 781845

1st edition November 2022

ALSO, BY GABRIELLE TARGETT

A Labour of Love – a guide to natural childbirth without fear

A Labour of Love II – Empowering through knowledge to create the birth you want and desire

Empowered Birth –A guide to Natural Childbirth Without fear

Birth Your Way – Empowering through knowledge to create the birth you want and desire

CONTENTS

Praise for Gabrielle Targett and The Power of Birth

I really wanted to share my birth story with you so you can share it with Mum's to be in this book, to empower and inspire them. When I read, you're a Labour of Love books, attended your childbirth sessions, listen daily to your hypnosis scripts, and positive birth stories it really helped me get into a positive mindset, and being emotionally ready. I cannot thank you enough for what you gave to me in that respect - it really is priceless :) What I now know is just how important it is for women to share their positive and powerful birth stories which highlight how women enjoy their births and really love the experience – as I came to do as well. However, I must admit I did doubt somewhat where they were coming from a little, but once I experienced my own birth, which was orgasmic, I totally got it and agree with them just how amazing, powerful and joyful giving birth can be.

Vicky 2021

This book is a must-read for women wanting to gain knowledge from women's innate wisdom and experiences of birth. It is a timely and gentle reminder about women's ability to birth, which helps women to have complete confidence in their bodies and to be fearless about the natural process of birth. In a no-holds-barred book jam-packed full of so many different experiences, one cannot help but be inspired.

Janet Thompson 2021

This book shares blissful natural births of new mothers totally focused and connected with successful outcomes, through to women who chose to have a medical induction with a powerful positive vaginal birth, to those that choose to birth breech babies naturally. I can't recommend this book highly enough as it just had so many great stories in it. This book truly is a wake-up call for birthing women of the world to understand birth and how powerful it can be.

Sara Jacobs 2020

I love this birthing book and Gabrielle's ability to deliver a gentle message of 'anything is possible if you just surrender, trust and empower yourself' and prepare yourself properly mentally, is testament to her 25 years of experience as a Doula and Childbirth educator, helping thousands of women/couples to birth their babies in an empowered way. Gabrielle attended many of the births in this book which highlights and captures the essence of her dedication to assisting women and her innate ability to educate, empower and teach her client everything they need to know to birth naturally. After reading Gaby's book, it is difficult to imagine that anyone would choose a medicalised hospital birth with a looming obstetric cascade of intervention (except in the cases of clear complications or emergency) A must read if you really want to feel into what birth is really about!

Mary-Jane Dodd

DEDICATION

For the wonderful women and their partners who have graciously gifted me their stories so they can be shared with the world, to inspire educate and empower others.

Deepest thankyou also to the many women and couples I have had the privilege of working with during pregnancy, labour, birth. You have taught me more than you will ever know, enabling me to bring these stories together based on what I have observed and learnt over my 25 years as a doula.

Thank you also to Hayley, my friend, soul sister and inspiration, pictured on the front cover. I witnessed you birth in the most empowered, open and honest way.

I feel so honored and humble having been able to be at so many births, witness the grace and beauty of women fully empowered as they bring forward their baby/s into the world.

Birth Your Way in Love Not Fear – because it is the only way!

Gabrielle x

ABOUT THE AUTHOR

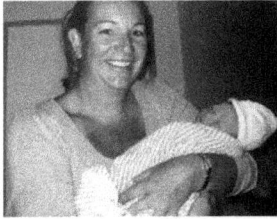

Gabrielle has been a doula witnessing the power of birth for over 25 years assisting over 450 couples bring babies into the world.

Her greatest achievement and inspiration came from her own three beautiful water births in 1995, 1997 and 1999. After the birth of her son in 1997, she was first asked to attend a birth as a support person. It was at this time she fell in love with the idea of supporting women in labour and assisting in empowering women.

It was at this time she realised the need for more childbirth education that was positive and empowering and trained as a childbirth educator and in Hypnobirthing practitioner.

Within three years Gabrielle realised the importance of the work she was doing as a doula (birth support person) and the impact it had on women and their birthing outcomes. It was at that point that she decided to document the births she was attending and write a book from her experiences of what really worked for women to create the birth they really wanted.

In 2004 Gabrielle's first book A Labour of love- a guide to natural childbirth was published and sold Australia wide. A year later Gabrielle was asked to write for the Australian Pregnancy and Birth Magazine and became an expert consultant and writer for the magazine.

A natural progression from training couples in childbirth education was to train more doulas as the demand and popularity was growing. In 2003 Gabrielle ran the first doula training course in Western Australia.

In 2005, Gabrielle launched her business, A Labour of Love, and became a well-respected speaker and presenter and many birth related conferences around Australia, all for the purpose and goal of empowering, educating and inspiring both birth workers and pregnant women to trust and believe in natural birth again.

INTRODUCTION

I dedicate this book to all the wonderful women and partners who have given me permission to share their most intimate and beautiful labour stories with you, the reader. Over the last 25 years I have had the privilege of working with thousands of pregnant women who attended my childbirth educational workshops, fitness classes, or came and had a massage or hypnosis session with me. Many of whom have kindly offered me their story.

Some of the birth stories in this book I attended as a support person (doula), and many stories are from women who just wanted to share their positive and inspiring story with others. This book is a collection of both. I cannot express enough the gratitude and love I have for all who have contributed and allowed me to offer these stories to you the reader, thank you.

I hope you gain as much enjoyment from reading this collaboration as I have in bringing them together to dissolve the epidemic of fear around birth, and show how labour can be enjoyable, empowering, positive and most importantly the most selfless, loving act a woman can do!

My wish for you...

Just as our ancestors once provided the next generation with valuable knowledge, we (the women who believe and trust in natural birth) can share our knowledge, wisdom and insight with one another for the betterment of childbirth.

It is this loving connection, attachment, caring and sharing that we have sorely missed in our society and within our communities for some time now.

My aim is to empower women to trust and believe in themselves and the power of their bodies in natural birth. Help women tune into the strength they have within, that they may not even know that they possess. Assist them to create, celebrate and prepare for birth as it was intended to be celebrated - as 'a labour of love'. May you go forth and create your beautiful labour filled with love, confidence and self-belief.

Love your way,

Gabrielle

How it all
Began – My Story

The waters off the coast of WA were warmed by autumn sunshine as heavily pregnant, I slipped into the ocean for my regular afternoon swim. At 24 years of age I was a swimming instructor and university student, studying Physical Education.

Paddling from my boat across the shallow waters of Australind WA, I could see the bobbing heads of my familiar `cheer squad'.

The pod of dolphins who had befriended me in early pregnancy had been greeting me with increasing enthusiasm as my rounded tummy grew.

But on April 18th, 1995 – the day before the expected arrival of my first baby, the dolphins were more playful and exuberant than ever, surrounding me as they jumped out of the water and performing tumble turns as they swam underneath me.

It was as though they sensed the baby was on its way.

I had recently returned from Japan where I'd been working as an Outdoor Education instructor to children and teaching baby swimming classes at the Pony Swimming Club just outside of Tokyo in Koshigaya prefecture.

Throughout my pregnancy they'd become more attracted to me – swimming past and being playful in a loving sort of way, for hours at a time.

But on this day they swam really close to my tummy, clicking and buzzing and making deep eye contact as if they were picking up on the baby inside me with their sonar.

I'd never seen them so frisky and playful – it was as if they were celebrating something.

The over-the-top antics of the excitable pod seemed to be telling me something!

After a full-on swim that lasted over an hour, I returned to the beach with my partner Jerome, aware of the growing twinges in my tummy.

Convinced now the dolphins were alerting me to my imminent labour beginnings, I returned home where I jumped into bed for a good night's sleep, only to be awoken with my membranes breaking at 4 am. By 4.32 that afternoon I had given birth to a healthy water-baby.

My little girl, Jaeosha, was born in a giant tub in Woodside hospital in Fremantle, Western Australia, with the assistance of a private midwife named Mary Murphy– almost swimming her way into the world.

I'd planned to have a water baby from the time I attended a lecture in Japan by European obstetrician Michel Odent, who was pioneering water births overseas. His videos of water births were amazing and inspiring.

My decision was compounded after meeting Estelle Myers, who had won the United Nations Media Peace Prize for her research into dolphin interactions with pregnant mums and water babies at New Zealand's Dolphin Research Centre.

Back in Australia - even before meeting my partner Jerome in 1993 - I had tracked down progressive WA midwife Mary Murphy, who was assisting women to birth babies in water.

She must have thought I was mad because I didn't even have a partner then, let alone a pregnancy!

Now on this long-awaited day, Mary Murphy was with me at my home as I laboured away. She was right by my side as we arrived at the Woodside hospital for my first water birth experience.

Although I'd really wanted to have a natural home water birth, I'd agreed to have my first baby in hospital. This was because I have a genetic blood clotting problem, and we were unsure whether this was going to present as an issue during birth. It turned out not to be a problem at all.

While blood plasma was on standby, it was not necessary as the birth was over in a matter of hours and was trouble free.

But because water births were illegal in WA hospitals, I needed special written permission to have my baby born under the water in a giant water tub.

Jaeosha's birth was permitted in this hospital because I was taking one of the most experienced Independent Water Birth Midwives in Western Australia with me. However, in other hospitals accidental water births are written up as an accident – for insurance purposes.

Jaeosha's birth was no accident!

News of Jaeosha's birth soon reached Japan - firing the imaginations of a Japanese film crew who travelled down-under to make a documentary on the little Aussie water baby.

They were intrigued to discover a child who had interacted with dolphins in utero....who was born into water, and within months was out swimming with dolphins.

At just four months old, tiny Jaeosha was filmed with her mum at Monkey Mia, being inspected by a pod of inquisitive dolphins.

News of the birth became a talking point at my pregnancy-specific Aqua-fitness classes where pregnant mums were also intrigued.

I'd been teaching at Fremantle Leisure Centre from the time I was two months pregnant. I kept fit for my own births through teaching pregnancy Aqua–fitness classes and general fitness classes, as well as participating in yoga.

Other women in my classes who had not had such positive birth experiences, or who had undergone caesareans, were very interested to hear about my natural water birth.

With mild pain, no stitches and a quick recovery, I explained to them how the water had been calming during labour and the birth was no more painful than a Chinese burn!

I told them about the dolphin interactions I had in Japan and here in WA, where I swam with my girlfriend Rowena while dolphins played around us.

I described how once we relaxed - and the dolphins began to trust us, and us them - I remember the feeling of complete peace, harmony and calmness as the dolphins played under us, spinning around and over us. On the odd occasion if they felt happy and very playful, they would make giant donut bubbles that burst on our tummies.

Another time a dolphin swam up and put its beak on my hand and looked me straight in the eye. It was the most magical and special moment.

Now, my water baby was learning to swim with dolphins! In 1997 and 1999 I welcomed two more water babies, sons Jarrad, and Benjamin!

Because my first birth was so straight forward, Jarrad and Benjamin were born in water tubs at home, and Mary was my midwife again. It seemed like the most logical thing to do as I laboured so quickly and with ease.

At the ages of two and then four years, Jaeosha watched her little brothers being born at home, which was a wonderful experience for her too.

By now, my girlfriend Amanda - who had been attending my classes - announced her second pregnancy.

Amanda had a caesarean delivery the first time, and after hearing about my births she decided she wanted to experience a natural water birth.

I agreed to support her along with another wonderful and experienced Midwife.

On the day she went into labour my son Benjamin slept in his baby capsule next to the tub as I supported her. Watching her birth her baby girl at home in a tub of water was one of the most exciting events of my life.

Thrilled to have shared the precious experience, I was asked to attend three more births that year.

I wasn't a midwife. And it took ten births and a year later before a midwife told me that what I did had a name.

I was told "You are a doula" - a woman who supports another woman in pregnancy, labour, and birth; whose role was recognized in traditional cultures. The Aboriginals called them 'Chalali', the Japanese 'Josanpu' and in other cultures they were referred to as the 'Monitrice'.

Loving my new work, I went on to train as an Independent Childbirth Educator, gaining an advanced certificate through the National Association of Childbirth Educators.

But my doula work with labouring mums revealed new issues which I spoke publicly about.

I realised I was seeing a biased, medicalised approach to birthing, where women were continually disempowered within a hospital system which offered few options for the enjoyment of natural birthing. I began lobbying the WA government to legalise natural water births in all hospitals. In 2010 Waterbirth in Western Australia was finally permitted in hospitals.

I began keeping notes – my journal being a reminder of the positive birth experiences I'd shared and experienced myself.

Today, 25 years on, those notes have been turned into a book called A Labour of Love - a guide to natural childbirth without fear, and new edition Empowered birth, inspired by Grantly Dick Read, one of the leading educators back in 1943. This modern-day book has since taken the world by storm, empowering, inspiring, and educating women everywhere.

A Labour of Love - an Australian guide to natural childbirth was originally self-published until overwhelming demand led Fremantle Arts Centre Press to re-publish it with the endorsement of the Australian College of Midwives.

From my own experience, along with being privileged to share in others' births, I know birthing can be calm, enjoyable and empowering. I have since launched my own hypnosis for birth scripts on itunes. The 'Hypnosis for birth scripts' were created to get into the minds of women to assist them to think and feel positively about their imminent labour journey. Listening to Hypnosis for birth scripts is one of the most positive forms of mental preparation a woman can be doing leading up to her labour, day or night.

Over the last 25 years I have been teaching independent Couples childbirth education classes, where women and their partner can learn vital 'hands-on skills for labour' and learn how to 'surrender' and 'breathe' into the labour sensations and contractions. This is the key to labouring.

I also published my second book in this time - A Labour of Love II – empowering through knowledge to create the birth you want and desire – a 618-page book power packed with fundamental ideas, pregnancy preparation tips, labour/birth suggestions and stories.

My business and website alabouroflove.com.au is aimed at helping women feel empowered and excited about birth once again, so that women and couples treasure their childbirth experience forever.

My family of water babies are always excited about the prospect of making a splash back in the natural habitat of wild dolphins who witnessed them swim before their first birthdays.

Not surprisingly, they have a natural affinity with the water. Jaeosha, Jarrad and Benjamin all swam before they could walk. Their full birth stories can be read in the beginning of A Labour of Love- a guide to natural childbirth without fear, and chapter three of this book.

1.

POSITIVE EMPOWERED FIRST-BIRTH STORIES

My first beautiful, natural, intimate, vaginal birth

As all mums do, I prepared for the arrival of my first baby, however I did it in a way that was different to lots of other mums. I didn't read all the normal books, go on the forums, watch births or listen to horrible birth stories. My husband and I decided to educate ourselves on what our rights were as parents and ensure that we had the birth that we wanted, and not what the doctors wanted. I read books like, A Labour of Love and Well-Adjusted Babies and learnt about the effects of drugs and managed labours. My husband and I did Gaby's couples birthing class and learnt a lot about what to expect during the labour process, how to manage the pain drug-free, what pressures would be put on us from the medical staff and how we could counter that. By the end of the class we both felt very much empowered and ready to have the birth that we desired. I used Gaby's Hypnosis for Birthing audio, listening to that daily in the last 3 months of my pregnancy.

I had a fantastic pregnancy and really enjoyed being pregnant. I had a lot of energy and felt great throughout. I was still able to run at 38 weeks! I am a runner, so it wasn't something new I had recently taken up.

On the 1st January 2017 my husband and I were at the Twenty-Twenty cricket at the WACA. I was 38 weeks pregnant and did a short 1km run to get to the WACA as we had to park quite far away and were running a bit late!! During the game I was feeling a little uncomfortable. I thought that was just because I was sitting down in a small space on an uncomfortable chair.

We got home from the cricket at 11pm and at 1am my waters broke spontaneously!! Luckily, it didn't happen whilst I was at the cricket!! My contractions started straight away, however they were not too painful and were well spread out. I laboured at home for the next few hours, trying to sleep but was unsettled as I felt like I had to keep going to the toilet. I used the fitball, a shower, massage and a bath to help with my contractions. At 6am we called the hospital to say that my waters had broken, and at 7am I left to go to the hospital to be checked. On the way to the hospital, we had to stop via the petrol station, as we had no fuel!

When they checked me at the hospital, I was 4cm dilated and was told to stay and get ready to give birth to my baby. My husband and I had written up a birth plan with Gaby's help, which included things like the natural pain relief options I wanted to use, as well as my desire to have a vaginal birth and physiological third stage for the birth of my placenta. We gave that to the staff when we were moved into our birthing suite. They agreed with most of what we asked for but were not keen on us birthing the placenta without syntocinon. My husband just let it go at that stage and figured he would deal with that when we came to it. My husband set the room as we had discussed, closed the curtains, dimmed the lights and lit our diffuser with clary sage, frankincense and peppermint.

I had asked not to be on the foetal monitor so throughout the labour they used a handheld Doppler to monitor me and only once did I have to go on the foetal monitor. I had my earphones in with Gaby's Hypnosis for Birth script playing for most of the labour. It felt like she was right there with me. We had asked that they speak to my husband and not me so as not to interrupt my hypnotic state. I laboured beautifully and calmly for the next few hours, using the fitball or sitting facing backwards on a chair. I changed positions regularly and received massage on my lower back from my husband and used the shower. I found it easy to be at ease with my oils burning and the hypnosis scripts playing in my ears. I breathed through the contractions and stayed in my zone. The contractions were getting stronger, and I guess closer together, although I don't really remember. The midwife checked to see how dilated I was however I didn't want to know. I was seven centimetres.

I began pushing as I thought I was ready to and spent the next two hours tiring myself out with ineffective pushing! I was getting really tired as no movement was happening from the baby. I took my earphones out and got out of my zone for about 40 minutes. I remember saying to my husband, "I can't do this anymore, I need some help, I'm not doing it right". My husband was amazing throughout the whole labour. The midwife asked if I wanted gas and my husband told her very firmly that NO I DIDN'T!! I was like, maybe I do!! Will it help? Since I was pushing, I felt that I wasn't doing it right as nothing was happening. I said I needed a rest and my husband said it was fine. He put my earphones back in my ears and I got back into my hypnotic zone. So, there I sat, squatting on the floor, leaning up against my husband for about 30 minutes just resting. I found this position very comfortable. The midwife was worried that I couldn't stay in that position as it would tire my legs out. Yet I found it very comfortable, and my husband assured her I was fine.

After what felt like a long time our doctor came in. We got on very well with our doctor - he really worked with what we wanted throughout the whole pregnancy and birth. This made us really happy. The doctor gave me some clear instructions on what I was to do which was to take a big breath in, hold it and then push as hard as I could four times with only a short breath in between each push. I had forgotten about these instructions; Gaby had suggested the same thing for when it came time to push. Once I had some clear instructions and something to focus on, I got back on track and began to feel the baby move. This was an amazing feeling. I was positive again and continued to focus on holding my breath and pushing.

I was lying on my back on the bed at this stage, as that is what the doctor had suggested. However, I didn't want to do this, instead preferring to give birth in an upright position. Once I ended up there, I just went with it. The pushing was intense but so encouraging as I could feel the baby coming. I was so tired but feeling my baby move was enough to keep me going. I changed position to lie on my side as my back was hurting from lying on it. My husband kept encouraging me and said that he could see the baby's head. I reached down and felt the baby's head, and this gave me a boost to keep pushing. I knew our baby would be out soon. The Doctor said that he needed to do a small episiotomy, one stitch to help prevent me from tearing as it was very tight down there. I felt the baby crown and at that stage, I let go and realised that I was birthing this baby! Our rascal of a child had managed to put one arm around his neck, which is why I was having trouble pushing him out. The midwife had to get in there and move his arm down from around his neck. As she did this, he put his other arm up around his neck, so again she did some manoeuvring and moved his arm. My husband caught our son as I did the final push to birth him. We delayed the cord clamping and my husband cut the cord.

He was placed immediately on my bare chest. Holding him in my arms and seeing my husband's face was the most precious thing I have ever seen. I was so tired and exhausted but elated and at peace, all at the same time. I put him on my breast, and he began to suckle. It was such a precious time with the three of us there sharing the moment. My husband had convinced our doctor to take a long walk whilst I birthed the placenta naturally. The doctor would rather have given me syntocinon. It took about 30 minutes, and the placenta came out without any interference.

One of my affirmations throughout my pregnancy was, 'I will have a beautiful, natural, intimate, vaginal birth' and that is exactly what I had. It was such an amazing journey going through the birthing process, and something that I treasure and feel very privileged to have experienced.

Allie's Empowered Natural Birth of Harper Ann Adamson

It took Ben and I 16 months to fall pregnant, and as this was our first pregnancy it was a blessing that throughout the entire pregnancy I was 'low risk' and felt great. I worked until

37 weeks and exercised throughout its entirety. However, my estimated date of August 3rd came and went and each day past made me increasingly anxious. Her head was very low, and she was in an optimal foetal position but did not want to grace us with her presence (I blame the bad Perth winter weather!). I was aware that often first baby arrives 'later' than expected but I had my family from the USA arriving two days after my estimated date in the forefront of my mind and I did not want them to miss out on meeting their first grandchild. I became increasingly impatient and uncomfortable and started to emotionally melt down that Harper had not yet arrived.

I became negative and started to lose the confidence and calmness that I had built up in anticipation of labour. I had three acupuncture appointments to try and get things moving, and the day I went into labour had an Induction massage booked with Gaby (that is always the way isn't it!?). I had done all the "tips and tricks" to bring labour on (exercise, intercourse, certain foods, acupressure, raspberry leaf tea, Chinese herbal medicine…) to no avail but I now realise that babies come when they are ready, full stop!

At my 41-week antenatal appointment at Fiona Stanley hospital, an induction (at 40 + 10 days) and stretch and sweep (at 40 + 7 days) was discussed. I had envisioned going into labour naturally throughout the entire pregnancy and the thought of potentially being forced into the 'cascade of intervention' by induction I simply would not accept. This also meant that if I was induced, my family may miss out on meeting Harper before travelling back to the States as inductions could take a couple of days. After this appointment I was quite upset so my family and I went for a big walk around the Claremont Quarter shopping mall to keep trying to stimulate labour. It was rainy and stormy that day in Perth.

Fortunately, at 2am that night (at 40 + 6 days), I woke up to the howling wind and rain and a strong sensation in my abdomen. This was unlike any other 'period like pains' that I had been feeling in the couple of weeks prior as it was prolonged and intense.

The sensation came again 4 minutes later, and I knew that something was happening. I told my husband (already woken up by the storm) that I knew this baby was going to come today! My contractions came on strong and regular from 2am ranging from 4-6 minutes apart and lasting from 30-60 seconds each (I highly recommend the contraction timer app for partners!). I tried to rest for one or two hours but then decided to use the tens machine. I did labour in bed for a bit longer, tried to eat and drink something and put together a few last-minute things in my hospital bag.

I was able to carry on a conversation with Ben at this stage but felt quite uncomfortable. Eventually I moved to use a fitball in the shower at home as the sensations became stronger. Being over the ball in the shower felt great and Ben was helping me to stay hydrated and nourished with food during this time. We ended up labouring at home for 10 hours before going to Fiona Stanley Hospital around midday. I believe that the midwives were a bit hesitant to tell us to come as they would not admit us unless I was at 4 centimetres. However, I was unable to concentrate on anything at this point apart from labour, so I knew it was time to go and this was established labour (I had not yet felt my waters break or have a bloody show though).

Once we arrived at FSH the walk to the birthing suite was a tough one. We had to pause several times and I think I nearly gripped Ben's hand off! I overheard the midwives talking about how busy they were that day, and I could see why - there appeared to be a full waiting room and agency staff everywhere to accommodate the high demand. In the assessment room, I was again advised that if I was not 4 centimetres, we would be sent home or sent for a walk around the Hospital to try and progress a bit more. After a urinalysis, blood pressure and listening to the baby's heart rate, to the midwife's surprise my internal exam showed that I was a GOOD 4 -5 centimetres dilated! However, the birthing suite was so busy we were still sent for a walk! Ben mentioned we wanted to use the bathtub at this stage as we wanted to have a waterbirth, however the midwife advised us that this was not an option on this day as there were not the staff to accommodate us. I only had a half of a second to feel disappointed because of being in established labour. I moved on from this idea as I knew I could still enjoy the shower in the birthing suite.

We went for a walk around the main level of FSH and it was borderline unbearable. I did not like the feeling of being stared at by people and I did not feel relaxed at all and quickly started to lose the ability to focus, breathe rhythmically and calmly through each contraction. We lasted 45 minutes before I said to Ben that I wanted to be admitted and use the shower straight away. After another hour of waiting on the ward in another busy waiting room, we were finally taken through around 2pm. Straight away I used the shower and fit-ball and stayed on all fours over the fitball in the shower for the rest of my labour, which ended up being about 3 hour).

My waters broke in the shower and the poor midwife (Beck- she was lovely!) was drenched! I was making very primal noises during this time and suddenly felt the urge to push or poo which I shouted out at Beck. I also asked to try the gas for a few contractions, so she brought me the portable machine (I think this was my transition period because I felt like I was reaching the end of my tether). The gas was only mildly helpful and once I felt like I needed to push, I did not use it anymore.

When it came time to push around 4pm, another midwife entered the room and I started to birth my baby's head while I stood in the shower. After a period of time being coached through pushing and listening to my body, the midwives advised me that her head had not progressed further through the birth canal, and they wanted to move me from the shower to the bed to push the rest of her out. I had to walk with half of her head birthed from the shower to the bed which was incredibly uncomfortable, but by the time I made it onto the bed, with the next contraction on all 4's the rest of her head came out! With one final contraction and push, her body was born, and she was passed through to me.

Harper Ann was born at 5:22pm. Unfortunately, I had a 3rd degree tear which required immediate attention and suturing as I was bleeding. Syntocinon was given and out the window went my physiological third stage, birthing the placenta with no drugs or interventions. I did however keep the placenta to eat frozen and raw - to give me a lift emotionally and energetically.

Our birth of Harper was a beautiful experience and I feel like it has been my biggest achievement in life to this day. What I learned the most from our birthing experience is that whilst our "birth plan" did not unfold 100% the way we envisioned it, feeling knowledgeable, equipped, staying strong mentally throughout labour, trusting and letting go had a profound effect on allowing my body to do what it is designed to do - to birth her naturally!

I attended Gaby's aqua classes throughout my pregnancy, as well as read "A Labour of Love II" and my husband Ben and I attended Gaby's couples birthing workshop. I feel like these really prepped us mentally, emotionally, and physically for creating an empowered, positive and natural birth. Ben and I went into labour confident and informed, which helped me to relax and be present to embrace each contraction as one step closer to meeting our little girl.

The three things I want to say to all ladies who are expecting their first child are:

1. Before I fell pregnant, I was 54kgs and Harper was born at 8.3 pounds- I encourage all women to trust that regardless of your size, your body can birth a baby naturally!

2. Gaby's couples birthing workshop was an invaluable experience for Ben and I. Since birthing Harper, Ben has admitted that he maybe did 5% of things that we discussed him doing to support me during labour (ha-ha!) but I have no regrets just knowing that he felt confident in the birthing process, and equipped to be my advocate if need be. He was amazingly emotionally strong, brave and present throughout.

3. If your "birth plan" does not go exactly how you envisioned it (in our case we did not have a water birth or physiological third stage for the placenta birth), the important thing is to focus on the fact that you did indeed BIRTH A BABY regardless of how he or she entered the world. And that is huge and something to be proud of! Born 9 August 2017, 8.3lbs 51cms at Fiona Stanley Hospital - 40 weeks + 6 days.

Celine's Empowered First Birth

Giving birth to my son was the most amazing, crazy and intense thing I have ever experienced. It was perfect, beautiful and transformative. I simply surprised myself. A part of me wasn't sure that I had what it took to keep the focus within, trust and surrender to the intensity, to have a natural birth (based on the assumption that the baby was well and healthy). The thought of giving birth naturally triggered me to feel so positive and helped to dissolve any 'Self-doubt' that arose. I had an amazing birth team, and with the yoga and meditation I had done over the years, I felt prepared to keep my mind out of the way and let nature take over. My baby and I were blessed to have had a natural birth.

I was big, slow moving but still quite active. Nine days passed from my estimated date and I felt great. However my relatives and partner started worrying. The hospital staff wanted to induce me but I was dead set against it; the baby was fine, it was moving and kicking as usual, and its heartbeat was perfect at every monitoring. I also wanted to experience a natural birth and was against forcing the baby to come out through induction, risking a cascade of interventions. So with the support of my doula I stayed strong and grounded. And I kept reassuring Mum that this baby had no choice but to come out, and if all was well inside why force things?

Nonetheless, the social pressure got to me. I decided to compromise and get an induction massage. The massage was very nurturing and at the same time confronting. Pressure points were being held down and it hurt like hell! But this was only a taste of what was to come....the following day I lost my mucus plug, and 24hrs later I had my first contraction. I had just jumped in bed and felt the very first wave of contractions. I got excited and hugged my partner real tight and we talked about how our life was going to turn upside down and we couldn't wait to meet Bub. The contractions stopped, and I fell asleep.

The next day the contractions came back from 9am and stayed with me until Bub came.

The first part of labour was relaxing and very enjoyable. I stayed at home the whole day, gardening a bit and attempting to make jam (for the first time ever?!) while a close friend visited. I was chatty, happy and relaxed and we took note of the space between my contractions. I was having them every 5 min and they were short. It was so amazing to share this moment with my girlfriend - so much love, excitement, happiness, knowing that this was it.

She left in the afternoon and at about 6pm I asked my partner to take me to the beach for a walk. It was so amazing. I felt my heart being completely open, the sunset was stunning, the full moon was rising, there was hardly any wind, and we were walking gently holding hands. Our last walk, just the two of us... I felt so much gratitude for everything.

Then I suddenly begged him to run and get the car! No, the baby wasn't coming (yet) but my bowels had to empty! I knew that this was a sign that my body was preparing, and that baby would come tonight.

Once home we had dinner with my step kids, but I wasn't concentrating on what was going on...I was quiet and very much connected to what I was feeling. The contractions were changing, they were intense and strong enough to take all my attention. I tried to go to bed but the discomfort was worse lying down. So once everyone retired to their room, I went to the lounge. I instinctively dimmed the lights, lit candles and played my birthing music. Changing the atmosphere helped me focus even more on my body. It must have been around 9pm.

I started breathing deeply, making sounds while breathing out and rolling my hips slowly. It felt so natural that I couldn't stop. The circular movements were so relaxing and connecting that I started to go into à trance, and it helped me to manage the surges and the pain in my back that seemed to be getting more and more intense.

But eventually the pain in my back became unbearable. Never have I experienced something like this. I started panicking because nothing that I was doing was easing the pain and I felt totally out of control. Fear took over me and I could feel every single cell in my body panicking. So, I called my doula. I felt that it was time to have her next to me because for sure the baby was coming soon. But to my surprise, she advised me to relax as much as possible, to try to rest, have some sleep, that I was doing great but there was still time before the baby would be born... I was shocked, so shocked that I didn't say anything and simply hung up. Relax?? Try to sleep? Have a bath?? Didn't she understand how much PAIN I was in? She simply said to call her back if the contractions were getting stronger after the bath.

I felt angry, abandoned and helpless. I had tried everything I knew to ease my state, but was yet to try the bath, so I did. I followed her advice and once again was taken by surprise! The pain eased off as soon as I got in and I even fell asleep. What she had suggested was exactly what I needed. It allowed me to have a break for a little bit, to fully prepare myself energetically for what was coming ahead and to rest. I must have slept for an hour. When I woke up the contractions had eased a bit. But they soon returned not long after when I left the bathroom. This time they were stronger than before. The pain in my lower back was excruciating and I started to think about death, that I was going to die...it felt all too much.

I called her back, my contractions were every minute and I was starting to lose awareness of my surroundings. My partner, who went to bed after dinner to be fresh for the active part of labour, got woken up by my moaning noises. I believe it was around 1am.

Before my doula arrived I spent my time on the toilet, emptying myself. Me who feared public pooping during labour got reassured instantly. There would be nothing left by the time we would arrive at the hospital!

My doula arrived not long after. I heard her voice and recognised her gentle perfume. I was on my knees resting my head on the couch and she started pressing on my hips during each contraction. The surges were amazing in their power, in their overwhelming nature. I cried, moaned deeply, shouted and screamed into the couch, and the more they passed the less aware of my surroundings I became.

Everything went so quick from that point on. My awareness changed, I had a need to focus deeply inside, to stay with the breath and to make as much sound as I felt for each contraction. I could hear Matthew saying, "we need to go, she's ready" and my doula would say, "no, not yet we need to wait a bit longer". The contractions were getting more and more intense, and I could feel how the time in between to recuperate was shortening.

I don't see myself as someone who can handle pain very well. I'm far from being a sportsperson, I hated any sports requiring endurance and stamina as a kid and never stretched myself physically as an adult. This part worried me while preparing for the birth because I kept reading how physical strength and being used to physical pain through any cardio work for instance will help birthing tremendously... well I'm not sure how I managed but I found a way to just stay connected with the breath and hold on to the last piece of rational thinking I had which was "this is going to end, and I will meet my baby soon" and somehow went with it.

The surges were very intense, uncomfortable and debilitating which makes me understand why they are referred to as being painful. However, surges are more complex than pain. The body is so beautifully designed that we are not left just with raw pain and bones opening up, but we also have amazing endorphins going through our blood which is a key point to handle "surge pains". I was so out of it that it helped me to fully let go and let my body run the show. I was so connected inwardly that I didn't really know what was going on around me. I hardly opened my eyes during the whole labour and time became warped. I was totally oblivious.

I was also fortunate not to know how dilated I was and therefore had no hard facts interrupting the zone I was in. This I believe helped me to put the ego aside and to keep trusting in my body's intelligence.

Once we arrived at the hospital after several massive contractions in the car, in front of the hospital main entrance and in the lift, I was astonished to find out after having a vaginal examination that I was fully dilated and that I didn't have time to jump in the pool!

It is true that once the cervix is completely opened, a new stage of labour begins. This is when I felt like pushing. At each surge I pushed down, once the surge passed, it felt like I was floating in space. My body would feel numb for an instant, I could only hear my breathing slowing down. I felt still, thoughtless, and it seemed that even the room got quiet. Then the next surge would come in and I'd hear everything again - the midwives, my partner, my doula.

At this stage, I was on the floor, on my knees resting against the bed pushing down. I was advised to bring the breath down at each exhalation. It was working, I could feel the baby's head making its way down my birth canal and into my vagina. I sensed the will and resilience of its soul, it wanted to come out and was making the most of each contraction too. We were working together.

Suddenly I felt wet on my legs and I heard the midwives saying that my water had broken. I turned my head around and saw this brown liquid over my legs and feet. It was explained to me that the baby had poo-ed and that it does happen sometimes and that it was time for the baby to come out. At the next surge I refocused and pushed as far down as I could. Then my partner, very excited, told me that he could see the baby's head coming down. My doula asked me if I wanted to feel it but I refused... I didn't want to feel how stretched out and open I was! I kept pushing down, kept pushing down and suddenly hit rock bottom. It didn't feel like I was making any progress, the baby didn't feel that it was coming down anymore. It felt stuck and I started to feel frustrated. I shared this with my doula, and she reassured me that I was doing great and that everything was going well but I felt so far from the end at that moment.

After a few more surges and focusing the breath further down (I reached the core of the Earth at that stage!) I suddenly felt a painful burning sensation!

"What is this???" I ask myself! Oh no! That's right, I'd forgotten about the crowning stage, the ring of fire! How could I have forgotten this?!

This part of the labour was the hardest for me. I was exhausted and although I was so close to the end, I felt miles away from it. It felt like I had finally reached the top of Everest only to realise that I had another valley to cross before climbing the last part of the mountain! The pain scared me also. My doula suggested a new breathing technique where I was doing "horse mouth" sounds while breathing out between my lips. I'm not sure whether it helped me or not, but I took her advice on board because I desperately needed something new to help me through this. Each surge increased the burning and I felt I was going to tear apart. My doula spoke softly into my ear telling me that I had to trust my body, that most first-time women birthing get scared at that stage and that I just needed to trust in my body.

So, I did, I visualised my vagina opening up, I spoke to it to tell it to open up, I even prayed and called on all my ancestors, guardian angels, spirits of all my girlfriends who knew that I was in labour and to assist me to OPEN UP! I really felt that I needed as much help as possible because deep down I wanted to give up, my stamina was running out and for the first time since labour started, I was doubting that I would be able to birth my baby naturally.

I started to hear in the background the midwives saying that the baby had to come soon because of the poo in my waters. They were concerned that the baby might get distressed, and wanted it to come out now, otherwise they would need to intervene. This freaked me out even more but was a blessing at the same time as it gave me a boost of stamina. I realised that I had to give all that I had now or all the amazing work I had done so far may eventuate into some medical intervention.

So I focused again, started pushing and prayed at the same time. I hoped for each surge to be the last one. But nothing... then the midwives said you have three surges before we intervene. Out of complete frustration I decided to change position. All that time I had been on my knees on the floor. I climbed up the bed, rested my head on the elevated pillow, had one knee bent and one knee down and at the next surge, the baby slipped out of me. Yesssss! We did it! What a relief. It was over, my baby was on my chest looking at me. HE was beautiful, I was in love instantly and I felt so proud, so proud of us two. My

Lenny ended up coming 12 days overdue, was 52 cm and 3.77kg and was perfectly healthy.

Half an hour later the contractions returned and in three surges I birthed the placenta which was like the icing on the cake! So warm, squishy and enjoyable. A great way to end such an intense journey.

A couple of days later, I was back at home, it was Mother's Day. Friends and family were there, and I suddenly felt really overwhelmed. Once everyone had left, I couldn't stop crying. A part of me was grieving the end of my pregnancy, the fact that I will never feel Lenny moving inside my belly again. It was such an odd feeling to experience, having him in the flesh in my arms but it was how I felt in that moment. This is when I decided to cut up my placenta. I had kept it to cut it in cubes and freeze, to take as a vitamin boost during my recovery.

I went into the kitchen and silently started cutting the placenta in little cubes. I was crying while doing it. It took me a good fifteen mins to do it all and this was such a therapeutic moment for me. No one could have understood what was happening for me, I could barely understand my own emotions! But it felt so nurturing to do so. I was honouring the end of a chapter and welcoming the new one all at once. Once I was done, I felt lighter and went back to the lounge to give the biggest cuddle to my little man. What a beautiful journey we had together.

Tanya's Birth of Olivia

It was only a mere five months ago but memories of my pregnancy, labour and birth have already been clouded by so many new memories, thoughts and experiences; a whole series of firsts.

As I sit here watching my little one roll and squirm after her toys on the mat I can't believe five months have already flown by!

My pregnancy, all forty weeks and 6 days, was relatively trouble-free. After my husband's shocked reaction at five weeks when we learned we were finally pregnant, and a short hospital-stay at 13 weeks for a retroverted uterus which blocked my bladder and caused significant fluid retention, everything went smoothly.

A few months into my pregnancy I found it challenging to keep up with the exercise classes I loved and had been attending routinely, so I sought an alternative. It was at this time that I met Gaby, when I joined her Aqua classes from 14 weeks. I loved these sessions. Not only was it a safe and effective method of exercise, but a great opportunity to meet other expectant mums, many of whom were 'first-timers' like myself. However, what I valued the most were the little 'nuggets' I would find I would leave each class with. Gaby has such a wealth of knowledge, and these sessions proved to be one of my main sources of education regarding pregnancy and labour.

I am so thankful I found these classes and met Gaby because what I learned from her, and later from the stories I read while editing this book, I used to build my understanding of what was available to me, what rights and choices I had as well as the possible consequences of the decisions my husband and I would make. Ultimately, I became informed and empowered as I reflected on the journey I wished to take with the remainder of my own pregnancy and labour. So despite being booked into a private hospital, and somewhat blindly choosing an obstetrician, I was confident in my pursuit of a natural birth.

As the weeks went by I attended all the standard tests and checks, each as perfectly boring and uneventful as the last. I continued to take care of myself, seeing Gaby for a massage, resting where possible and watching my diet. I did however enjoy the opportunity to indulge my cravings for 'naughty' foods each time I went food shopping; lamingtons here, donuts there... I attended Gaby's aqua classes at least once a week, if not twice, as well as her fit ball classes on a Saturday morning. Together with exercises at home I was conscious of doing my best to ensure my baby was in an optimal foetal position as the due date approached. Getting comfortable in bed became more difficult and I would snore ridiculously loudly at times, often waking myself up! Sleep was regularly interrupted with trips to the toilet.

With the due date fast approaching, I ensured my bags were packed, the OB had a copy of our birth plan and that my husband was schooled on my wishes. To his credit, although my husband's state of shock lasted the whole nine months, he stepped up when it counted. After attending Gaby's birth education class we discussed our options at length and somewhat surprisingly were on the same page. Furthermore, my OB was very supportive of our wishes. All of us were striving for a natural birth; one without intervention, all being well.

In the final few weeks some mucus and blood would pass. Each trip to the toilet I'd begin to wonder, "Is this it?" "Is this the beginning of labour?" At this stage, I never wanted to travel too far from home 'just in case'. However, any pain I experienced wasn't regular or particularly intense.

By this stage, visits to the OB were weekly and despite putting on approximately 20kgs, my blood pressure and protein count etc remained fine. Bubs appeared to be in a good position, just not fully engaged yet. I would book my next appointment not knowing if it would be necessary, but bubs proved to be perfectly content, and the due date came and went.

Naturally each day would be peppered with text messages and phone calls from concerned family 'checking in'. I continued to assure them that no news meant nothing to report. If indeed I was in labour they would know soon enough.

On Thursday evening, at 40 weeks and four days, I began to experience what I thought were contractions. Dinner was interrupted as I paced around the living room. My husband began timing as I rocked on a fit ball. Now that it seemed imminent, my husband rang the hospital to get their advice as to when to come in. We were advised to stay home for as long as possible.

I was unable to sleep and by 2am I woke my husband as the 'contractions' became closer together and more intense. I really didn't want to go to hospital only to be sent home again, but I was sure (or as sure as I could be) that this was it. With the car loaded we drove to the Emergency department at SJOG Murdoch. Once we were escorted into one of the labour suites, Baby and I were monitored. After about an hour we were informed I was fully effaced but only one centimetre dilated. Were you kidding me? I had to endure hours more of this. The nurse outlined that, in general, dilation occurs 1cm per hour, so with another possible nine hours we would probably be best to go home and rest. However, she was rather confident we would be back later that day.

After returning home about 4am Friday morning, we decided to go to bed and try to get some sleep. Surprisingly I found that I could. When I woke a few hours later I realised my contractions had stopped. We tried to carry on as per normal but by Saturday afternoon I was becoming frustrated. Any contractions were intermittent and passed quickly. To pass the time, distract ourselves and to bring on labour, we went food shopping and for a long walk. If it wasn't going to happen quickly we needed to eat! In the evening we decided to go out to a local Indian restaurant. Perhaps the spices would help! Funnily enough, around 7pm, as we entered the restaurant, I felt the contractions start again.

From then on the contractions were very regular but not as intense. By early afternoon on the Sunday my husband rang the hospital again to see what we should do. The nurse encouraged us to come in again to get checked; after all, what did we have to lose?! After all the checks I found out I was 3-4cm dilated. You mean, after all this time, I wasn't at least 7cm?!? Although disappointed and frustrated I was pleased that I didn't have to go home, even if the birth was still hours away. I took comfort in knowing I was in hospital and had medical professionals close by.

Every four hours my OB would come and monitor me and each time I was only about 1cm further along. My contractions were very regular, but I wouldn't say they grew in intensity. Although, once I agreed to have the OB break my waters, it was harder to breathe through the pain. I used the fit ball for a small period, as well as crouching on all fours on a cushion to get baby to move down and into an optimal position. Most of all I stood and walked slowly around the room. With every contraction I did my best to pause and breathe through it. I found hot showers helped immensely, especially before my waters were broken. I even convinced some of the lovely midwives to heat up a heat-pack so I could use it on my back. Only when the OB came in did I ever willingly lie down on the bed because I found each contraction particularly uncomfortable when lying down. My husband was a terrific support merely just by being present. He would help me shower, rub my back and hold on to me. I found I would just look ahead to the next time the OB was due as a way of getting through.

Although three midwives were present during the day, the final one, Cathy (who happened to be the one that monitored me on the Friday morning) was particularly supportive. She gave us so much of her time and would just stand next to me and remind me to breathe. For some time after the birth, even now if I think about it, I can hear her say, "that's it my love…good girl…just breathe my sweet…" She was so present. Often, she would be chatty and joke, but when she sensed I was having another contraction she would be still, calm and speak softly to me. I couldn't have done it without her either.

Come 10pm, some nine hours after being admitted and 27 hours after my active labour started, the OB visited and said I was 7cm dilated. I was getting closer but still a way off. He said he would be back around 1am (Monday 24th). It didn't look like bubs would come that day. However not long after I felt the need to go to the toilet. Now I knew this was possibly a sign of transition, but I also wondered, 'what if I actually need to go?'. While on the toilet I had an intense contraction and noted that I passed some blood. The nurse assured us that everything was fine, and this was simply a sign that the labour was progressing.

As I walked back into the suite I was reduced to a shuffle because the pain had amped up considerably. If it wasn't the midwife I was holding on to, it was my husband. He was very understanding as I hung off him, screaming in his ear in pain!! The midwife encouraged me to pant; "If you pant, you can't push". Now, if I was only 7cm dilated a short time ago, I thought, [insert swear words here] "I have a long way to go…I have to learn to deal with this pain". Well despite my efforts to pant and not push, I felt things were moving along. Let's be honest, I couldn't help but pant, pant, pant, SCREAM!! I felt pressure bearing down and said (somewhat naïvely), "What's that pain?" to which the midwife replied, "probably the head…after this contraction, we'll get you on the bed and check. You can then push". Well, before we could do that, while standing and screaming blue murder, (heaven help anyone else on the labour ward that night), baby decided it was now ready to arrive.

With my husband on one side and the midwife on the other, and as I stood there half-dressed, hunched over the moveable table, baby shot out, springing into my undies before slamming on to the floor, headfirst. What was my first reaction you ask? Pure relief!! It was like passing a big poo, and after about 28 hours of active labour, I was tired and relieved to not

29

have to breathe through any more contractions! Meanwhile the midwife hadn't realised the baby had come so quickly and my husband wondered what was among all the blood and 'goop' on the floor…oh, just the baby! He quickly scooped it up. Fortunately, seconds later our baby screamed, and we established 'baby' was in fact a girl. I was just so bloody happy for it to be over!! Our baby daughter was swiftly wrapped up, nurses came in to begin cleaning the floor (whoops!!) and the OB was rung. I was finally happy to lie down.

After everything, it could be argued that I birthed my daughter on my own; without help from the midwife or my OB. I really didn't even push…I was actually trying to avoid pushing. I guess it just shows how quickly transition can progress! Safe to say we have a head-strong and determined little girl on our hands!! When the OB did arrive we joked that we might as well put him to work and get him to stitch me up. The speed and force with which she arrived did leave me with a second-degree tear. We also laughed about how we wouldn't tell anyone that the OB wasn't there to deliver the baby nor that my husband wasn't quick enough to 'catch' the baby! Again – whoops, so much for keeping that a secret!

So much for the delayed cord clamping that we wished for as the force of her arrival broke the umbilical cord! However, as requested, we were able to hold our daughter almost straight away. In fact, she fed for about two hours! My husband then enjoyed some skin-to-skin time as I showered with the help of the midwife. Thankfully, there were no ill-effects of her birth and she is now a completely healthy and happy five-month-old. On top of which, we were able to achieve our goal of a vaginal birth without intervention. Our bodies can do amazing things!

Olivia May Ferraro was born at 11:06pm on 27th July 2017 at St John of God, Murdoch. She weighed 3.385kg and was 50cm long.

A Wonderful Experience of Labour

As I sit here and write this birth story, I look over and see my seven-month-old looking back at me with his beautiful big eyes. It is sometimes hard to believe that he grew inside of me and came out of me through a natural vaginal birth. He was a little over ten pounds in weight, rather a big boy out of my rather thin, small-framed body. How the time after you have a baby flies, it really does. I remember women saying to me to really enjoy this short, precious time with your baby, because before you know it they will be toddlers, running about.

Back to the birth. During my pregnancy I travelled along knowing that I would possibly be having a C-section. I thought this because all my friends with babies had had one, so I expected I would also. The only information or understanding I had about birthing came through these main friends of mine. I did have one other friend who told me about a doula who had attended her birth and how this person also ran aqua classes at the pool. With total amazement I learned about the one and only natural birth experience out of all my friends. Somehow a natural birth really started to appeal to me. So when I met Gaby through her antenatal classes at the pool I began to question the possibility of not having a C-section. I felt I was being challenged about my belief systems every time I attended the class at the pool, and the concept, and my belief in my own ability to birth naturally, started to become a reality.

With only six weeks to go before my estimated birth-day, I asked Gaby to attend the birth of our baby. Gaby had been the doula for my friend, who'd had a big healthy boy naturally with no tearing. This intrigued me, and I was reassured that women just like myself can birth in a natural way.

As the last six weeks went by I tried really hard to block out all of the really negative birth stories and outside influences and listen to positive birthing stories only. It was not long before I realised I could birth naturally if I wanted to, as there was nothing really stopping me making that decision. Over the next few weeks I invested my time wisely and tried to prepare myself mentally by learning specific labour/birthing meditations, visualisation and relaxation with Gaby. I also worked at physically preparing myself by attending the deep-water aqua running classes, toning relaxation aqua classes, and pregnancy-specific fitball sessions, all of which helped me to stay toned, aerobically fit and more flexible.

On my due date I went into labour at about four in the morning. At 7 a.m. I rang Gaby to let her know so she could plan her day. She came over for her usual 'check-in' session just to see where I was at and connect with me on various levels to suss out what exactly was going on. Gaby had explained to me that she would not stay for long if it looked like there was nothing really going on. This way I would be free to really go into labour without her watching me and possibly causing what she calls 'performance anxiety'.

As it turned out I'd had a false start, and by 9am my contractions had completely stopped. As Gaby described it, nature had been really kind and had given me a taste of what labour actually feels like, and a little introduction to warm-up labour. As planned, Gaby went home and I just plodded around the house doing a few jobs, trying to sit down and rest when I could. I actually had a reflexology appointment booked at 11am that I was determined to attend, so maybe this is why my labour stopped?

After attending the reflexology session, which really stirred everything up, I went home and jumped into bed to have a cat nap. As I lay there in the bed the contractions became stronger. The time was now 2pm and Gaby arrived to find me half-asleep, moaning in the bed, unsure whether or not to get up or stay put. I decided I needed to get up as the intensity was definitely getting stronger the longer I lay there.

One of my biggest worries was about my waters breaking on the couch, as I thought the smell and mess would ruin it completely. So it came as a complete shock when my waters totally broke on the couch at approximately 2.30 in the afternoon. I guess our thoughts really do create our reality! At that moment I jumped up to run to the bathroom and left a trail of amniotic fluid all the way through the house. As I stood in the shower still more fluid came out of my body. I said to Gaby, 'Geez, how much of this stuff comes out?' I just could not believe how much there was. I was sure that it was at least a bucketful! I left Gaby and my husband to the unenviable task of mopping up, while I stayed in the shower to labour away. Things were happening now and I knew this was the real thing.

After a major clean-up, including the couch - which we all laughed about - Steve assisted me back to the lounge room. I sat on a fitball, then I moved to the bed on my hands and knees. I tried to get comfortable but felt restless so Gaby suggested a walk around the block. It was almost dark at this stage so it didn't bother me to be labouring away outside. I just needed some air. Before Gaby and I headed off I had some rescue remedy, which really helped to keep me calm.

At 10pm we all decided it would be a great idea to head for the hospital as the contractions were really getting strong. The only problem was that one of the worst storms to hit Perth in ten years was occurring as we drove from Fremantle to Mount Lawley, a forty-minute drive. It was an interesting trip to say the least. I laboured away very peacefully, unaware that the water from the Swan River was being thrown over our car, as lightning flashed overhead and the thunder roared. Steve just turned up the Pachelbel's Canon louder to drown out the noise. And I was in labour heaven, oblivious to all of this - well sort of - I was aware but not aware! Steve decided we would call our baby 'Thor', after the god of thunder!

Arriving at the hospital, I got into the shower to warm up and relax a little after our trip. This gave Gaby the chance to fill up the bathtub, which I was dying to get into. All was going well till the lights went out! A complete blackout of the hospital occurred while I was standing in the shower in a small bathroom with the door closed. Thankfully the midwife was able to locate a torch to come and check on us to see if we were fine. I figured it was just as easy to stay put and not move, as I was happy where I was. It did take a good while before the lights came back on, after which we had to put up with alarms going off, bells ringing and all sorts of buzzers for the rest of the night.

Finally, I stepped into the tub. It really was as great as I had heard it would be. Instantly I sank down and relaxed. Gaby talked me through a few meditations whereby I actually slept in between my contractions. I stayed in the tub for four hours (as I learned the next day), and yet it seemed like it was only half an hour. I was really surprised to learn that information.

Birth hormones really do distort the way a woman in labour perceives the time.

After four hours in the tub I started to feel a little urge to push, and wanted to go to the toilet, so I hopped out of the tub. I instantly felt very cold and shivery, so Gaby and Steve raced around to get me some clothes I could throw on, as well as socks to keep my feet warm. After a while I started to feel much warmer, and with the help of more rescue remedy I remained calm and focused.

Gaby had prepared the room by getting a mattress for the floor, with a big bean bag and lots of pillows, and it was here that I continued to labour away. After a period of time labouring and feeling like I wanted to push but couldn't, I opted for a vaginal examination to see what was going on. It was at this stage I found out I had an anterior lip, so I needed to stop pushing and breathe through, to try to assist it to push over and away from the baby. For the next twenty minutes I breathed and panted my way through lots of contractions. It was bloody hard work.

After another internal where the midwife actually flicked the lip away, I was able to start pushing my baby out of my body. It was now that I started to feel the full extent of hormonal activity as I again began to feel restless and wanted to move about in between the contractions — when I squatted holding on to the back of a chair. When each pushing urge was over I would then stand up and walk around the room. I was a woman on a mission, possessed by mother nature. Nothing was going to stand between me and my baby. I was getting pissed off now and demanding to know how much longer, as little by little my baby moulded his head down and through my body. It was hard but rewarding work, as I could start to feel the movement downwards towards mother earth.

The midwife I had at this point had been with me all night and had stayed over her shift to assist me the best way she knew how. She was really brilliant as she honoured me in every way, by accepting Gaby's presence at the birth and reassuring Steve. We were a team effort, all working towards the same goal and purpose. The only time I felt pressure to be doing something the 'right way' or more quickly was when my ob (obstetrician) came into the room demanding to know if the baby really was moving down. As if we had conspired to make up the story! He demanded the midwife be accountable and truthful, and he just looked at Gaby as if to say, 'And who the hell are you?' It was an interesting turnaround in every conceivable way from the wonderful supportive night that I had just had.

The pressure was on me now to get up on the bed, as my ob was not happy with the length of time I had been pushing. Thankfully, when I hopped onto the bed my baby's head was sitting just under my perineum, and so my ob assisted my baby out, trying to prevent a tear to my perineum. Although I was on my back with my legs up I did find this position helped to really push my baby out. Having my feet firmly on someone, pushing, seemed to give me an extra bit of energy and strength.

After sixteen hours of labour I brought into the world the most beautiful big baby boy, who was over ten pounds, with just a little tear and no painkillers at all. All I could think about after the birth was 'I did it, I really did it' and I couldn't wait to tell my friends and family about my wonderful experience. I really felt alive and like I could do anything and handle any situation from that day forward. Thanks to the help of Gaby I achieved the type of birth I set out for, in every way possible. I say never underestimate what the presence of another woman with you at your birth can do.

I truly believe that having Gaby attend our birth allowed me to relax, enjoy and therefore focus on breathing through the contractions and relaxing. As a result of doing this I didn't once feel as though I needed any form of pain relief. Steve was just able to focus on me and the birth and not worry about other issues like what to do or when to say something.

Sean and Sally's Birth Journey

The old adage is true. Go on holiday, relax and you'll come back pregnant. Sean and I were in the last eight weeks of our six-month world tour when I discovered I was pregnant. We bought the test on my twenty-eighth birthday in Oxford, England. After dinner and a movie we sat in a beautiful bed-and-breakfast in shock. Although we wanted children, we thought I would fall pregnant after our holiday. Needless to say we were overjoyed. We continued travelling but came home a couple of weeks early. Our bank balance was suffering and so was I with morning sickness. Sickness that lasted all day and all night.

It was great to be back in Australia after being away for six months. Travelling really showed us we were lucky to live here. With no money it was straight back to work for the both of us. Not so easy when one is vomiting all the time! Luckily I only had to endure that for sixteen weeks.

Through an old work colleague I learned there were aqua-aerobic classes for pregnancy at my local swimming pool. My first lesson was during my fourteenth week of pregnancy and although I still felt very average, the class lifted my spirits and made me feel great. It was the relaxation, being towed around the pool by another person, that had me hooked. In fact this was the first time I had actually relaxed since Sean and I had returned from overseas.

At the classes run by Gaby I found out that she also ran ongoing Active Birth classes, which I started to attend. They opened my eyes to a whole new world in which I met other women who - like me - wanted to know about birth and had little idea of what to expect. Even though I was myself a nurse and I had attended many births previously, you really do see the birth process through different eyes when you are the one who is pregnant. Not only did I make some wonderful friends,

39

but I found someone I could trust to support me in bringing my baby into the world in a loving, supportive way.

As my tummy began to swell, I started to think about my birthing options, and Sean and I made the decision to have Gaby as our doula. We thought it would be helpful to have guidance through such a positive life-changing experience and really gave our thoughts lots of time and attention. I am a good organiser and wanted to be really well-prepared for the birth-day and not just leave it to the mentality of 'We'll just see what happens on the day'.

I loved being pregnant and loved the way I looked and felt. I have never been one to show off my body but I believed I looked fantastic and was happy to show off my belly to anyone who wanted to see it.

As the birth-day drew nearer I kept in close contact with Gaby, who allayed so many of my fears. Fears of becoming a parent, fear of birth and just the feeling of being plain scared.

I had experienced a couple of antepartum bleeds, which fortunately didn't amount to anything — in fact I found out through talking to lots of other women that they are quite common. On this particular day I thought I was having another one, however this turned out to be my 'show'.

On 26 August I awoke at 6am after a rather unsettled night, to empty my bladder, and experienced my first contraction. So that is what they feel like, I was thinking, and I felt so excited. After hurrying back to the bedroom to tell my partner, I then asked him to open the curtains so we could watch the sun come up together. It was so beautiful being able to experience this moment with just the two of us knowing that on this day we were going to have our baby.

The contractions were three minutes apart from the beginning. I was handling them really well. So well, in fact, that when Gaby arrived at 9 a.m., I said to her, "This feels really great, bring it on!". With that Gaby smiled with an amused look on her face. Gaby was pleased to hear that I was so accepting and enthusiastic about the contractions and later commented to me how wonderful it was to hear a woman talk like this prior to going into more established labour.

Soon after, I was moving about the house from station to station. I had a great position on our bed, leaning over the bean-bag and pillows, then I moved to the shower, followed by the bath, then onto the fitball in the lounge. It was a happening thing. I moved between these stations in between the contractions, really utilising what each station and position had to offer me. This really helped to pass the time and to cope with the intensity. Having Sean and Gaby at my side also made a huge difference as I felt so supported and strong.

By about 2 p.m. we decided it was time to go to the hospital. I was petrified I would have contractions in the car on the way to hospital and no one would be able to assist me in any way. I feel that because of this fear I stopped my labour temporarily on the way to hospital, as I did not have one single contraction in the time it took to get there. Getting out of the car and into the hospital was a whole other matter. As soon as I stepped foot outside of the car I had three contractions in a row, right in front of a group of visitors to the hospital. They disbanded in various directions and disappeared as soon as they could, thank goodness.

It was a long walk to the labour ward and I had to stop many times and lean on Sean, the wall or Gaby to get through the intensity, as they were coming on thick and fast at this point. At this stage I felt the need to start using the visualisations and breathing Gaby had taught me and this really helped me to keep myself and the contractions under control.

The next few hours went past in a blur. I do remember having an internal examination just prior to getting in the shower. An internal was something I really did not want to have, so I had one but requested that I not be told how dilated I was. Thankfully the midwife did not tell me. The next day I actually found out that I was four centimetres at that stage, but it took me less than four hours from then to have my baby.

I found myself giving birth on a mattress on the floor, leaning over a bean bag with pillows on top. It was funny really, as I had always pictured myself semi squatting on the floor, but when the time came this felt just right. With every contraction Sean and Gaby would apply pressure and lots of it to my lower back, which felt fantastic at the time. As the baby came down and started to stretch my perineum I requested a hot flannel down there, which felt wonderful and really took the sting away. I felt like I was screaming at this time but Sean tells me I was reasonably quiet, all things considered.

At one point an anaesthesiologist accidentally walked into our room, and Gaby and Sean called out, "I think you have the wrong room, we don't need you here" and all I was thinking to myself was "Come back, come back, I need you". In the next moment I was telling myself, "No I don't, I'm a strong woman having a baby now". It was like having an angel on one shoulder telling me I can do it and the devil on the other shoulder trying to convince me to have an epidural. The angel triumphed, as it was nearly all over and I was starting to push my baby out of my body.

After just thirty minutes of pushing with Gaby's guidance and support I was able to push my beautiful baby out and into the waiting hands of Sean and the midwife. They then slowly passed my baby through my legs, where I held him skin-to-skin on my chest. I then turned around slowly and sat down so that Sean and I could discover the sex of our baby.

And there he was. Dark blue eyes blinking, staring up at me. His hair darker than I had anticipated, glistening in the light. His perfect hands clasped together. His body moist and soft. Wow, what a moment.

I tried him on my breast but he was more content to be cuddled. I was awash with emotion. Love, glorious love. Amazement. How could two people create this perfect little angel? Thankfulness — he and I were both healthy. Exhaustion — labour is tough, no doubt about it, but you live to tell the story over and over of how wonderful it is — that, I guess, is the irony.

This is the beginning. We knew having a baby would change us forever and it has, for the better. For this reason it was so important to have our baby in a calm, loving and unobtrusive environment. We wanted to start our new life together in the best possible way. We are eternally grateful that our dream and wishes were granted.

The Birth of Vincent

Such a perfect pregnancy, no real hiccups apart from having gestational diabetes and not being able to eat any of those delicious cakes and a big bowl of pasta when I wanted! Then, at thirty-three weeks, I had to start being monitored twice a week, strapped to machines and waiting to see if the baby moved sufficiently enough for the midwives to be happy that he/she was not stressed. This was kind of tiring but really nothing bothered me as I knew deep down that the baby was fine and moved around non-stop. I was still doing Yoga twice a week and Gaby's prenatal aquatic classes once a week. I was totally content with my baby and my body physically generally.

I was due to give birth on the 12th January 2007 but knew I would go into labour early. Bag packed, Christmas came and went, along with New Year with many a comment like; "my goodness you look like you are about to pop". Days went by and then I woke up on Saturday 6th January feeling very chilled out and wanting to potter around in the garden. I went for a swim down at the beach and came home and just really wanted a warm bath to submerge in.

My husband (Carmelo) popped out for a few hours and I was very happy just feet up, reading and flicking around the TV...... then around 4.30pm I started getting a little strange feeling, one that I had never had before, but it seemed ok and I thought it was just one of my many Braxton hicks. Around 4.45pm it happened again but a little more intense this time, and then it went away. I didn't really know I was in labour as it was of course my first experience of anything birth related. This feeling happened twice more, and I started to think that something might be happening. So, I got a pen and paper and started making a note of the time, how long each contraction was and how intense they were, using a scale of 1-10. I could see a pattern forming, shorter time in between and longer contractions which became more intense with the need to lean over and breathe.

At this time the story becomes a little funny.... I called Cam and said to him, "I am not really sure what is happening, but maybe you should think about coming home, and by the way could you grab some food on the way?" When he got home and saw me taking deep breaths and bending over, he started grabbing my stuff and moving towards the door, to which I said, "have a plate of food, it might be nothing", to which he responded, "I think I will have a beer then".... well, the inner mother exploded in me and I told him "what are you thinking".... blah blah blah blah ..... he couldn't believe my change in temperament. At this moment he realised that tonight was the night to get his shit together.

By this time it was around 7pm and the contractions were every five minutes, so I called the hospital (Murdoch) and they said to come in. By the time we got to the door they were every four minutes and lasted for one minute. The lady behind the desk at the front of the hospital said, "are you ok, you look like you are about to have a baby?" to which I replied "I'm not really sure. I may be sent home soon". She then went on to say, "I really don't think so, would you like a wheelchair?"

"A wheelchair? Don't be silly, I will be fine". The very next second I was totally stopped in my tracks and couldn't move with the next contraction. Now Cam was trying to get me in the wheelchair, and I was fighting him off and getting pretty wild.... I eventually gave in as it took us fifteen minutes to get from the hospital front door to the lift!

Straight into the birthing ward I got taken and examined (which I was dreading) but to be honest, it was nothing at all. The nurse said "You are 3cm dilated and your cervix is paper thin. Expect to give birth within a couple of hours, get your clothes off and make yourself at home". I looked up at Cam and just smiled - it was the first time I believed that I was about to give birth. By nine o'clock I was 6cm and was trying many different body movements to try and get as comfortable as possible...... I remember saying to Cam "If the pain stays like this, it's no problem at all". I think he just looked at me in total shock as he had seen me groan and breathe through the contractions every three minutes for the length of one minute. He was quite concerned I was not coping and in too much pain.

It was now around 10pm and yes, the contractions were getting way more intense. I couldn't get comfortable, but I was now 9cm dilated. I tried having a bath, but it just didn't feel right, and it was making the contractions feel way more intense, so I jumped out after five minutes and just made my way back to the bed thinking that I may need some intervention soon, if not straight away! I told Cam and he let the Midwife know. After another examination, I was 10 cm dilated and about to go into the pushing stage of labour - no time for pain relief as I would be giving birth within the hour!

I remember feeling quite relieved and then I just zoned out of everything around me. I was lying on my back, quite happy and relaxed between the contractions. Cam told me I was totally in my own world, doing a semi dance with my hands and swaying between contractions.

The obstetrician was called with what they thought was fifteen minutes to go. After lots of pushing and relaxing and pushing and relaxing, the next thing I remember is hearing the Obstetrician say "You have been pushing for two hours and your baby hasn't moved. You are going to have to move positions to allow the baby to move on through the canal". I was not happy with this and resisted as I felt totally chilled, in my own way, but it did hit me that I was getting very exhausted. I carried on laying there for a while and then a beautiful midwife came over and said "Why don't you just move your knees right up onto your chest and it will tilt your pelvis and I'm sure the baby will move on out".

I was very happy with this advice so with each contraction I pushed my feet into each midwife's hip and soon I could feel the baby crowning. It was an amazing feeling. However, it was another half hour of hard labour pushing before my prize arrived...at 12.45am on 7th January.... and what a prize he was.... a perfect boy of 3.1kg. I was totally exhausted after two and a half hours of pushing but it really didn't matter at that moment as I had him in my arms, the gift of life. I was so very proud of myself and Cam for getting through this experience with such a positive tale to tell, and very happy not to have had any pain relief. I also loved the fact that immediately I could get up and walk and go and have a shower... bit wobbly mind you, but I felt euphoric. Ashley, Carmelo and Vincent Miragliotta.

Hugo's Birth Story

Having Gaby as my doula was one of the best decisions I have ever made in my life (besides getting married and having two children – but even that has its moments!). Anyway, it's true. Let me tell you why.

I moved to Perth from Byron on 7 April 2006. Hugo was due on 19 May. I originally contacted another Perth doula, who was no longer practising. Just as well, as I never would have met Gaby (maybe, we can thank fate regardless). She gave me Gaby's number. Over the next few weeks, I became anxious, as I didn't hear from Gaby, not realising she was away in New Zealand. I felt time was running out and that it might be too late to feel comfortable having her as my doula. After all, you want to feel safe with someone who is going to see you at your best and worst. How wrong I was!

When my partner Justin and I met Gaby, I felt like I had known her all my life. She understood me and was extremely supportive of my decision to have a natural birth. I thought I was a bit of a guru on natural childbirth from all the books I had read. Well, I only had the knowledge. Gaby had this innate wisdom and knowing. Gaby's stories opened my eyes to the world of birth, and to top it off, she had written an amazing book on birth. Gaby gave me the courage to approach natural childbirth without fear. I knew that having Gaby as my doula and having my child naturally was the right choice.

Gaby was also my one-stop shop. Not only had she written an amazing book, but she also gave massages, antenatal classes (much better than the classes through the hospital) and relaxing aqua classes (oh, how I used to look forward to the hot pool, floating in the water to the sounds of the rainforest – it made the pregnancy more bearable!). I also had some very powerful hypno-birthing sessions with Gaby, visualising the birth I wanted and even experiencing my own birth. And boy, did we have some laughs! During one massage I laughed so hard, I thought I was going to have my baby then and there (unfortunately, I didn't!).

I was five days over my estimated due date when the fear started to creep back in. The thought of medical intervention was daunting. Gaby reassured me that my body would be ready soon and that the baby would birth into the world when they were ready and that I wasn't to worry. Medically, I had fourteen days before they could induce me. I was getting impatient and decided to hurry up the process anyway; Chinese herbs, castor oil remedy (which was hideous, but highly recommended for cleaning out the bowels!), curries and sex. Still no baby! Ten days passed, with an appointment to go to the hospital to organise an induction, I was now getting desperate. In the end, I sat on the toilet and prayed. Low and behold, five minutes later while bouncing on the fitball, my waters broke. It was 12pm on 29 May. A 'gush literally!' of excitement came over me. It was game on!

I would have opted for a homebirth but living temporarily with my mother upon arriving in Perth, I didn't feel comfortable, and she didn't have a bath. I had to have a bath, but I wanted to labour at home for as long as possible before going to the bath at the birth centre. When my waters broke, I called Gaby. She offered to come over straight away, but I told her that I was fine and continued bouncing while watching a bad action movie. When the bouncing became too much and the sound of guns was doing my head in, I knew it was time for a change in scenery. Justin and I decided to go for a walk with my towel over my shoulder (a great recommendation from Gaby, as strange as it looks). By the time I returned home, I was finding it very uncomfortable to walk, so I called Gaby who was there in 20 minutes. She was a wonderful comfort. As hard as it was, she encouraged me to stay on the fitball to help open my pelvis (she also knew it was a good distraction from the contractions). Within the hour, my contractions were four minutes apart. I was ready to go to the birth centre. I wanted to get in that bath.

When we arrived at 6pm the bath had just finished being used. The room hadn't been cleaned and another lady had rocked up to the centre also wanting to use the bath. Gaby was amazing. She sprang into action, cleaning up the bathroom and got it ready for me to use. She even bought a large piece of foam to line the bath, so my knees wouldn't get sore. It was complete bliss when I entered the warm water. I instantly relaxed and the intensity of my contractions reduced. I leaned over the side of the bath with my head in my arms and Gaby softly talking to me, while I focused on my breathing. For the next four hours I was lost in the moment. During this time, Gaby and Justin massaged my back with lavender oil, kept me hydrated with plenty of water and cordial, dabbed my head with a cool face cloth and told me what a wonderful job I was doing. I think I was oblivious to all of this at the time, but subconsciously every little bit helped.

Just before 11pm the sensation of contractions suddenly changed to something different. I felt like I had to stand up. Gaby asked me if I felt a bearing down sensation. I think I did. I wasn't quite sure what was going on. I had become so used to the feeling of contractions that this new feeling was weird. It was overpowering. Gaby reassured me that it was nearly time to push. The midwife, Janine, suggested I get out of the bath. The next hour and half of pushing would be the hardest work I have ever done in my life. I tried every position possible – pushing standing up, pushing leaning against Justin, pushing on all fours, and pushing on the birth stool. At one stage, the midwife had to tell Justin to stop pushing! His bright red face made him look like he was about to have the baby! (Unfortunately, that wasn't going to happen).

Justin's small talk analogy of me coming to the finish line at the end of running a big marathon, was meant to be encouraging but fell short of the mark as there was still an hour of pushing (at one point I think he said, "I've decided to go for another lap" - just as well I wasn't really listening). I had done breathing exercises with Gaby for the contractions, but I wasn't prepared for breathing while pushing. The midwife and Gaby told me that if I put as much energy into my pushing as I was my vocals, then the baby would come out. Easier said than done. Finally, Hugo was crowning, but I was having problems getting him past that one point. Gaby suggested looking down into the mirror so I could see how close I was. It was too confusing....focusing on the mirror, pushing, breathing, having a baby....so she took photos instead. That didn't help either, but I'm so glad she took them. Even two years later I can look back at the photos and recite my birth, word for word. What really spurred me into action was when the midwife cheekily slipped the word 'episiotomy'. She knew full well I didn't want one. With that visual clearly in my mind and with every inch of force and breath left in my body I pushed - not twice, but three times - Hugo's head, shoulders and body came into this world.

And boy, what a relief it was! Hugo was born weighing 9.5 pounds at 12:23am on 30th May. I was so exhausted I could barely hold Hugo, but I was so proud that I had laboured naturally for 12 hours and only had a graze.

Straight after the birth Gaby helped attach Hugo to my breast so he could start feeding, as I was almost too weak to hold him. For the next few weeks, she became my angel. She was there for me when I needed advice on feeding, sleeping, immunisation… and also checked up on me to ensure I was looking after my own health

When Hugo was two and half month's old we moved back to Sydney. It was sad saying goodbye to Gaby - she was not only an amazing doula but had become a close friend.

I want to thank you Gaby from the bottom of my heart for helping me bring a beautiful boy into this world. Even as I write this story, it brings tears to my eyes knowing what an amazing person you are and what a wonderful job you do; assisting mothers like myself experience the most beautiful and natural birth possible.

Birth Story of Rawiti Elias Crawford 12th March 2017

We went to bed as usual on Friday night. I later woke up as I thought I was peeing the bed. Then I realised I had no control over it - it was in fact my amniotic fluid pouring out of me as my membranes had just broken. I quickly woke my partner Dylan and he jumped up and grabbed some towels. We were both excited as the anticipation of meeting our baby was close. However, Dylan fell back asleep! I lay awake with a million thoughts running through my head, as well as irregular contractions keeping me up.

I moved to the baby's room which was right next to ours and knelt on the floor with a blanket over me; this position felt comfortable, and I could nap in between contractions. Between now and 5pm Saturday we went into the family birthing centre a couple of times, but I was not dilated much, and they encouraged me to continue back at home. I was happy to continue at home but dreaded the car ride each time, the only comfortable position was kneeling behind the passenger seat with my arms on the back seat. My housemate and good friend Lucy supported me during this time by rubbing my back and giving me sips of water.

At 5pm we went back into the birth centre as my waters had been broken for 18 hours, which meant a cannula and a dose of antibiotics to help stop any infections. By this stage my contractions were gaining strength and were very regular, so we stayed and got comfortable in our room at the birthing centre. I spent much of the time kneeling on a mat on the floor with my arms resting on a bean bag and pillows. My support-team - Dylan, Lucy and the midwife did an amazing job keeping me hydrated, putting cold cloths on my neck and forehead, feeding me nibbles of paleo bars and massaging my lower back.

At 9pm my contractions were very strong, and I got in the shower. It felt amazing spraying the water on my lower stomach and back during contractions. Around 11pm I asked to get into the bath. They did a quick check, and I was 8cm dilated so they filled it up and I was able to hop in soon after. The feeling when I got into the bath was indescribable; it really helped with the contractions and I felt that things were starting to happen. Lucy, Dylan and the midwives all supported me with words of encouragement, sips of water and cold cloths as I pushed through each contraction. I soon felt a strong urge to push so the midwife checked, but I was still only 8cm dilated. She suggested that some gas may help me focus on my breathing rather than pushing, as it was still a bit early. I waited for a while but was finding it hard not to push, so I thought I would try with the gas. I found the gas helpful for me to focus on my breathing but not so much for the pain; I think Dylan found it more useful than I did!

About 15 minutes later I threw the gas and said I needed to push; my body was strongly telling me it was time and I listened. After what felt like a long time pushing the baby was crowning, and I tried to slow down my pushes and follow the directions of my midwife. It was amazing to feel the baby emerging, especially when the midwife told me to reach down to receive him and put him straight on my chest.

At 2.03am on Sunday 12th March 2017 our baby boy Rawiti Elias Crawford was born, weighing 3.9kgs/8.6lbs and measuring 51.5cm in length. The feelings were instant: relief, love, fulfilment and empowerment. As I was losing quite a bit of blood the midwife suggested an injection of oxytocin, which

I said yes to, and the bleeding quickly eased. Soon after, I hopped out of the bath and went back into our room. I lay on the bed, still with Rawiti on my chest. Once the umbilical cord stopped pulsating Dylan cut the cord. I started having contractions again and soon after gave birth to my placenta.

The birth of Rawiti was the most challenging, painful and empowering experience of my life. I would do it all again tomorrow if it meant holding my boy in my arms as it was worth every minute. We were so glad to be able to give birth at the family birthing centre. The midwives were amazing; they are so passionate and provide such great support and guidance. I could not have achieved a natural active birth without my support team and I will forever remember this as a positive and empowering experience.

I'm Kyra Swift and I Had the Most Perfect Natural Birth

Without the knowledge and confidence I gained from Gaby's classes I wouldn't have been so prepared and ready for the birth. THANK YOU GABY!

On the 7th April, 2007 I started having regular Braxton Hicks contractions that were a lot more uncomfortable than normal. They were fifteen minutes apart and lasted over a couple of hours. On the 8th April, my due date, they were eight minutes apart and also lasted a couple of hours. On the 9th April they were six minutes apart.

The Braxton Hicks were always in the late afternoon and stopped when I went to bed. On Monday the 9th April I went to bed as normal and the contractions stopped. I woke up at 2am, Tuesday 10th April to use the bathroom. As I was getting back into bed, I had the sharpest pain in my tummy that made me stand still and hunch forward. I was unsure at first and went back to the toilet thinking I had a stomach-ache. As I sat there it happened again, so I went back to bed. As I was getting into bed, my stomach tightened and it happened again. It felt like really bad period pain that stretched over my tummy, reached a peak then eased off.

I was scared, excited and unsure of what was happening to my body. Were they contractions? Would they go away when I lay down? As it were they didn't, they just got stronger and were so painful I couldn't move. So I decided to wake my husband. We sat there not quite sure of what to do. We decided to time them, to see how close together they were.

The contractions were four minutes apart, so we decided to get ready. I called my mum who was going to be with us through the labour. She came straight over. The contractions were so close I decided to phone the hospital, and because I hadn't felt the baby move, they suggested we make our way there.

The drive to the hospital felt like it took forever. I had no idea how far apart the contractions were. My husband was keeping track while my mum drove, but they felt very close. In between each contraction I would rest my head on the back of the car seat as I was rather exhausted.

We arrived at the hospital around 3.30am, and in between each contraction I walked to the maternity ward. I was taken to a private room where I told the midwife that I didn't want any pain relief, so therefore there was no need to do an internal at that stage. The midwife listened to the baby's heartbeat and everything was fine.

I was then taken to the labour room where another midwife asked if I wanted any pain relief. I told her 'No, I wanted a natural birth.' I asked her not to offer me anything again. As the midwife got the bath ready, I laboured away on my knees, leaning on the lounge or on my husband's knees. When the bath was ready I stripped off and got in. The contractions felt a lot softer at first, but they soon were just as painful. I had no idea how long I was in there for but I soon got too agitated and had to get out.

I went back to the birthing room, labouring on my knees on the floor, leaning on the lounge. I then decided to have an internal examination because I wanted to see if the pain and contractions were getting me anywhere. I had to climb up on the bed for the internal examination. I was 3–4cm dilated. I couldn't stay on the bed as I had lower back pain.

I went back to labouring on my knees, on the floor. My Mum was very supportive, holding the heat pack on my back and taking turns with my husband to rub my back and remind me to breathe. I had a sheet draped over me, which felt great. I felt less exposed as my bottom was in the air.

My contractions were now unbearable, and I felt the need to push, so I decided to have another internal examination. I was 5-6cm dilated and therefore was not able to push. My membranes were bulging which caused that pushing feeling. We decided not to break them as my cervix could retract back down in dilation. We decided the best thing was to wait until they broke naturally or until I was 10cm dilated.

My mother-in-law arrived and I welcomed her in.

I was so frustrated; I wanted to push but wasn't allowed. I was hot and sweaty, but cold at the same time. I couldn't sit still or even get a little bit comfortable between contractions. As each contraction approached, I was saying, "I can't do this anymore", and my husband, mum and mother-in-law were all telling me that I could. They put up with a few nasty comments from me, but they were all there helping and supporting me in so many different ways.

I then got to a point where I couldn't help but push, so I decided for another internal. I was now 10cm dilated and all I wanted was to meet my baby and for the pain to stop. I was now on the bed. My mum and the midwife decided it was now time to break the membranes as the pressure they were causing was unbearable.

When the midwife eventually broke my membranes she informed me that my baby had pooed inside, so then she called in another midwife to monitor my baby's heart rate and get the suction tube ready to clear my baby's airway of any mucus and amniotic fluid. When the membranes were broken I felt instant relief. The bed was soaked, but I didn't have a care in the world. It just felt so good - until the next contraction started. I was still on my back from having the internal, so as soon as I could I turned over onto my hands and knees. With each contraction my lower back burned with pain and I rocked to help ease the sensations of the contractions.

The contractions now had a completely different feel. It wasn't just getting to each peak of the contractions anymore but now my body was making me want to push. I was scared to do so and wanted to cry but couldn't, but instead I laughed. With the support and encouragement from my husband, mum, mother-in law and midwives I was able to start pushing. It was now about 8am.

As soon as I began to push I felt the baby's head moving down. Even though it burned it also felt really good because I knew it wasn't long now, which encouraged me to push for longer during a contraction. As the baby's head was crowning I followed the midwife's instructions on when to push or pant.

The head was then finally out - the only way to describe it was as a pop!

I was exhausted and slumped forward onto the upright bed head. It wasn't long and I was pushing again. As I was pushing the shoulders out, the feeling inside my pelvis was incredible. I felt the shoulders move as I pushed, which was scary but amazing at the same time. Then with a few more moaning and grunting noises from me and one more contraction my beautiful baby boy, Samson Granville Swift, was born at 8.42am. He was 10lb 5oz and 58cm long. Labour was approximately 6hrs and 42mins and I was pushing for 50 minutes.

I felt incredible but really exhausted after the birth, and I'm so proud of myself for not having any pain relief. Samson was so alert when he arrived. As soon as he was on my chest he took to the nipple and sucked for about 15 minutes. I had no grazing or tearing which was such a relief. I prepared my body for the birth and stretched my perineum every second day for about 3 weeks before Samson arrived.

I recommend natural childbirth to everyone that can, and don't be scared!

Christy's Labour and Birth Experience

We had been waiting ten days past our baby's estimated date for our little one to arrive in the world to meet us. This period between the estimated birth-date and the birth-day was really hard for me as everyone we knew was asking us daily if the baby had come yet. I felt this pressure because she was 'overdue' (I hate that word!) and should have been with us - therefore something must have be wrong.

Once my estimated day came my partner had some time off. At first, every day together was a bonus as we love spending time with each other as a couple, even though we were looking forward to meeting our little one. But after a few days, each day felt like – 'here we go again; a new day and still no baby yet' and we were going for yet another big walk, another curry and more......

Another big stress was that I didn't want to be induced. This was the one thing I was dreading all through my pregnancy. But as time came closer, we had to face the fact that I might actually need to be induced if my labour did not begin anytime soon. I then got a booking with the hospital to be induced and I had to come to terms with it.

On Monday 1st October 2007, after a morning at the hospital to monitor the well-being of the baby, I went home to clean the house. Later that evening we had fish and chips at South Beach before going home to watch a DVD. We went to bed late. When I woke up to go to the toilet before midnight I started to feel some strong period pain, but I was not totally sure if labour had started. Anyway, I woke Christy up which was quickly followed by putting the lights on, boiling the kettle for Chamomile tea, spraying lavender in the air and taking rescue remedy drops. Then I began labouring away on the ball. We called the hospital who said we would have plenty of time, but after two hours of intense contractions it was definitely time to go! Christy was timing my contractions and they were one minute and a half or one minute straight from the start. I particularly remember the last three contractions on the way to the hospital as they were really full on. By the time we arrived I was kneeling half on the concrete and half in the car in the hospital's car park, yelling away to the moon as Christy described it.

I could hardly talk to the midwife when she asked something. She told me "You don't have to walk if you have a contraction" so I quickly turned to the first thing I could grab or lean on (a crib) and yelled again. I walked directly to the birthing room instead of the assessment room as suggested by Christy. I remember hearing the midwives saying, 'This sounds promising...' In fact once I was in the birthing room, the midwife did an internal and I was 6 to 7cm dilated. I laboured away on the bed in the recovery position for just over an hour before the midwife asked me to change position. She suggested I go on all fours on the bed for a little bit because the pushing was not really happening. As soon as I got on the birthing stool things progressed really quickly. 50 minutes later, with some good pushing and panting as soon as I felt the burning sensation, Lucia was born.

This stage was amazing for Christy as he sat right behind me, his head locked on my left shoulder by mine. He saw the head crowning and our baby being born, thanks to the mirror the midwife placed on the floor.

With a lot of preparation – physically, mentally and spiritually - I could not have wished for a better birth experience. The midwives were fantastic and respected our birth wishes, but also Christy, my partner, was there each step of the way. Thank you Gaby for your support all the way through my pregnancy, you were a big part of why I had such a good birth experience due to all the preparation you gave me.

Vicky's Birth of Rhys

Little Rhys and I are still figuring each other out, so I am on the computer while he is having a sleep in his swing! He is nine weeks old now and I cannot believe where the time has gone. I cannot express enough how much I am enjoying being a mum. Yes, it's hard but when he looks up at me and has a little smile and a giggle, my heart melts. Garth and I couldn't be happier! Garth has gone back to work so Rhys and I are spending lots of time together, and the days just roll into each other.

I really wanted to share my birthing story with you. When I read Gaby's A Labour of Love books, it really helped me get into a good mindset about being emotionally ready. I always knew I would go into labour with a positive attitude and disregard all the negative words or stories people had shared with me. This was mainly due to spending the time with Gaby, other gals in the pool at Gaby's Aqua classes and listening to Gaby's powerful Hypnosis for Labour scripts.

I cannot thank Gaby enough for what she gave to me in that respect, it really is priceless. Other women that shared their stories in Gaby's books talked about enjoying their births and really loving the experience. I must admit, I did doubt somewhat where they were coming from, but once I experienced my birth I totally agree with them and know it can be a joyful and empowering experience.

The one killer for me was that I experienced back labour: starting whilst at home and lasting through to the transitional phase! Rhys was in a posterior position, so I was an unlucky trouper. Unlucky because I have been blessed with a healthy back throughout my life, so to experience labour intensity in that area was quite full on. However, everything I had learnt and practised helped me through it. If it wasn't for the back pain, I would agree with some of the other ladies in the books; the experience was almost orgasmic!

A rundown of our birth:

A few days before I went into true labour, I had the worst wind! I have always been a 'gassy' person being wheat and gluten intolerant, so I was well in tune with that part of my body. It was quite incredible! I had seen my OB, Hugh, on Thursday (10th) my estimated due date, and he was great. He wasn't in a rush to induce which was wonderful and we made our wishes very clear to him, talking through our birth plan early on which made all the difference. I never felt under any pressure, but we did talk about what would happen if I had to be induced as I wanted to know.

About 1pm in the afternoon on Monday 15th I started to feel a bit out of sorts and had a few period-like twinges (I had had a few of these in the preceding two weeks but just a 'tweak' and then nothing). As Monday went on, I felt quite tired and then later that evening, about 10pm, had a show (then another show at 4am). We went about our business making dinner to-gether and watched some TV before going to bed at about 10pm. By this stage I was having contractions every hour for about four hours and come 12pm they were every half an hour. I contracted in bed holding my lovely husband's hand (he was asleep, as I told him to rest while he could as I was in bed resting between contractions!) By 5am I couldn't stay in bed any longer and the contractions were about 10-15 minutes apart! We got up and Garth made me some food and we watched episodes of 'Will and Grace' and a movie 'Kiss the Girls'! We laboured away together in all sorts of positions that we had practised to see what worked the best - on all fours was great for me! By 1pm the contractions were about 7 minutes apart, but we were going ok.

I called the hospital just to let them know it might not be long, and they were great to encourage us to labour away at home for as long as we could and just keep an eye on the baby's movements. By 2pm I was 5-6 minutes apart and had noticed a slight change in baby's movements, so I called the hospital again and they suggested we head on in as it was time.

We jumped in the prepared car and I had two contractions on the way in and then one outside the hospital waiting for Garth to park the car! I wanted to wait for him and was quite calm, however people around me were not! I was asked about a dozen times in the space of two minutes – "are you ok love?" I replied "Yes, thank you. Just in labour, but all good!" They were all a bit freaked, but I just calmly told them to go about their business!

Garth ran from the car park and we went in. I was thrilled to hear that no one else was birthing so I had access to the bath suite! Yeah! However, I didn't end up using it. It was 2.30pm by this stage. The baby hadn't moved too much, which I mentioned to the midwife, and they said let's just whack on the monitor and have a listen and looksee. They were not in any rush to do a vaginal examination at this point, which was great, so they just let me settle in. The wait to have the monitor popped on was the longest wait of my life and this is when a little fear started to kick in. However, when monitor went on and we could hear a very loud and healthy heartbeat! Bubby wasn't moving and responding the way the midwife was happy with (not too overly concerned but enough to ask if I wanted to check in with our doctor).

I replied "Yes, no worries" and he was called. They spoke over the phone as he was in theatre and said he would pop down when he got out. He popped down and saw the monitor output and then said "Why is she still hooked up?" Before I got off the bed they did a VE and about five minutes later my membranes broke. I came off the monitor for a while and laboured away and then went on a mobile monitor, just to check bubby was going ok. I went in the shower for a while. When I came out I thought 'Wow! It is really getting full on now in my back area', so I opted for some gas just to try and take my mind off it. It worked well for me which was great as I was worried it would make me feel sick. Then at about 8.30pm I really had the urge to push!

We moved through the last phase quite nicely. When they first checked me, I was only 3 cm dilated but they didn't tell me which was great. So I went from about 3cm to 10cm dilation in just under five hours. I was happy with that! Rhys was about to show himself to the world and then decided to turn his little head a bit which made everything slow down, to the point that he did not come out! I had a bit of suction and some good pushes he was out. I had two stitches afterwards and that's it.

Rhys was so alert and came straight onto my chest before looking up at us. We looked at each other and said "We did it!" My husband was a real gem and I really felt like I loved him more after than before. I didn't think that was possible! He was just so supportive and knew exactly what to do before I even asked! He kept chanting waves of bearable intensity and helped me visualise my OB trying to boogie board (as he was going to go on a family beach holiday that weekend)! Hugh is a wonderful man, very tall and slim so imagining him boogie boarding helped me ride my labour waves with a bit of humour!

Also, the midwives were so happy for us; they were thrilled we did it naturally as many women don't at that hospital. And as we were the only ones in there, they all came to see us and visit Rhys after he was born which was lovely! I also was a bit noisy in labour and when I was transitioning I may have sworn a bit. They told me afterwards that they were just giggling at me as I would swear and then say, "I'm sorry. I'm sorry, that was rude!" I didn't really remember that at all!

And here we are, 9 weeks on with little Rhys William! A cutie pie!

An Empowered First Labour using Gaby's Hypnosis Scripts

I just want to say a huge thanks to you Gaby. I feel really lucky that I met you and had some time with you to help me prepare for my birth.

I had a lesson and hypnosis session with Gaby back in 2013 before the birth of our son, Reuben. The information you gave me that day was invaluable. It taught me there is no need to fear childbirth or take any notice of the horror stories many like to offer. I listened to your hypnosis scripts religiously every evening.

My waters broke at 12.30am. I had tested positive for strepB and was told to come straight in when this happened, so we called Murdoch Hospital and headed in there. By the time we arrived, checked in etc it was 3am. I was hooked up to the antibiotics and had blood taken due to my low platelets. The nurse told me to lay up on the bed and get some sleep as it would be hours yet. Ha-ha... She just left the room and the contractions started. I headed straight for the shower and the fitball.

The nurse came back, and I said to her, please don't offer me any drugs, I will ask for them if I need them. She replied, 'We'll see' with a tone as if I couldn't possibly do it without. Well, that just made me more determined. I stayed in the shower for 4.5 hours just thinking of you saying each contraction is just a wave closer to meeting your baby.

Your hypnosis script was playing on repeat in the background. It was painful but the time flew by. It got to the point where the pain was so bad, I felt like I was going to vomit so my husband helped me out onto the floor and a new nurse asked if I would like to be checked. I was 9.5cm! I started

71

pushing in a squatting position on the bed. My husband and I still joke how uncanny it was that you seemed to be dictating our labour as you were in sync on the cd talking me through 'bearing down' etc at the exact same stage we were at.

Bub's heart rate started to drop so our Ob asked me to flip over onto my back for the final pushes, and she did give me an episiotomy which unfortunately took a very long time to heal. But overall, we had the most amazing birth experience. I knew how I wanted it to go and was open to the fact anything can happen on the day. I feel truly blessed that we were able to have the natural birth I'd hoped for and I absolutely believe that the sense of calm that came over me from the time my waters broke through to holding him in my arms was thanks to the tools you had given me. I cannot thank you enough. Carlee.

Our Birth Story is Indeed an Amazing One, Full of Little Miracles

Our original plan was to birth at the Family Birth Centre (midwifery-led care), because the peaceful and natural birthing environment appealed to us greatly. It was important to feel safe and 'at home' during the labour and birth because we had decided to aim for a drug-free birth. We felt that the place in which this was most likely to be achieved was the FBC.

Unfortunately, because I tested 'just' positive for gestational diabetes, the birth centre could only take us if I went into labour before my 40-week gestation, after which we would be transferred next door to birth at the main King Edward Memorial Hospital.

My 40-week gestation came and went with no sign of our baby. We were disappointed that the Birth Centre was no longer on the table, but promptly put this behind us to focus on the new plan! At 40 weeks and one day we had an ultrasound to check the baby and make sure she was still happy inside of me, as we really wanted to avoid an induction if possible. However, the scan results showed a couple of not so favourable variables, so we decided to go ahead with an induction the next day.

I was all booked in for an induction at KEMH on the afternoon of 26th February at 40 weeks and 2 days gestation. However, my body was already getting ready to bring my little girl into this world; my contractions started on the 26th at about 5:30am! I was able to make breakfast and tidy up the house but as soon as I started vacuuming (about 8:30am) the contractions amped up big time. I texted my husband and told him to come home from work as I really needed him. My doula Kristin soon arrived at about 9:30am, and I was in another world by that stage.

We had been told several times over during the pregnancy to 'labour at home as long as possible', so this is what I did. I laboured at home with my two amazing support people, with only soft 'spa' music, cold face washers, and back massaging to ease the pain! To say it was intense is absolutely an understatement - I've never felt anything like it in my life. The way my body worked to bring her down through me was incredible. The way I was zoning in and out and using only a few words when talking was interesting. The way I felt my body was going to explode and knowing I was far away from pain relief (even though I wanted a drug-free birth) was entertaining! The comfort my husband brought when he whispered, "You're doing great, babe" was so reassuring.

At about 1pm, after telling Mic and Kristin I wanted to go to the hospital 'NOW!' (I think I was making a beeline for pethidine or something) we were finally on our way. The 25-minute drive to the hospital went by quicker than expected; I was kneeling on the backseat facing oncoming traffic and half-way through the drive my contractions changed from unbearably painful to a slightly less-intense feeling with the need to bear down. I knew then I was close! Prior to that, none of us knew my progress. We all assumed, being a first time Mum, that the labour would go on for hours. No one knew, including me, how much pain I would tolerate before going to hospital.

My waters broke halfway through the drive, and I casually said in between contractions "My waters just broke". Kristin promptly jumped over to the backseat, and I now know, it was because she was getting ready to catch a baby! Mic rang our Birth Centre midwife who instructed us to meet her, not at the hospital, but at the Birth Centre. She knew there was no time

74

to get through the corridors and elevators of a hospital. If I had to have done that I would have had the baby in the corridor for sure! I remember hearing Mic say, "We're meeting Claire at the Birth Centre now," and being so relieved that I wouldn't have to navigate through the hospital in my condition!

We arrived at the Birth Centre at 1:30pm and (apparently) I did an awkward almost run to the door and met Claire, my petite 25-year-old midwife, who took one look at me and promptly started barking orders at everyone inside. She knew we had little time!

I made it into the labour room and had her at 2:01pm, kneeling on a mattress in a beautiful room with my husband in front of me and Kristin and Claire behind. Because there was meconium in the waters there were two paediatricians gowned up ready to help our baby if she needed assistance. However, there was no need as she came out and within seconds started to cry. I was instructed to reach underneath myself while still kneeling and bring my baby girl up to my chest. What a moment in time.

I sustained a second-degree internal tear and so was admitted up to the hospital for aftercare. What an amazing day and amazing sequence of events, considering we went from birthing with the Birth Centre, to being asked to transfer to the hospital for care, to being booked for an induction, to finally end up birthing at the Birth Centre after all! We could not have planned it that way if we tried.

Ava Beth certainly knew how to make her grand entrance into this world of ours!!

Thanks Gaby :)

An Inspiring Story from Stef

We got pregnant easily; very very easily in fact. Under normal circumstances, it would be a pleasant relief to not have to wait for months to get the positive result so wanted by a couple who were trying to have a baby. For me it was such a beautiful confirmation of the belief I had in my body being able to conceive. My circumstances were not entirely normal because 12 years ago I received a serious, permanent spinal injury in a very serious car accident. Throughout subsequent weeks, months and years of contact with various medical professionals related to my injury, I received many projections relating to my ability to conceive, carry through till term and give birth. Some examples were: I probably wouldn't be able to conceive (told to me two weeks after my accident by a nurse when I was 19 years old), if I could conceive, I would end up in a wheelchair or in a hospital unable to walk in the latter stages, I may not be able to carry to term, and finally, I will definitely not be able to birth naturally.

Like I said, we got pregnant very easily, so that "truth" was dispelled. The rest I decided was up to my body, which up until that point had given me no reason to believe I could not have the drug free, natural birth I wanted for my baby and myself. The problem was that all of the negative information I had received over the years had had an effect on my belief that I could do this the way I wanted to. Also, I had no real understanding of the stages and processes of pregnancy and labour, therefore I had no idea what to expect, and I was nervous.

As my pregnancy progressed I felt great physically. Relaxin was helping in ways that no physio, chiro or osteo ever had! A few symptoms of my injury were exacerbated, but I took measures to manage those as best I could. I finished work earlier than I had planned and began pregnancy aqua classes where I had the good fortune of meeting Gaby. Through her classes I got to meet other pregnant women. I had never spent time with other pregnant women before, and the exchange of experiences and the casual question and answer sessions held during the classes were a priceless source of information. It also made me realise how nervous I was about "b" day.

I doubted my body's ability to do what it was designed for, giving birth. I managed to identify that my nerves were also due to the fact that I had no idea what labour and birth were about. So, I decided to get educated. And since I wanted Adrian, my partner, to be my birth support, he was going to join me on that journey! The hospital that I wanted to birth at had absolutely no qualms about me wanting a natural birth; they saw no hindrance from my injury despite all of the information I had been given in the past. The only problem, therefore, was me.

I attended antenatal classes at the hospital but found them to be lacking. So I jumped online, not sure what I was looking for. After a bit of research, I found something called 'Hypnobirthing' and decided that was for us. It educated us on every stage of labour, different relaxation techniques and the power of believing in yourself and your body to do what it was designed for, as well as the importance of reclaiming your pregnancy and birth from the medical community. We completed and cemented our education with a daylong seminar run by Gaby. This was the icing on the cake!

Prospective Dads were given practical, hands-on guidance on what to expect during labour, what their role was and how to be present. Mums-to-be were given information on what to expect, in a practical way, that focused on the complete naturalness of the process. Adrian and I walked away from the session feeling empowered, excited and completely focused to go through this experience together as a team. Now the waiting began.

The Wednesday before I gave birth I went to have a massage with Gaby. She asked me when I thought my baby was going to come. The hospital had given me my estimated date, which was two weeks away. I said exactly these words, "I think I will go into labour next Wednesday night and give birth the next day". And I did. Six days before my estimated date, I went into labour at home. After labouring there overnight, I went to the hospital when I felt the time was right. I gave birth six hours later, without any drugs and without any major hindrance from my injury. I loved our birth experience. My midwife was fantastic, and Adrian was essential to this wonderful outcome. We now have an 11-and-a-half-month-old girl who is chilled out, relaxed and easy going. Anything is possible when you "Believe you can" and you have the will to do so.

Megan's Beautiful Labour Journey

My contractions initially began in the early morning of the 11th August, coming 10 minutes apart for about an hour and then fizzling into nothing. This was enough to keep me awake and get excited but not enough for the baby to come. By the next day they had almost completely gone until that evening when the same thing happened. I tried not to get my hopes up and tried to get some sleep as I knew I was going to need rest.

At around 3am on the 12th I awoke with contractions every 10-12 minutes apart and they continued until morning. By 9-10 am the contractions increased to about 5-8 minutes apart. I took a long hot shower which seemed to ease them slightly and made me feel better with the lack of sleep.

My partner and I decided to proceed to the birth centre at around 11:30am as the contractions had increased to 3-5 minutes apart. When I arrived, I was 3cm dilated and my waters had yet to break. We got comfortable, heated lavender and sandalwood oil and both tried to relax as much as possible. I enjoyed every contraction as I knew it was one closer to meeting our baby. I used many tools such as the shower and fitball to my advantage and made sure I was in the zone when the contraction started. They were intensifying but I just breathed deeply into my body and pictured our baby moving downwards.

At around dinner time the birthing pool was prepared and just before I got in my waters broke. I was 6-7 cm dilated. Once I got in the pool I felt so good, but the contractions got so strong! Even with the contractions intensifying I could not help but be so blissful about finally meeting the baby. Some time passed and I remember just before going into transition was the only time where the contractions got the best of me and I thought to myself, 'Why did I choose to do this without drugs?' Then as quick as that thought came, it left me with the urge to vomit.

After that moment, my whole body was on a mission to get the baby out. According to my partner I grunted very loud and very deeply; I guess that's when the primal being within me took over. I cannot remember the contractions at this time, only intense pressure. I started to get very warm, but I wanted to stay in the pool to keep the momentum going. No sooner had I had that thought, I was told to get out because the baby's heart rate had dropped. I felt her head right down on my vagina and it was awkward, but I got out so quickly and onto the floor on all fours for the last two big pushes, one for the head and one for the body.

At this stage there was such a relief and overwhelming joy to hear her cry and find out that it was a healthy girl. She was so alert on my chest; I could not believe it. It solidified my strong belief in a natural birth for sure. Whenever possible I tell everyone about how amazing it was. I am so happy that I was able to have such a wonderful birth. It was more amazing than I could ever have imagined, and I am so happy with the way the birth went.

Liljana Marie was 3.355 kg born at 21:34 on the 12th August.

A Wonderful First Labour

My estimated due date had come and gone, and I was trying every 'old wives' tale there was to try and bring on the labour. My obstetrician had advised I was only allowed to go ten days over, but with some careful negotiation I managed to get the weekend as well, which allowed me a couple of extra days to myself and for my body to do what it needed, naturally. I had been attending Gaby's Aqua classes right throughout my pregnancy, one of the few things that I really enjoyed. Tuesday's class was my favorite, so I worked really hard with Gaby's positive affirmations swimming through my head while running up and down the pool. I went home to listen to my hypnotherapy session and thought, 'It has to happen soon.'

The following day I was booked in for a massage with Gaby, a truly beautiful experience whereby I visualised my birth, all the while remembering her words from her hypnotherapy sessions. She then worked on my points and began speaking again but this time it was quite a different feeling having Gaby actually there rather than listening to her words. I left feeling ready to surrender to my body and felt quite floaty as I drove home. That evening I had minor contractions and had a little more show. An early night to bed but awake quite often, I could feel something was happening. I awoke in the morning feeling tired, not wanting to get out of bed. I told my husband Ravi that I would stay in bed a little longer and fell back to sleep. I awoke suddenly to a small gush of water coming out of me. I jumped out of bed and got to the bathroom where my waters ran down my legs to the floor.

I stayed in the bathroom thinking about what to do and how to relax while Ravi cleaned up and got my things together for the hospital. I didn't want to rush there, instead heading downstairs to have some breakfast in between some controlled breathing in the kitchen. My mum had been staying with us, visiting from Queensland and was oblivious to what was going on as I didn't want her to get too excited just yet. Mum was talking to me and then my head would go down and eyes would close for a time before re-joining the conversation. Mum asked what was wrong to which I replied, "I am in labour." I spent some time in the bathroom having a shower and mentally preparing myself. Gaby's words from her hypnotherapy filled my head and once my contractions were ten minutes apart, Ravi suggested we start making our way to the hospital.

We settled into the birthing suite. Not wanting to be on the bed, I headed out into the courtyard, listening to the birds and the water flowing in the nearby water feature. It was such a hot day, with summer temperatures still around in March that I had to go inside to stay cool. Being in a hospital, there were people coming in and out and the midwife wanted to monitor me, and requested I lay on the bed. I told her I didn't want to stay there long; she smiled and promised it wouldn't be long. But twenty minutes felt like an hour on that bed. I soon became frustrated that I couldn't do things my way. She wanted to know all about my birth plan...I stated I didn't have an official plan as I wanted to take each step as it came, as naturally as possible. However, I was adamant that I didn't want an epidural and asked for her not to mention it again.

She disappeared for a while and I was still on the bed when she came back into the room wheeling what looked like some sort of drip. When I asked what it was, she mentioned quietly that it was an epidural for later on. The previous woman hadn't used it and it would be in the corner just in case. I immediately became tense and threw Ravi a death stare, meaning I didn't want that thing in the room! The contractions started getting deeper and more full-on and I began to feel nauseous. The midwife gave me a sick bag and suggested I have some gas to ease the pain. "No! I didn't want pain relief" I stated, but I was beginning to think I should have it. I was disappointed and upset that I wasn't going to last and told Ravi that I wanted a different midwife.

He came back to say that her shift was ending and that maybe I should get off the bed. I went to the bathroom, a dark and small space with no interruptions and sat on the toilet and immediately felt better. I decided I was going to stay there before the midwife came bursting in, to which I asked her to leave and locked the door. Time passed and Ravi came into the bathroom to tell me there was a new midwife from Mauritius and she seemed lovely. He had filled her in on what I wanted, and she had got rid of the epidural from the corner of the room.

She came and introduced herself and suggested I get in the shower. Why didn't I do that earlier?! What a relief! All this time I had not used water to relieve me. Ravi held the handheld shower on my lower belly, and I stood with the water running on my lower back for what seemed like minutes; I found out later it was for four hours! My legs had become tired and shaky from standing and the midwife suggested I move to the bath.

It seemed as if the bath was too far away to get to, so I rested on the floor and leaned on the fitball. It wasn't very comfortable but it gave my legs a rest. Ravi assured me the bath wasn't too far away and he and the midwife helped me across the corridor to the steaming bath. As soon as I was in, I felt relieved and again wondered why I waited so long. Contractions came and went, getting stronger and closer together. The midwife told me I was nearly at the transitional stage and I would need to get out of the bath once the pushing began. They left me alone for a short time and I could feel the pushing start. My body was taking over, and I had no control against that pushing feeling. I imagined I was just listening to Gaby's voice on the hypnotherapy scripts and tried my best to "welcome each contraction as if it were a friend". I had listened to this affirmation one hundred times over, over the last few months and now it was really happening.

It was time to get out of the bath. I fought not to get out, but it was hospital policy. By this stage I was too tired and focussed on getting this baby out to argue; I became quite subdued as I lay on the bed. The midwife helped me to change positions so I wasn't lying down, and she whispered that the baby would be here soon. The obstetrician arrived and the real labour began, with Ravi by my side breathing with me and cooling me down with wet cloths. I kept my eyes closed and imagined being in Gaby's massage room and each contraction was just my points being pressed. It would soon be over.

The pushing continued and became harder and harder with no end drawing nearer. When would this end? I kept my eyes closed and took a huge breath and pushed with everything I had in me. How much longer? The midwife told me to push

85

as hard as I could as the baby's head was in sight. My eyes stayed tightly closed and I didn't respond to anyone, instead imagining my baby's head coming out of me. This continued for a long time and I was growing tired.

The obstetrician acknowledged that I was giving it all I had but that she would need to perform an episiotomy for it to be over. She explained that the baby's head was traveling down my birth canal as I pushed, but as soon as I stopped, it would recede back up. I didn't want an episiotomy and continued with all my might. When would this be over? In the end I agreed. With the next contraction, the obstetrician did what she did, and the baby's head moved out of my birth canal. Then I had that tight burning feeling and had to stop pushing which was the hardest part of all. I still had my eyes closed even though Ravi kept telling me to look at the head. I was silent and in deep thought about all I had heard over the last few months. I felt another contraction coming and heard them say "Push!" I pushed as hard as I could and felt the rest of the body slip out of me. They lay the baby boy on my chest and I felt an absolute sense of relief. I opened my eyes to see a healthy baby boy lying on me and looking at me with squinty eyes. Ravi kissed me on the forehead and said, "You did it". Wow, I really did.

Jacqueline Spencer Birth Journey

Excited at the prospect of the birth of my first baby, I wanted to do everything possible to make it a safe and wonderful experience. I asked Gaby to assist the birth, as my partner, David, is extremely squeamish and didn't feel up to being present during the entire birth. Also, we had moved to Western Australia only a few months before the baby was due and I didn't have anyone else with me. As I was 36 at the time, I also felt quite anxious about the possibility of things going wrong and wanted someone there with Gaby's experience. Gaby and I had a few long talks about my birth plan, and I told her I wanted a natural birth, and I hated the idea of having a needle put into my spine. I didn't want to interfere with the birth process knowing that it would make further intervention more likely.

My contractions started at about 9.30pm with mild cramping pains. By about 12 pm the pains were getting a bit more intense, but I still wasn't quite sure if I was in labour. I began timing the pains and realised they were 5 minutes apart. About an hour later I had a show, and the pains were quite gripping, so I woke David and told him the baby was on its way. We rang the maternity hospital and the nurse I spoke to suggested I take a Panadol and go back to bed. I don't think so! David made me a cup of tea and I slowly got my bag together and then decided to go into the hospital. When we got there they put us in a little room with two beds and David tried to get some more sleep.

I lay down, but when each contraction came I had to stand up and pace the floor. After a short while Gaby met us, and David decided to drive home to drop off the dog (she had come with us to the hospital and was waiting in the car). To be honest I was glad to see him relieved of his duty. He obviously felt a bit out of place, and I really only wanted to be among women who understood the birth process. It was a big relief to have Gaby there who immediately set up some pillows on the bed and gave me a fitball to sit on. I think I stayed in this position for quite a while, and just put my head into the pillow during each contraction. Gaby massaged a special essential oil into my back during each contraction. After a while it felt time for a change and Gaby showed me another position, leaning against the wall with my arms above my head. That was surprisingly comfortable, and I had all my other contractions in that position.

I breathed through each contraction and that allowed me to focus on something else rather than the pain. When the pain increased Gaby and I went to the shower and she held the hose over my back or my tummy for each contraction. I stayed in the shower for what seemed like a long time, until eventually I felt a bit waterlogged and we went back to my room, which smelt beautiful due to the massage oil. Every now and then the midwife came in to see how things were going. Gaby had let her know that I didn't want to have an internal examination until it was really necessary and that I had chosen not to have pain relief (unless it was also really necessary).

After changing to the standing position for my contractions, they came on more intensely and more frequently. I sometimes had a shorter contraction (with no peak to it) followed by another shorter one about two minutes later. When things got too hard to bear, Gaby and I went to the shower again. Later when we got back in the room I started feeling a bit anxious about how much longer the labour would take. Gaby asked me to visualise the size of my cervix and I had a really clear image of a circle with a diameter of about 4.5 centimetres. More time passed, with me standing against the wall, breathing into each contraction (they were pretty intense at this stage) and Gaby massaging my back. David came in at one point after returning to the hospital and wished me well before going off to the waiting room.

Several hours later I started to feel anxious and worried about how much longer the labour would take. Gaby asked me to do another visualisation and this time the circle was about 9.5 centimetres in diameter. Shortly afterward, at about 8am, there was a change of shift among the nursing staff and a new midwife came in to introduce herself. She said she would like to do an internal examination soon as they weren't sure that I was in established labour – this wasn't what I wanted to hear! The midwife decided to give me more time and about half an hour later, as I was getting ready for another contraction, Gaby was telling me what a wonderful job I was doing. Then we heard a loud splat as my waters broke onto the floor. Poor Gaby ended up with amniotic fluid all over her as the impact of the fluid hitting the floor and the wall made it splash upwards and all over her. The midwife came in at that very moment and said "What have you two been up to?"

We were in fits of laughter, hysterically laughing as it was so funny and spontaneous - a real serendipitous moment. Neither of us could move from where we were as we were surrounded by amniotic fluid. The midwife ran out to get a mop and bucket and some towels. As the next contraction came, I squealed "Gaby please don't make me laugh, I'm having a contraction". Somehow, she managed to and from that time on I coped really well as everything changed.

The feel of the contractions changed right at that very moment. I could now feel the bulk of the baby in my pelvis. The midwife came in and asked to check the baby's heartbeat as she said there was a small amount of meconium in the amniotic fluid. The heartbeat on the monitor was strong and steady though and I felt a huge relief knowing that the baby was doing well through all of this. Gaby was wonderfully supportive and calm and kept talking to me in a gentle, soft voice. I felt anxious after my waters broke. Gaby suggested to me that I was probably in transition at this stage. I told her I would agree to an internal but that I only wanted to hear the results if they were good. As the midwife put on her gloves, I had another contraction and had to jump up off the bed. There was no way I could cope with a contraction lying on my back.

After the internal Gaby and the midwife said it was time to go to the labour room (shortly after Gaby told me I was 10 cm dilated and the head was 1 cm through my cervix, so much for not reaching established labour!). Once there I had about two more contractions against the wall and then they set up pillows on the bed for me to lean against. During the contractions I felt an urge to push and at the same time, open my mouth wide and let out a noise (David tells me it was VERY LOUD, and he could hear me all the way down the corridor). I think I expected the baby to pop out pretty quickly but as it took a while, I had to ask if the baby was stuck. I was told it wasn't, and after 20 minutes of pushing, out it came. I think I slumped forward onto the pillows until I heard the baby cry. I turned around and there was my little baby girl. I certainly had a wonderful experience. I felt so grateful for Gaby's presence, which was like having an angel watching over me. Finally, David came in and got to meet our little miracle!

A Positive First Birth

Well, I'm just so happy my boy is so amazing. He only cries for a feed and if we change him; he does not like having his clothes off and being naked! However, even that is getting better as he must be getting used to our dress sense. This is how my labour went ...

At 1:20am on Wednesday 21st, I woke up with something going on and wondered if it was the curry I ate or if it was contractions. I started timing the sensations/contractions and they were coming every five minutes for about 15 minutes, then down to 3 minutes apart for the next 15 minutes.

In next to no time, it seemed to be that I was having two contractions right on top of each other followed by a one-to-two-minute break. It was now that I decided to call the birth centre. Gaby's lovely friend and midwife, Fran, answered. I had not met her yet as she wasn't in my labour team, but Gaby had spoken about her one day whilst at class. Fran listened to me having a contraction and said it sounded like things were getting going so it was into the car to labour away for an hour whilst hubby drove me to Subiaco where the birth centre is located.

I listened to Gaby's hypnosis scripts on my i-pod and even though my contractions were coming faster than she guided me, it helped me to really remain focussed on opening and going with each contraction instead of freaking out about their closeness...

Going over the Canning Bridge freeway exit Matt said, "I think we might need petrol" which was very funny but he quickly said, "Oh no, I think we can make it". We got to the birth centre and Fran greeted us at the door. I had about four contractions from the short walk from car to room and Fran said, "Ok, looks like things are moving along nicely".

Once we were settled, she then asked if I wanted a VE. She explained that it was not just dilation they were looking for, but the thinning of the cervix too. I agreed to go ahead. It was tricky to do the VE with my contractions so close together, but it wasn't too bad and when she said to me, "You are 5 centimetres dilated." I stood up, looked at Matt and started to cry. I couldn't believe I was really about to have my baby and not just a bad case of curry tummy! This was my baby's due date as well which was really special. My waters hadn't broken which was wonderful as I wanted them to go when they were ready and not be broken by anyone. Everything was really going amazingly well.

Things got moving along even more so, and before long I was experiencing two contractions with a 30 second break. Matt was feeling a little useless as I was walking around not wanting to be touched or massaged. I got in the bath, but it didn't work for me, so I got out. I then decided to go in the shower. Matt sprayed the water on me and really reminded me to breathe through each contraction and make low noises. It was very intense at this time and I did wonder when I would get a break.

My Obi boy really wanted to meet his Mum and Dad ... I then went through transition when I called out, "OH MY

GOODNESS!" and went to sit on the toilet jumping up quickly saying, "MY BABY IS COMING!" I then walked over to the mat on the floor and went down on all fours, leaning over a bean bag and cushions, and started to push. Matt spoke words of encouragement and Fran kept me up to date with what I should be doing and what was happening. I could hear in Matt's voice a sense of amazement at what he was seeing, and I knew I was doing well... Obi's waters (membranes) were still intact and after about an hour of pushing he came out looking squished behind his stocking (as Matt described it). Three more pushes later his body was out, and Matt received him and handed our miracle to me... "Wow, what an experience!"

Lisa and Trent's Birth of Sana

"This baby is huge! It's at least 10 pounds!" These are the words said to me while having an ultrasound nine days past my estimated date. I however, was not convinced and not in the least bit concerned. I felt good, I felt healthy, and I was confident that whatever size my baby was, it was the right size for me.

Perhaps if I heard these words before I read the book 'A Labour of Love- a guide to natural childbirth without fear', it would have sent me into an absolute panic! As I was now nine days overdue, I was booked in for a routine induction at 15

94

days over. I told my midwife that there was no need because this baby would be born before then.

I am 32 and having my first baby. My pregnancy journey has been an interesting one. I have been paying for private health cover for well over 10 years, always imagining that I would give birth in a lovely private hospital and see an obstetrician. I had lists of names of Obstetricians to choose from and had an appointment booked with two of them.

However once I fell pregnant a new life journey began, not only for my new baby, but for me too. I decided I wanted a natural birth; no drugs at all. It felt right for me and the best for my baby. I wanted to be in an environment which was supportive of my choices but one which I also felt safe in. This is how I came across The Family Birth Centre. I can't speak highly enough of my experience there. Even though I knew that I wanted a natural birth, I still felt that I had to boost my confidence and really believe that I could do it. I borrowed 'A Labour of Love' from my friend and finished reading it as early as 10 weeks pregnant. It was an inspiration for me! I then went on to the website and completed two courses on offer- the 'Couples Childbirth' support workshop to empower my partner and 'The Four Week Journey for Women'. I also listened daily to positive affirmations on Gaby's CD as well as her hypnosis for birth prep scripts.

By the time I was ready to birth my baby I felt so confident and relaxed, it was truly amazing! I also kept fit and healthy through my pregnancy with yoga, aqua classes and walking regularly. My husband had also experienced his own journey and was equally confident in both my ability, as well as his own as a birth support partner. He also read Gaby's book.

On the day I went into labour I felt different; heavier, with more pressure down below and period cramping- like sensations, yet I felt very relaxed. I think to myself, "This baby is coming tomorrow (Saturday) and will be here for Father's Day on Sunday". I am booked in for a massage with Gaby. My eyes looked glazed over, and I felt like everything was happening in slow motion. Gaby says that I have that labour look about me. Gaby concentrates on my pressure points to encourage labour and we finish with a visualisation/meditation. It is very vivid, and I could see my baby being born. A tear rolls down my face with happiness.

At 3am the next morning, I go to the toilet and come back to bed whispering to my husband, "It's showtime, the show is here". We laugh and are both excited. My period cramping seems to be happening more often now and it is definitely stronger. I try not to get too carried away as I know that this does not necessarily mean a baby is coming soon. I wake up the next morning around 7am and my husband and I take our dogs for a walk. I feel like I am walking with a melon between my legs, as the baby feels like it has dropped.

I go about my day leisurely but keep busy and moving doing a few house chores. I send my husband off for a massage and a haircut. About 12pm I feel like there is a bit of a pattern to my cramping. I ring Gaby and tell her that I am not sure if it's labour because it feels too easy. She laughs and says, "Our bodies very kindly warm up slowly to labour, especially when it spontaneously starts on its own".

About an hour or two later, I am having to concentrate and stop to breathe. Ok, I think something is happening. At 3.30pm my husband comes home. I ask him to time what I think are contractions; five minutes, three minutes, four minutes, three minutes. At 5pm we are on our way to the Birth Centre. We call the birth centre to let them know. I have six contractions on the way and listen to Gaby's hypnosis scripts for labour. I have two contractions from the car to the front door of the birth centre.

I feel good, relaxed and am going with the flow. Sharon, our gorgeous midwife, shows us to our suite with a smiling face. It's the suite I had visualised being in. After a while I am feeling a little shaky and there seems to be some blood. Sharon is not concerned. She runs the bath for me. I am feeling like I want to make noise and now have to really focus on each contraction. My husband stays with me at all times, but this really is time for me to focus inward and on my own. His presence is enough to make me feel safe and supported.

At 7pm, a new midwife, Debbie arrived. I tell her that I am feeling pressure, like I almost need to push. She looks at me and says ok, but I can tell she is not totally convinced. To be honest, I am not sure that I am convinced either. She asks me if I would like to be examined. I wasn't sure because I didn't want to be told I was only one or two centimetres dilated. I feel confident in what my body was doing, so I agreed to it. I was eight centimetres! Hooray!!

I feel it is time to get out of the bath and get on to the birthing stool. I think I can feel the baby's head, but my midwife then tells me it's just my waters bulging. I move to all fours, leaning over the bed. A few contractions later and I feel like I'm slowing down.

I can feel irrational thoughts creeping into my head - I don't want this baby anymore, this is too hard, I want to go home and rest. I observe these thoughts and realise that this must be 'transition'. Our baby will be here soon! I feel determined again. Contractions have now spaced out to five minutes apart. I ask for help, but I am not sure what I want. I definitely don't want any drugs. Deb suggests that she can break my waters. I want to think about it and ask for three more contractions. I change positions in order to lie on my side. Deb goes to check my membranes and instantaneously, after my 3rd contraction, they break naturally and explode all over Debby…oops!

Wow! I feel the burn now; the head had been cushioned on my membranes but was now pushing on my perineum. I knew I was close, not long now, I think. However, I also think I could be pushing here for another hour or two as this was my first baby. A few more pushes. The baby is crowning. I have so much energy now; I want this baby to be born. Deb and my husband talk me through calmly. Breathing throughout labour has been an incredible way to focus. As Gaby taught me, in for the count of four through my nose and out for the count of six through my mouth. I push hard and the baby stops at its forehead with eyes just showing like it's stuck. My eyes are tightly shut. I feel panic around me, but I remain calm. I know I am in control, and I know the baby knows what it's doing. Deb tells Trent that this is a big baby and to get my legs up around my ears. Deb runs for the emergency button to call in the other midwife.

Our baby had decided to come out two shoulders at once instead of one at a time. One big push with all my might (I did not care if I tore) - this baby was coming out now. I thought to myself I must look so unattractive right now with my face so squinted. It's funny the thoughts that pop into your head. I felt my baby slither out and then she was plonked on my chest. She was beautiful, just as I imagined - big, long and chubby with a mop of dark hair. Looking all around, so alert and so beautiful. So much for two hours of pushing, it was all over in 26 minutes!

My husband and I sat there looking at our little girl, Sana Amelie. We were amazed and so emotional; she was just so beautiful, so perfect. I felt incredible... so full of energy and on the most amazing high!! My placenta then just plopped out like a big jellyfish; no tearing at all! My midwife was truly amazed! For anyone who is reading this, buy an EPI-NO. Look it up on the internet! My midwife tells everyone about them after witnessing my birth.

I felt like I could do anything after having a natural birth with such a big baby - 9 lb 1 oz . It was a truly wonderful experience, and for me, mental, emotional and physical preparation was the key.

I would do it all again tomorrow and wouldn't change a thing!

The Birth of Zac – Right on Time!

As a midwife I've seen the good, the bad and the ugly sides of childbirth. I knew what I didn't want to have happen, but I was unsure how to get the type of birth I really wanted. During my pregnancy I tried my best to do the right things. I ate well and avoided all alcohol, then started exercising more to ensure a healthy baby (and Mum).

That's how I met Gaby. I was looking for a local water aerobics class and I ended up meeting an honest and empowering woman who really helped give me the edge on getting my head around what it would take to have the natural childbirth that I had always wanted and deserved!

I chose a birthing centre attached to a main hospital as my place to give birth. I received professional care from a team of midwives and would only need to see a doctor if there was a problem. To my delight, all my appointments went well, my baby was growing nicely, and I was enjoying a straightforward pregnancy. My birth preparation included daily walks, swimming and water aerobics, the odd yoga class and listening to Gaby's CD's often which helped me get into the space needed to have a natural childbirth. I also drank raspberry leaf tea from 32 weeks and felt really amazing.

The night before my estimated due date I went into labour at 8.15 pm. At first I thought it might be a false alarm, but within a few hours I was doing the breathing I'd learnt on Gaby's hypnosis scripts and was cleaning the bathroom between contractions! At 1am, I really wanted to go to the birth centre. I'd had a bath at home, tried a hot pack on my back, but was becoming restless. We arrived at the birth centre at 2am, and on examination I was already four centimetres dilated open.

I went straight into their big bath and got comfortable. I relaxed, did the breathing and enclosed myself into my own private space that I needed. At 4.30am I became very, very restless and could no longer focus as I had been. I felt lots of pressure and suddenly my waters broke. What a relief! I asked to be examined and my midwife said, "I already know you're fully dilated because your behaviour has changed!" but if you want me to examine you I will. She examined me and I was fully dilated!

I stayed in the bath for another 30 minutes. Then at 5am I got out and laboured on my hands and knees. I started using the gas at this point; it made me feel like I'd had a couple of glasses of wine, and just took the edge off the final stages. I never did any formal pushing and was so glad my midwife wasn't screaming at me to, 'push, push, and push'. It was quiet (except for my noise), private and the lights were dimmed. My husband was by my side the whole time giving me sips of water, brushing the hair out of my eyes and sitting quietly, waiting for our baby.

I became tired of being on my hands and knees after a while and my husband sat on a bean bag and I leaned into him on my side. Then all of a sudden the midwife asked if I'd like to feel my baby's head as it crowned! I reached down to feel a warm wet wrinkled head. With the next contraction at 5.47am, I had a warm brown-haired baby plopped onto my chest. He let out a small cry then my husband and I had a little cry too. He was perfect and I was deeply in love already.

This experience was the proudest and most beautiful moment of my life. I will never forget it and hope to do it again and again.

2.

TWO BIRTH'S
- ONE MUM

Erin's Birth Stories
Birth Story of Alice, Baby No 1

On Tuesday morning, I woke up at about 5.30am with tummy pains, but just thought I was constipated or that they were muscle pains - I'd experienced quite a few of those lately. It didn't even cross my mind that they could be contractions!! So I rested for another two hours on and off, and ended up getting up with Cam. He went off to work and I pottered around. I was finally able to go to the toilet ... then couldn't stop number twos at all! I thought it might be Braxton Hicks because I had read that if you have to ask, you aren't in labour. Plus, I hadn't had any type of bloody show or mucus. Around lunch time I spoke to my Mum. After describing them as bad period pains and telling her about the diarrhoea, she suggested that perhaps I was in labour! I had a raspberry leaf tea and waited a few more hours, timing the contractions (five minutes apart) and then told Cam to come home and called the Midwife. She said to stay at home as long as I'm comfortable, so I kept pottering around packing our bags, only stopping to deal with each contraction. I was just using breathing and positioning to help out.

When Cam got home I started to use the heat packs and at about 7pm we decided it was time to think about going to the birthing centre. We called up the centre and Sharon was on shift. Sharon was the midwife I'd seen the most throughout my pregnancy. She had predicted that I would go into labour Monday, Tuesday or Wednesday of this week because she was on nights. I was so glad we got her. I was still coping fine with the contractions but knew that the car ride would be awful and desperately wanted to get it over and done with.

We arrived at the Family Birthing Centre at about 8pm. At first, I found it harder to cope with the contractions at the centre. I had to find new positions to relieve the pain and found it more difficult to relax in between. Then I got in the shower and Cam put the handheld shower head on my back. I coped in there for another hour or so and about 10.30pm, I opted for a vaginal examination. I was nervous because I didn't want to hear that I was only a little way dilated and get despondent, and also because it required me to get on the bed on my back which is the worst position to be in during a contraction! But curiosity got the better of me, so I climbed up on the bed and Sharon did the Vaginal Examination and told me I was 8cm! It felt so good to hear that. I knew it meant there was only a small chance of needing the epidural I so desperately wanted to avoid, as I still had the bath and the gas up my sleeve.

Sharon then went off to run the bath while I got back in the shower for another hour and started to transition my baby down into my birth canal. I was starting to feel the urge to bear down by the time I got into the bath. I leaned on the edge and Cam used the handheld shower head on my back again. After a little while, I decided I could do it with the gas. It helped take the edge off the pain and gave me something to concentrate on during the contractions. It also helped me relax in between as I felt all woozy and drunk in between as a result of sucking on the gas. I soon felt the urge to bear down and could feel her moving down the birth canal. She was moving down and back up and I started to get frustrated. I was so ready for her to be born.

I made a joke and asked the midwife if there was another way for her to get out. (She didn't think it was funny. I guess they have to take those things seriously in case I was asking for a c-section. But at that point if they had suggested I get out of the bath for ANY reason I would have punched them!) Cam was so brilliant. I didn't have to ask him for anything, he just knew what to do and what to say. He was constantly reassuring me how much of a good job I was doing at birthing our baby etc. He didn't even complain when I made him repeat the

SAME songs for two hours. It was amazing to see how your body just does what it needs to do. I wasn't really consciously doing anything; it was like being a zombie. I would just move into another position and involuntarily start pushing.

After what seemed like an eternity, she started to crown. I had thought she'd been crowning earlier but Cam informed me later that this was the first time they'd all seen her head. As they weren't permitted to have water births in the centre, Sharon had slowly been letting out the bath water, so I was in the empty bath leaning forward onto Cam who was on the outside. Sharon asked me to pant my baby out, but I was so eager to get her out that I pushed instead and then OUT SHE CAME in a rather dramatic entrance!!! As she came out in one push, she broke her (unusually short) cord, hit the pillow on the bottom of the bath and flew around the bottom of the bath like a little luge competitor!

Sharon called out for the other midwife and grabbed hold of Alice's tiny cord stump. It snapped about a centimetre from her! This was only the second time in 20 years that Sharon had seen this type of thing happen. So much for all my plans about leaving the cord until it finished pulsating! I looked at Cam and said, "I made that!!" and grinned. Once they'd clamped Alice's cord, I got to pick her up and hold her to me. After a few minutes, she had to go out to see the paediatrician. Cam went with her and I got up and birthed the placenta naturally, as I had wanted to.

We then went back to our room and I showered and got sutured (just a 2nd degree tear downwards and a tiny graze upwards.) The sutures were almost as painful as the birth! Then we got to have a cuddle. Alice wouldn't feed so I expressed some colostrum and they syringe-fed her. She then had to have a rest under the heat bed while we got a few hours sleep. Alice was cold because she was so small, just 2.77gram (6 lb 2 oz) and 46cms. No wonder she just flew out! After we'd all had some rest, she attached well to the breast and fed away.

Birth Story baby No.2 – Lucy

Lucy was estimated to be due on either the 24th February (LMP) or the 6th March (ultrasound) so I was either 39+3 or 40+6 weeks pregnant when I went into labour. All day on Tuesday I was feeling very crampy, and I had a feeling that I was going to go into labour that night, or the next day. I went to bed around 10.30pm and tried to listen to my hypnosis scripts. However, I couldn't concentrate as I started to have regular sensations within half an hour of going to bed and I just couldn't relax. I got up and took some paracetamol before trying to lie down again. Again, this failed, so I got up and watched the UFC (of all things, I hate UFC!) with Cam. After some time, I realised this was probably labour, but I didn't want to get my hopes up, so I sent Cam to bed to get some rest before I needed him.

I loved that we didn't have to worry about driving anywhere, so he could get some sleep. He dozed for the next hour and a half while I sat in the garden, came inside and sent some emails and just generally tried to keep distracted in between. The contractions were pretty intense and required my full concentration, but as I couldn't sleep I didn't want to sit around waiting for the next one. About 1.30am I tried to lie down again, but as I had to be somewhat upright for the contractions I found that fumbling out of bed at the beginning of each one just wasn't worth the effort. Eventually I found that I could sit on the ground and put my head on the bed and that let me get some rest in between. I was actually able to sleep in between a few contractions for about half an hour. Then I needed to lean against the wall with my heat pack on my back. I started to say to Cam that I didn't think I could do this because they were so intense. The pain was in my back (so I thought maybe she was posterior). I thought, based on my previous labour and her position, that I could still have seven hours or more to go, and I didn't think I'd be able to cope that long. After each contraction, I thought I was going to vomit, but I never did.

Sometime after 2am, I moved to the other side of the room and put on Gaby's hypnosis scripts. I sat on the bed in between contractions and stood with my hands on the wall during the contractions. The contractions seemed closer together, but I still wasn't timing them – I didn't want to get caught up worrying about time or anticipating the next one. I started to change my pelvic movements during the contractions to more of a squatting motion. Then all of a sudden my waters broke! I hadn't had them break at all during Oscar's labour and Alice's were just a trickle in the shower, so the huge splash was a surprise for us!

Luckily, Cam woke up straight away and moved the impeccably placed vomit bucket to catch a great deal of it. The carpet was soaked and there was a heap in the bucket. The midwife was amazed by how much there was when she saw it. I felt such a huge sense of relief once it happened because I knew then that I had to call Melissa and I didn't have to worry about calling her too early. I also knew this was definitely the real deal now. I also knew that I must be quite far along because my noises started getting low on my outward breath and I could feel more pressure. I actually began to feel like I was managing better because I understood why it had been so intense earlier, as my body was actually working really hard, and at a faster rate than my previous labours. I felt better about how I was coping.

Cam called Melissa and my Mum to come watch the kids, and then rolled the pool into the room. Melissa arrived at about 3am and I immediately wanted to get into the pool. It was the longest 15 minutes of my life waiting for it to fill. The contractions were about three minutes apart now and it was really hard work. Melissa's presence was so calming, and she stayed with me the whole time, without ever seeming like she was imposing. It took her a while to get a foetal heartbeat because I kept moving around, but she never made me feel like I was bothering her. I heard her tell Cam that she thought I was 'holding off' to get in the pool and I knew then that I was getting really close. I didn't want to believe it though because I remember the midwife at Oscar's birth surmising, he was almost there and letting out the pool water only to have him take hours longer!

Finally, the pool was ready, and I hopped in. Bliss! I think the best thing about the water in labour is how much more I can relax in between. It really helped me cope plus Cam could finally just stay with me. He was busy organising up until then. We had really held off doing stuff because we thought we still had so much time. My Mum arrived just after I got in the pool and I wouldn't let Cam go and see her. She lay down on the bed we'd set out in the lounge room. She didn't bring Kate my sister because she wasn't sure if she should wake her, and she too thought we still had hours to make that call.

By this stage I was clearly in transition and started to push. Cam was really fantastic at this stage. I think that Melissa's support really made a difference to him. He said he was so reassured that she didn't leave the room and she just stayed down "the business end" and he could really focus on me and help me with my breathing. He did think I was going to break his fingers though. I was lying over the edge of the pool, holding his hands. I could feel her coming down the birth canal and I was so astonished that we were there already! To be honest, this was easier than the earlier contractions because I knew the end was in sight and I knew I could do it! I kept saying I needed to go to the toilet because I couldn't believe the sensation could be her being born already, and then I felt her crowning and I was like, OH MY GOD!

Melissa got me to put my hand down and feel her and I felt so strong and capable. I worked so hard on the breathing and out she came. Her head was under the water and I expected her shoulders to just slip out like they had with the other two, but in fact they were much harder. I was unaware but she had her hand up against her face, so I had that extra width to get out. She didn't come out the next contraction and it was so hard to not push in between. I eventually had to stand up for the next one, so she wasn't a water birth, but I really needed the gravity as well as some twisting and wriggling from Melissa. And then she was here!! It was only 4am!!

My mum had heard me pushing and snuck up to the door just in time to see me pick her up. I just kept saying, "Oh hello baby, hello baby, hello baby". It was so emotional. She was a bit lazy with her breathing; I had to blow on her face and Melissa had to rub her feet a bit. Apparently, that's quite common with home births and water births – they can be a bit too relaxed!! Like her big sister, she had a ridiculously short cord, and I could barely lift her above my belly button. Thankfully, I birthed the placenta really quickly and said "here's the placenta" and kind of floated it towards Melissa; she was a bit surprised! I stayed in the pool a bit and then hopped into bed. She lay on my chest and had a feed. She wasn't interested in doing baby-led attachment, so I popped her on and she fed away. I was a bit sad she didn't do it but she did the next morning, yay!

Alice woke about 5am after wetting the bed and was very upset. Once she'd calmed down, Cam bought her in to meet Lucy and she was ecstatic, jumping around and just grinning. She and Melissa inspected the placenta together and I was glad she was able to do a 'job' and be involved. It didn't feel right to wake them up for the birth and I feel like everything was exactly as it needed to be anyway. Alice went back to bed after a bit and Oscar woke at 6am, and he too was thrilled. He just wanted to kiss her and look at her. He wouldn't go back to sleep and only wanted to lie where he could 'see the baby'.

Positive Birth of Freja - Baby No1

I'm writing my birth story on the third day after the 'birth' of Freja, and thinking about the birth brings a proud tear to my eye. I feel so lucky to have experienced two natural births, but in some ways I think luck is only a small part of it. I always wanted a natural birth (I knew my Mum had four!) but I had to work for it as I feel women these days are often led to believe they need an obstetrician and ultimately, many of their pregnancy and birth choices are decided for them.

So, I religiously attended antenatal yoga and water classes run by pro natural birth instructors (Gaby was one of them) as well as kept active by walking 10 minutes to and from work every day. I read Gaby's book 'A Labour of Love- a guide to natural childbirth without fear' over and over again, and listened to her affirmation script, went to her couple's childbirth education workshop as well as the Family Birth Centre classes. I wrote a birth plan and most of all had confidence that my body would do what it was designed to do; birth my baby. I also thought that the anticipation of not knowing the sex of the baby would help boost me through the labour.

I had a beautiful couple of days warm up to Freja's birth. First there was a show and then the next day, very mild contractions that started in the morning and continued throughout the day at various times. I went with my partner to the licensing centre then to the movies. I wasn't sure if it was the real thing as I hadn't experienced any Braxton Hicks during the pregnancy, so I went about my day as usual. When we got home from our afternoon out, I thought it would be good to go for a walk around the block to get some fresh air and help my imminent labour along.

We then sat down for dinner, but I didn't feel like eating much. I went to bed early but couldn't sleep as the contractions kept me from wanting to lie down, so we rang the midwife. She asked me when I was due and I said, "tomorrow", feeling very silly as I didn't want her to think I was calling her because I was due! She said to have a shower, take some Panadol and go to bed. I was still finding it very difficult to sleep because of the consistent contractions but I kept trying to rest as the midwife had suggested.

I moved from my bed into the lounge room to sleep. My partner slept on the floor with a million blankets and fully dressed as it was a cold winter's night. Here I was throwing my blanket off and on, half naked and turning the heater on and off as I experienced contraction after contraction. Early in the morning, we rang the midwife again (I kindly waited for a suitable time, I don't know why, they are on call for a reason) as my show was very bloody and I wasn't sure if this was normal. At around 8am, when I woke up for the hundredth time as I got up off the sofa, I heard a loud snap, and my waters broke.

The contractions really kicked in from then on. This time when I was speaking to the midwife, I had to literally throw the phone at my partner as I couldn't hold a conversation and have contractions at the same time. Apparently this is an indicator to come in! The midwife said to have some breakfast and that she'd meet us there at 10am. I couldn't believe she made an appointment. I tried to eat some toast, but I couldn't. I grabbed my bag, and we went earlier than arranged. I did one last lean against the wall outside and got into the back of the car. We decided not to fit the baby car seat so I'd have plenty of room to move around. I laboured away in the back of the car, oblivious to the watching eyes as we stopped at the red lights. When I got to the FBC, the internal showed I was seven to eight centimetres dilated!

I laboured away in our private room with what felt like just my partner and I (he said the same and was wishing afterwards that we'd decided to have a doula!). The midwife was practically not there, only coming in occasionally to see if we wanted anything and to check that everything was progressing ok. I remember screaming out very loudly for no reason, just so the midwife could hear me and not go too far! I don't know where I thought she was going to go! I kept my eyes closed the whole time and focused within. When my partner kindly suggested a labour position, I remember yelling at him, "No, I get to tell you what position I want to be in!" Maybe this was transition. He kindly massaged my legs in between contractions.

I couldn't wait to get into the bath. However, once I got in, I couldn't wait to get out as there was a strong chlorine smell and it was hot. I liked leaning over a pillow on a bean bag or bed the best. I got onto my hands and knees for the pushing stage, but to help things along the midwife suggested the birth stool. I spent a long time there pushing, but to honour my wishes the final pushes were done on my knees, leaning over pillows on a bean bag squeezing my partner's hands. I really felt the support from him through our hands. My partner had thought he'd just stay at the top end, but he kept letting go of my hands and running around to watch the head appear. Freja was born at 3.15pm weighing a healthy 6lb 12oz on her due date!

Birth of Matias - Baby No2

I woke at around 5.30am to two intense contractions quite close together. I got out of bed and happily thought to myself, "Today we're going to meet our baby!" Again, we didn't find out the sex beforehand and so we were even more excited about the birth. I went and lay down next to my partner. He was sleeping in the lounge room as our 2.5-year-old daughter came into our bed during the night and together with my BIG belly, forced him out. I happily woke him with the news that something was happening. It was three days before the EDD, and we anticipated every little niggle from week 37. I'd had a lot of Braxton Hicks this pregnancy, but this sensation was different. I tried to go about my day, but I wasn't getting much done as I kept having strong, bend over furniture contractions quite close together. I had my partner time the contractions at the same time as he was running around frantically doing washing, having a shower and packing his bag! But then I had to take over the job myself as he wasn't always around when I needed him!

I wanted to stay home as long as possible but was also aware that second births were quicker, sometimes very quick, and I didn't want to leave it too late either. So, at about 8am we rang the Family Birth Centre because the contractions were getting stronger and coming three to five minutes apart. The midwife gave me the option of going straight in or staying home. I chose to stay home. We also rang my mum to let her know that we would need her to take care of Freja sometime that day, but no rush right now we told her. But half an hour later I was ringing the midwife again and telling her that we were on our way as the contractions were getting stronger and closer together! I called my mum again to say, "Please come over as soon as possible as I need you now!" When mum arrived an hour later, I was making a snack for Freja in between contractions (I was really determined to keep moving about to help the baby along!) By now Freja knew her Mamma was having the baby and was content seeing me leaning over chairs and bench tops, breathing slowly in and out. She happily left me alone and ran off to play with her Nanna.

The car trip was similar to Freja's labour as again it was mid-morning, but this time we had two baby car seats in the back so I had to squish into the front seat. I sat down but every time a contraction came I'd jump up, turn around and lean over the seat. Thankfully the Family Birth Centre was only 20 minutes away and there wasn't any traffic. We arrived at 11am and I walked calmly in. I was feeling so fit and ready for what was to come. However, I was worried the midwife might send me home again after the vaginal examination. Thankfully the internal confirmed that yes, I was in established labour and was in fact five to six centimetres dilated. I had passed the test and could now stay! As this was a second birth the room we were put in was set up ready for the actual birth (paper sheets on top of a mat on the floor, towels, midwife equipment etc. etc.). This was exciting for me to see as it reminded me that the end was near. However, it was not until five hours later I really needed to be down there on the floor!!!

I laboured away, firstly leaning up against the closest wall, then kneeling against the bed on my hands and knees, leaning over pillows. I felt very primal moving about the mat hoping that being in the position I finally wanted to be in to birth my baby would somehow get my baby out quicker! However this wasn't the case as there was a lot of pushing to come. The midwife had a student (aka home birth mum of four – pheww, I wasn't her first birth) with her and they came in to observe me a little more often than they would have if there wasn't a student learning. My waters broke with a loud snap and gush towards them, and because I was on my hands and knees, I managed to get both the midwife and the student with amniotic fluid!

I found the pushing stage really long and hard because I kept thinking it shouldn't take as long the second time round and the midwives were kindly saying so too! I was put in a squatting position with my partner holding me as I leaned back against a bean bag when the head finally appeared; but then the contractions halted, and everything went quiet. I could feel something wasn't quite right, but I was in a calm birthing state with my eyes closed the whole time and I was content and confident that the experienced midwife would assist our baby safely into this world. It turned out his shoulder was stuck. The midwife called another midwife to help and the three of them, plus my partner, worked together to tilt me back, legs pushed wider apart, pushing on my stomach and pulling our baby boy out. I was thankful that I prepared my perineum by stretching it as I did not need any stitches at all; there was just a small graze. I was relieved to have my baby boy in my arms and despite the sense of urgency at the end, he was ours straight away to touch and cuddle.

Matias was born at 4.15pm weighing a healthy 7lb 12oz.

Teneale's Labour Journey of Baby 1- Emmanuel

I know I was incredibly naive during my first pregnancy - I didn't finish a single book, as I was worried about reading all the contradictory information. All I knew was I wanted a natural as possible birth but wasn't going to be a 'Martyr' either and if I needed an epidural I would have one, that's all the information I had.

Thankfully a friend put me onto Gaby's pregnancy Aqua-fitness class, so it was also at this time I knew I had to wise up!

My husband and I ended up employing Gaby at about 33 weeks into our pregnancy to be our doula. I had purchased her books and read them, and the following week finished work and all I had left to do was get through Christmas shopping, baking, and cooking, attend Yoga, Aqua, get the packing done and then have a baby. Our little boy had other plans.

I guess in my heart I knew I had started to 'warm up' as on the last day of my work my 'Braxton Hicks' were so intense I had to breathe through them to not let anyone know how intense they really were. Then one of my clients piped up and said, "It looks to me that you are actually in labour". I responded with a "No I'm not" adamantly, "I've still got six weeks left". In my mind however, all I kept thinking was I need to get through Christmas then the baby can come. This was my secret Mantra that I kept saying to myself over and over through all the Christmas shopping, airport drop offs, the baking etc etc.

My husband had just started a new job that Christmas as a butcher which was a crazy time of year as it was just so busy! All the while I was drifting along not really thinking about the baby too much as I was thinking I had plenty of time - my full gestation was still weeks off, hence I had not packed a single thing into a bag.

I made it through the week leading up to Christmas, but on Christmas day I began to have contractions in the morning starting at 9am. As the morning went on I was trying to get ready for Christmas lunch, but the contractions were so intense it was difficult. I had to contact the family to excuse us from attending lunch as this was really happening and I needed to just rest. I contacted Gaby in which she said, "Well you are either in true labour or this is just a warmup, and it may die off a little later, just keep me informed". She also went on to say "Try to get as much rest as you can and see how you go."

By 11 am the contractions had eased but I was getting horrible sharp pains in my pelvis, so I made a quick call to King Edward where I was going to have this baby. So, we decided to go in for a quick check up. We were in total denial at this point that labour was really happening, so we got dressed and left with nothing except ourselves. After a long drive going over every bump in the roads leading us there, we arrived.

When we arrived we were taken straight upstairs where they did a quick vaginal examination, and I was 2 centimetres dilated - they said I was not going anywhere. My head was spinning, I could not believe I was about to have a baby and that my life was never going to be the same again. I had mixed emotions of feeling nervous and having sheer excitement all at once.

The next 4 hours were a total blur as it was very, very slow and by 6pm I was 4 centimetres dilated and was moved to the labour ward. Shortly after my amazing friend arrived after collecting from home all my birthing needs with Gaby following. I felt a huge wave of release as I now had my support team with me. Unfortunately the next 12 hours were uneventful, except for the fact I thought I was transitioning and was given another vaginal exam only to discover I was still four centimetres dilated and felt this huge urge to push. The baby was Posterior facing which made me feel like I just had to push. It was just so overwhelming.

Gaby and Guy took turns to sleep while I laboured on and on, and by 8am in the morning it was suggested that I have my membranes broken to see if we could speed things up. I decided to go ahead and have my membranes broken which meant for the next 4 hours I had back-to-back contractions which was exhausting, after already having laboured all through the night. So I made the decision to have an epidural which was bliss but did lead to me needing an assisted forceps birth by a wonderful doctor, as I was just so tired and due to the position. During the birth of my boy my drip somehow had stopped working and due to total exhaustion, I started coming in and out of consciousness and felt very disorientated. Bub's heartbeat started to drop due to my blood pressure drop as well, so all in all it was a very dramatic entrance into the world, but I did get to do skin on skin whilst my boy was checked over.

Our little premature baby was in perfect health but weighing just 2.6kgs. He attached quickly latching onto my breast for his first suckle.

After 5 days at King Edward Memorial Hospital, we went home on New Year's Eve to celebrate our preciousness with friends and family, and we were on cloud nine with our little boy. Without Gaby's presence at our birth, I truly believe our experience would have been very different.

Baby No.2 Sampson's birth 13th June 2016

After having Gaby at Emmanuel's labour, we just had to have Gaby for our next labour journey, and upon conception I contacted her.

At 20 weeks we got together to do a debrief as I was quite worried about having another preterm baby again, plus I had a few unresolved issues relating to how things went the first time, which were totally out of my control. I really needed to talk through these things to get clear mentally for this next labour, so I was completely prepared.

Once I had my debrief things were pretty much smooth sailing for the rest of the pregnancy. As I got closer to my estimated date I started to experience 'warm up' period cramping which started on a Sunday afternoon. I clearly remember the rain; it had barely stopped all afternoon and was so heavy and very windy. While I was mildly anxious, I felt very prepared and confident this time around and the rest was up to God.

Gaby arrived just after dinner sopping wet which was hard to avoid considering the amount of rain still falling. After a quick chat and an observation of my contractions she decided to hang around as my labour looked like it was underway.

We turned the lights down and I had candles lit everywhere and I could still hear the wind and the rain which I really enjoyed. It wasn't long before I felt things gearing up and that familiar feeling of needing to push came on again. So, we began to quietly discuss our options as I was thinking that maybe this baby was about to come, and I was about to have a home birth. As we were discussing what we wanted to do my membranes broke, and I thought to myself this is just like in the movies, this can't be, it feels too easy!

We decided to wait it out a little longer and see what was happening and thankfully the contractions eased off a bit and we decided to quickly drive to the hospital in the crazy stormy weather. We made it safely and I was wheeled up in a wheel-chair as the contractions were so strong. Upon arriving upstairs, the Midwife did a vaginal examination in which I was told I was four centimtres dilated. This was such a blow as I thought as did Gaby that I was about to have the baby!

As it turned out this baby was in a transverse (side lying position) which was making me feel like pushing all over again and to top it off I had an Anterior lip. After a while of wallowing and a bit of sleep I felt so much better. A had a wonderful Midwifery team who were trying to keep the doctors at bay and to do everything to make this labour happen including using the expressing machine to bring my contractions back on.

Not long after this I had the urge to go to the bathroom where I stayed sitting on the toilet. This was when I (finally) went through transition and felt ready to really push. The Mid-wife and Gaby had to coax me off the toilet and into a sup-ported squat position to really get pushing, which was comfortable. The position I was in would have looked comical to an onlooker and Gaby suggested that I move to an even better position as I literally could have birthed the baby into the toilet at any moment. So, with the help of Gaby and the midwife I moved to the bean bag where I leant into my husband's arms and I was ready to push.

I remember that I gained great clarity all of a sudden, desperate to protect my perineum from tearing. I focused as hard as I could on each push downwards and it was beautiful to feel such control of this pushing stage which went so quickly. At 9am my beautiful 3.6kg baby boy came into the world on his due date, straight up onto my chest and went straight onto my breast. I was in shock, I was so present as the first time around I was so out of control and out of my body, so this felt so amazing and I just couldn't believe I had just given birth with no intervention.

Due to the speed at the end and the adrenalin I did shake for a good 10 minutes but still managed to laugh my way through that also. Eventually I moved back up to the bed and birthed my placenta which came away easily.

Whilst my labour was long and not what I had imagined it was beautiful and most importantly I was in control and felt like it was a huge success. I truly believe a good support team is essential and what ultimately gets a woman over the finish line.

My husband was clear and focused making sure I always had snacks and water and intimate physical touch when I wanted it, making sure the music was always what I wanted to settle me down and just generally tended to all my needs. Gaby was giving me continuous encouragement, she was my cheerleader. Guy's support when the night drew on was amazing, all of which I am forever grateful for-thank you team.

The midwives were impeccable, dedicated and supportive of me and my want and need to have a beautiful labour journey buying me more time when the doctors got pushy.

As I am now pregnant a 3rd time, I must also mention that I thank God during my labour, crying out in prayer and reading scriptures supported me immensely to feel strong and believe in myself.

So now I feel confident for my next arrival knowing the entrance into this world will also be a beautiful and empowering experience.

My Natural Birth Experiences, Mother of Two Boys - Ethan and Darcy

I pause for a moment while I take my mind back to the birth of our first son, Ethan, in November 1999. I had just turned 24. We were expecting our first child, both eagerly anticipating the birth (we chose not to find out the sex of our baby, leaving it as a surprise). I must admit I was a little naïve thinking it would take months, maybe even a year, to fall pregnant. I fell pregnant the month after I stopped taking the 'pill', so we were slightly shocked to say the least. Thinking that I will be giving birth one day... that scared me just a little! For one, I can't stand pain. I have a low pain threshold. I usually go queasy at the thought of having blood taken. I don't handle cuts or needles very well at all.

For the first half of my pregnancy the last thing I thought of was reading books about labour and birth! But as my pregnancy progressed, slowly but surely I changed my way of thinking, partly due to getting over the shock of the pregnancy. I began to embrace it. I always believed that knowledge is power, so as I grew to love my new body and enjoy the pregnancy, I began to read books on childbirth, water birth, what to expect during the birth process, changes to a woman's body during labour (and every other topic in between!). Throughout the pregnancy I did a lot of yoga, meditation, walking, swimming, had aromatherapy massages, listened to calming relaxation music and drank traditional raspberry leaf tea (Hilde Hemmes) to maintain my fitness, health and wellbeing. However, I always kept an open mind that if I required intervention of any kind during labour, that I would use it.

As I was considered a low-risk pregnancy, my doctor at the time pointed us in the direction of the Birth Centre at King Edward Memorial Hospital (we were also public patients as we did not have private health insurance), so we chose to give birth there. I felt comfortable having midwives looking after me during my prenatal care and to guide me through the birthing process, after all, I thought, birth IS natural; should I need hospitalisation, it was only a short walk around the corner. This is where I believe that maintaining an open mind is so important. This way I was not adding more stress and pressure on myself, or at least, no more than was absolutely necessary.

[A note from my personal pregnancy diary: 3rd October 1999 -... I believe I can get through the birth without the use of drugs, pethidine or an epidural. All I have to remember is that the contractions are only for a short time; they are not forever and that they are helping my body prepare for the birth of our baby. Relax whenever I can].

I am also a firm believer of the power of affirmations. I particularly like the last affirmation as this is

the one I was focusing on through the contractions. During my 36th week of pregnancy

I wrote the following in my diary:

MY AFFIRMATIONS

Be a hollow tube, let the baby come through: be open to dilation.

Find your inner strength, become centred and let your body take over.

I am totally surrendering to my body's forces, knowing that it will do what it needs to do.

A contraction is a wave: it builds slowly, reaches a crest, then fades to a gentle end.

Let the wave carry you and set you gently on the beach.

During the afternoon of October 18th, 1999 (exactly one month before the birth of my first child), I wrote the following:

... I feel that throughout this pregnancy I have connected with our baby spiritually, yoga helping me enormously, both physically and mentally. I think it also has to do with listening to your body, being aware of the changes that are taking place and understanding why these changes are occurring.

The 'estimated date of birth' arrived (8th November 1999) and our baby was showing no signs of wanting to be born. At the eighth day overdue, I began to dread the thought of being induced (I was really hoping for labour to start on its own!). Little did I know that 24 hours later I would go through the worst case of diarrhoea imaginable, to the point of nearly fainting. I have vivid memories (still all these years later) of kneeling on my hands and knees, feeling cold and clammy. I was a wreck! (Maybe due to the homoeopathic remedy Caulophyllum 6C, prescribed by the naturopath that I took the day before.

However, my instincts tell me it was most likely due to drinking a mixture of castor oil and orange juice – something I would not recommend!)

After two hours of complete and utter exhaustion, on and off the toilet, mostly kneeling on the floor as I physically could not make it back to bed, my contractions finally started (3:31am in the morning of 18th November 1999 according to my pregnancy diary). Phil rang Rosemary (my extra support person and aromatherapist) at 4am; then the Family Birth Centre at 5:30am; finally, my waters broke at 5:50am. We left for the Birth Centre just after 7:00am. During the time spent at home before we left for the Birth Centre, I was continually changing positions. When my waters broke, I was kneeling on the floor leaning against the side of the bed. I then moved onto the bean bag leaning forwards. I was experiencing a tremendous amount of lower back pain – Phil was fantastic, providing me with some face clothes soaked under hot water. By this stage I was rolling around on the bean bag trying to get comfortable whilst also remembering that gravity will assist with contractions and help the baby move into the birth canal.

On the way to the Birth Centre I experienced about five contractions, each one becoming more intense and painful than the last. When we arrived the contractions seemed to be coming very fast and taking over my whole body. I tried to remain focussed, allowing each contraction at a time, and remembering to concentrate on my breathing and visualisation of our baby moving lower into the birth canal. When the midwife examined me to see how far dilated I was, to our surprise I was 8cm dilated! I was in the transition stage! Even now I can't believe I went through most of the labour at home – what an achievement! I spent the next hour and a half relaxing in the warm bath. I absolutely loved that bath! It was a deep bath, unlike a standard bath in most houses, so I was able to fully immerse myself, allowing the water to remove the force of gravity and take the edge off contractions. I had my husband, Phil, holding my hands and providing loving support and strength, my mum and my extra support person (and aromatherapist) Rosemary, who I am forever thankful for all those lovely aromatherapy massages I received whilst pregnant.

Finally, at 10:14am I gave birth to our son, Ethan Joshua (after a seven-hour labour), sitting over the toilet. What an amazing, empowering, emotional experience - one that I will never forget!

It is so empowering to think that considering I cannot handle pain of any sort and felt somewhat nervous that I would have to go through labour, I gave birth to a 7-pound 7oz (3.3kg) baby (AND after nearly two hours of diarrhoea!). My eyes were closed for the most part, as this was my way of focussing, meditating and flowing with every contraction, being in-touch with my body and my baby.

Nearly eight years later, in September 2007, I was due with my second child. My pregnancy and imminent birth of my second child had been a little more stressful as I was on this journey solely by myself, as a single parent. Phil and I had separated after three years of marriage and divorced late in 2006, although we always have remained good friends. I had numerous challenges, both emotional, mental and physical, to come to terms with during this pregnancy. I was an emotional wreck after my fiancé (at the time) asked me to move out of his home after I told him I was pregnant. I was about nine weeks pregnant when I moved into a place of my own. After having a bleed at ten weeks, an ultrasound confirmed my baby was okay.

"I have to calm down; I have to rest, everything will be okay, I am a strong woman" – these are the words I kept on telling myself over and over again. For the first couple of weeks after moving out of my fiance's home, I cried myself to sleep just about every night. It was horrible, so very stressful for any pregnant woman to be pregnant and living by herself with no supportive partner by their side... so thank you Mum for being there when I needed you!.

I was determined to travel along the same path as when I was pregnant with Ethan. I continued to exercise (again, mainly walking with a little bit of swimming here and there), drink raspberry leaf tea (two to three cups per day) and the occasional aromatherapy massage. What I found noticeably different was the limited time I had now that I had another child attending school, which meant scheduling in massages and appointments during school hours. Not having a supportive husband or partner really hit me emotionally; there was a part of me that felt empty inside as all I had to compare this pregnancy to was my first pregnancy, a time when I was married. I can truly say I have experienced both sides of the coin.

I really looked forward to massage time; this was my time to relax totally! Massage was a way for me to release built-up stress and emotion and quite often I could feel the tears well in my eyes. I always felt at peace and so relaxed leaving Roslyn's place! I highly recommend pregnancy massage (by a suitably qualified masseuse) – there are so many benefits for you and your baby. What made my massage experience even more special is the trust I placed in Roslyn and the friendship that we made, and still have to this day.

I chose to birth my second baby at Joondalup hospital, again as a public patient. The only reason I chose there and not the Family Birth Centre was the proximity; Joondalup is only five minutes by car. I remember when I had given birth to Ethan, the midwife at the time said to me that if I have another baby I should get to the hospital as soon as the contractions start (as it was a relatively short labour for my first baby and given that when I arrived there I was eight centimetres dilated). Gosh, it could have ended up as one of those emergency stories of, "lady gives birth in the back of the car!" Also, I took into consideration that I didn't have a partner who could drive me to the hospital at the drop of a hat, as well as having a son to take care of (so a bit of juggling was required with my parents' help!).

My labour with this pregnancy was completely different to my labour with Ethan. The estimated date had arrived, and I had been feeling the Braxton Hicks (or tightening); they were painless for me, but I was aware they were happening. I had a 'show' (the mucous plug had discharged) about one and a half weeks prior to my estimated due date which made me think I could give birth before the due date (however this was not the case). On the estimated due date the doctor gave me the choice of 'sweeping my membranes', hmm, what was that?

I hadn't heard of that before – no thanks, I thought, I want my labour to start naturally. Around my estimated date (I can't put my finger on the exact date), I had started to feel more discharge coming out; this came on gradually. I definitely thought that things were starting to happen at this point, little did I realise that my waters were slowly leaking! Two days after my estimated date on the evening of the 13th September 2007 I phoned my parents, to let them know what was happening and to ask them if they could come over – Dad was to stay at my house as Ethan was asleep, and Mum was to take me to hospital "just for a check-up" to find out what this extra discharge was all about.

Little did I realise that early the next morning I would give birth! It was just after midnight when we arrived at the hospital. I said to mum not to worry about bringing in my hospital bag as this was "just a check-up", so she left it in the car. Well, to my shock, I found out my waters had been leaking, and as I estimated and told the midwife, it had been for at least the previous 24 hours. After she did a test with some sort of cotton bud that came back positive for amniotic fluid, she promptly told me, "I'm going to have to break your waters, so you'll be having your baby tonight!" I looked at mum in shock (I think my body started trembling from nerves). Psychologically I wasn't ready – this was not meant to be happening now!

It was about half an hour later when I felt my first strong contraction. "Oh yeah" I thought to myself, this is what it's all about (eight years later!). The bath was in the ensuite of the birthing room, but it didn't enter my mind to use it this time. It was a standard bath and did not even compare to the bath at the birthing centre. I knew it would not be of much help in relieving the pain of contractions. Instead, I opted for the bean bag, the mats on the floor and the fitball. I told them I wanted an 'active labour' and the last thing I wanted was to be flat on my back, no matter how fast the labour! So, I kneeled, I rolled, and I leant; I did whatever I could to help my baby move further down. I remember it got to the point when I did say I wanted an epidural. The pain was becoming too overwhelming.

In the back of my mind, I remember thinking, "you've done this before; you've gone through seven hours of labour and given birth without any drugs!" Part of me was scared; I did not have Phil here with me and I did not have a supportive partner. I was so thankful to have my mum being with me, by my side (although poor mum had not eaten, and a couple of hours later felt faint.) I particularly remember a time when I was kneeling on the bed in an upright position, in between contractions, saying to mum, "it's okay mum, I'm okay, go and have a cup of tea and something to eat!".

The midwives told me to lay on the bed when the doctor came in so he could examine me and said that he needed to put a drip in my hand, 'just in case'. "What!" I said to mum, "why is he doing that?" They were doing it as a precaution apparently. That annoyed me and took my mind off focusing on each contraction. There was certainly more noise and more distractions during this labour compared to my labour with my first baby (and unfortunately I did not have my eyes closed for this labour at all). Having to lie on my back, whilst waiting for the doctor, was excruciating to say the least.

Finally, it was time to push my baby's head out and it took me about an hour! I was exhausted. It took ALL my strength. The doctor then told me she had to do an episiotomy and use the vacuum to assist with getting the head out. I remember feeling the needle before they cut me – "ouch," that really stung! I was not too happy to have an episiotomy as I would have preferred to tear (like I did with Ethan's birth), but at that point I was exhausted and just wanted my baby out. I had a quick peek in the mirror and couldn't believe how much dark hair my baby had! And there he was, little Darcy Jacob, born after a four-and-a-half-hour labour, weighing 3.4kg (about the same as his older brother, Ethan).

I was so proud of myself – I did it. I gave birth again and resisted the urge to have an epidural. I was considerably emotional at this point in time. Such an emotional rollercoaster of a pregnancy and a labour which did not go entirely how I thought it would, but never-the-less, a healthy baby boy to hold in my arms. Note: six weeks after giving birth I had to go back to hospital to remove excess tissue that had remained after the episiotomy. That was extremely painful and almost like giving birth all over again, having a needle to numb the area before the doctor cut it out.

I feel truly grateful, honoured and thankful to Gabrielle Targett for allowing me to share my birth experiences. My reason for sharing my personal experiences of pregnancy and birth is to inspire YOU! Too many women fear birth in today's society and given that the rate of caesarean has risen dramatically, we need to change our way of thinking. Birth is a natural process. Make informed choices! YES! You CAN have natural, drug free labour – believe in your body and believe in yourself!

As I reflect back on the past nine and a half years since becoming a mother, now as a mother of two beautiful boys, I think of how my birth experiences truly were amazing, emotional and spiritual journeys – and they can be for you too!

"Do not fear birth. Knowledge is power. Make informed choices and trust in yourself"

Natalie Garmson, 2009

Simone's Amazing Labour Stories - Piper Luxe O'Brien Baby No1

Your due date 8/8/2014 came and went.

Mum and Dad were so looking forward to meeting you. Your nursery had been set up and ready for you for months. Each day after the estimated due date we would sigh and say, "When is this lady going to come?"

On Saturday 9/8/14, only one day past your due date, I was off to have an induction massage with my doula Gaby. I then sat all afternoon watching movies waiting for labour to start. But it never did. Daddy was in Joondalup playing football for East Fremantle. He had the coaching staff waiting by the phone so that he could rush home if anything started. He was happy to be able to finish his game. For the next few days, I tried everything to get you to come - bouncing on my fitball, drinking raspberry leaf tea, going for long walks and jumping up and down, and still you showed no sign of wanting to meet us.

On Tuesday 12/8/14 we went to see our Obstetrician, Dr Gunnell, at Attadale. He gave me a stretch and sweep to see if that would get you moving. I hadn't felt you moving as much as usual, so he also did some monitoring of your heart for a few hours. That was all fine, but just to be sure; he booked me in for a scan the next day. We came back for the scan on Wednesday 13/8/14 to check how you were going. Duncan, the sonographer, told us you looked healthy and well, but he was concerned about the amount of fluid surrounding you as it did not appear to be enough. We went straight over to Dr Gunnels' rooms and he too was concerned about the scan. He recommended we get you out sooner rather than later and booked me in for an induction on Thursday 14/8/14 at 8.00am.

Although I was so excited to finally have a date that we would be meeting you, I burst into tears in fear of having to be induced. Since meeting Gaby, I was finally not fearing the birth. I wanted a natural drug free labour and birth. There was no other option in my mind because I hated needles, and the thought of having an epidural in my spine frightened me to death. I had also done lots of research about perineal tearing and did NOT want to have any of this. This is why throughout my pregnancy I did everything possible to keep fit, healthy and try to get you into optimal foetal positioning. This meant being conscious not to recline – instead always leaning forward where possible, sit on my fit ball, do Pilates and aqua classes for fitness, use an Epi-no to stretch my perineum ready for birth etc. I listened to Gaby's hypno-birthing recordings, read positive birth stories and visualised my wonderful birth.

I called Gaby to tell her about the induction and thought my chances of a natural birth were now over. The word on the street is that if you are induced you NEED an epidural because the intensity is so strong and fast when syntocinon is administered. Gaby once again encouraged me and supported me. She told me this was untrue, and I definitely still could have the positive natural birth that I wanted. That afternoon, Daddy took me for a long walk along the river to get some fresh air, and then to the hairdresser for a wash and blow dry. (This is the funniest part of my story - I thought I would have lovely, clean, straight hair for when you arrived. I had no idea that I might get wet from the bath/shower or want to tie up my hair in a bun whilst in labour. Let me tell you, keeping your hair straight during labour is the LAST THING ON YOUR MIND he he).

That night Aunty Renae and Uncle Josh came over to have curried sausages. Aunty Nae's curried sausages are yummy, and I was also hoping the heat may bring you on naturally. Puppa was also with us and Nanna was coming over bright and early to see me before I went to hospital. We spent the night talking about what you might look like and how excited we all were to meet you.

Thursday 14/8/2014- YOUR BIRTHDAY!

I slept pretty well last night (again thanks to Gaby, I didn't fear your birth; instead, I was empowered and strongly believed I could do this!). I woke up about 5.30am – like a kid on Christmas morning. I was relaxed and feeling positive. Nanna arrived at 6.30am and we all ate French toast for breakfast. Puppa is the best at making French toast. I then had a bubble bath and got dressed ready for the big day ahead. At 7.30am we left home and headed for Attadale Private Hospital. Nanna, Puppa and Daddy walked me through to the birthing suite and we chatted to the midwife who would assist you - Sharna.

At 9.30am my waters were broken and the syntocinon drip was administered. Having my waters broken was not comfortable at all; so much so that I didn't even worry about the needle going into my hand for the drip. Thank goodness! The contractions started immediately - very bearable, just like a period cramp. I had portable monitoring so that I could move around the room to the toilet, sit on my fit ball etc. My doula Gaby arrived at about 11am. I was very pleased to see her as things were starting to 'amp' up.

I met Gaby when I was around 20 weeks pregnant. Gaby runs Pregnancy Aqua classes at Oceanic Water Babies in Success. At these classes we talk about all thing's pregnancy, labour and birth, as well as mostly positive natural birthing stories, which really interests me. I did a lot of research and decided that natural drug-free was the way I wanted to go. Gaby came to our house to do a private antenatal class. This is when

Daddy realised how involved childbirth is when you want it to be drug free. There is a huge importance on massage, positive affirmations as well as knowledge to be able to make informed decisions in the hospital etc. So, we decided that Gaby should attend your birth to support me and give me the best chance at having the birth I wanted.

Gaby supported me to have a natural, positive birth experience that I will never forget. She made sure I was always as comfortable as possible, suggested best positions, applied heat packs, arranged for things like my bath to be run, liaised with the midwives to ensure I was receiving the best care and my birth plan was being followed as well as much, much more. Gaby truly was amazing, and I believe she is the reason my experience of giving birth was nothing short of wonderful.

I laboured in the birthing suite until about 12pm. I then decided it was time to hop into a nice, big, warm bath to help ease the intensity of the contractions. Monitoring and the syntocinon drug had been stopped to allow me to be free to go in the bath as my next form of natural pain relief. The midwife found a handheld monitor to listen to your heart rate, so I was allowed to stay in the bath for about an hour. To me it only felt like 10 minutes. I found it so strange that I had no perception of time whilst in labour. After about an hour, it was my choice to get out of the bath and return to the bed in the birthing suite as I felt like I needed to push and felt I would be more comfortable on the bed. I was on my hands and knees holding on to the bedhead for a little while. I started pushing which was such a relief.

The final stage of labour feels like you need to push, but when you do, there is no relief until you are ready to give birth. By this stage I was getting small bits of relief after each push. I was moved onto my back for the midwife and doctor to examine me, and weirdly, felt comfortable in this position so I decided to stay on my back. I never envisioned giving birth on my back but that is the way I felt comfortable. Your head was now crowning so I listened very carefully to the midwife, doctor and Gaby about when to push and how hard, and also how to breathe and let go. At 1.42pm you slipped right out and were placed on my chest. I didn't even graze- I had the perfect natural birth that I had planned.

Meeting you was the most amazing, overwhelming moment in our lives. We couldn't believe we had made this beautiful little girl and she was all ours. You were chubby and had a full head of thick black hair. You were frowning and looked just like Daddy! The love we instantly felt for you was unbelievable. Nanna, Puppa, Grandy, Poppy, Aunty Nae and Uncle Josh all came into the birthing suite to meet you and they all couldn't believe your hair and how much you looked like Daddy. You were perfect - you didn't have a mark on you.

Everyone left the room after about 15 minutes so that you could breastfeed, and Mummy could shower and refresh. Daddy stayed with you and cut your cord whilst the midwife monitored you. He then helped them dress you and wrap you up. I had a very large clot around this time which caused me quite a bit of discomfort. Dr Gunnell sorted this out by pushing my stomach until it came out. I then had an injection in my leg to ensure I wouldn't clot anymore. After this was done, Gaby helped me shower and get dressed, and by 4pm we wheeled you down to our room which was number 21, just like our home address.

Your name wasn't decided until about 8pm that night. We couldn't decide out of Pepper Luxe, Peyton Luxe or Piper Luxe. Daddy decided Piper was his favorite and Mummy agreed because it was your great Nanna Eccles's maiden name. We both thought Piper definitely suited you. And there our journey as a family began. We could not have been happier bringing you home from hospital three days later, on Sunday 17/8/14. We drove a black Jeep Grand Cherokee and lived at 21 Coleman Crescent, Melville. You are perfect, beautiful, strong, and everything we ever dreamed of. You are our daughter, and we will love and protect you forever. Love Mummy XXXX

Simone and Brock's Labour Journey of Madden, Baby No.2

On the 7th of April 2017 at 7am Simone, Brock and I arrived at Murdoch hospital for Simone's membranes to be broken so she could go into labour. At this stage, she was ready and was now seven days past her estimate and had a lot of warm up labour but nothing that really lasted any longer than a few hours. I was also going to Bali on a holiday on the Monday morning and Simone really wanted me there to assist her once again on her labour journey and couldn't face doing it without me present so therefore decided to go with an induction to avoid me not being present. This is something I would never encourage at all as going down the induction road can be seriously hard work, however both Simone and I thought once her membranes were broken, she would be in the swing of labour very quickly due to all her warm up. We were right on.

At 7.30 am Simone's membranes were broken and by 8am Simone was experiencing regular sensations like clockwork. There she was bouncing and rocking on her fitball, breathing and surrendering and laughing occasionally at my terrible jokes! All was going along as we planned. Her obstetrician came and said, "I will examine you at 2pm this afternoon and see what is happening with your cervix, unless you have the baby by then" and off he went.

The midwife and the student midwife were amazing assisting Simone in any way they could. Simone walked around a little, leaned over the bed, sat on her ball and just closed her eyes and let herself go to where she knew she needed to go. Simone is one of my beautiful friends and clients who labours so well. She just gets on with the job at hand, stepping aside and letting her body do what it needs to do. Brock was funny this time around as he kept wondering how much longer it was going to be as we were all sort of thinking that being number two baby it was going to go quickly.

At 2pm Simone's Obstetrician came in and did a vaginal exam to state to us all that Simone cervix was 4 centimetres dilated open. I could feel Simone's disappointment with that announcement. She thought as did Brock and I that she was going to be around 8-10 centimetres and ready to push so we were all a little taken back. Simone being Simone was like "right put the Synto up in the drip I'm ready, bring it on!" And with that the Midwife swung into action and before we knew it the drip was running and on came stronger more powerful contractions in which Simone handled so well as the strong woman that she is.

It was now she decided to use the shower as the bath at this hospital is not allowed to be used for some ridiculous reason that did not make sense to any of us at all. The shower worked so well for Simone as she went down on the floor and kneeled leaning over a plastic chair, towels were under her knees for cushioning and Brock held the hand-held shower head on Simone's lower abdomen, as the main shower water fell over Simone's back as I massage her lower back using oil and lots of pressure. This was the benefit of not having an epidural in which Simone could still go wherever she wanted to go and use whatever position she desired.

This kept Simone labouring away beautifully in a relaxed way till she started to breathe loudly and started to make a bit of noise. At 3.20pm she got out of the shower to have another vaginal examination in which it was announced she was 8cms dilated. Now Simone was smiling as she was moving along nicely. I stated as words of encouragement "Only 2 centimetres to go, you can do this, you are doing this right NOW, you're amazing and so strong". I looked at Simone and I could tell she was really listening and once again she had to dig deep to find the strength to surrender as the contractions were now one upon the other and pushing her mentally as well as physically. Contractions brought on with the drug Syntocinon are really hard work and not very nice at all.

At 4.05 pm Simone started to feel the urge to push. Once again, her Ob decided to do another vaginal exam to discover Simone had a rather thick Anterior lip and asked her not to push at all. The urge to push was very overwhelming and this is when Simone asked to use some Gas to distract her from pushing. Every cell in her body was saying 'push' and I was telling her not to push as it can make the Anterior lip a lot more swollen and thicker. Simone was amazing and tried so hard to focus on her gas sucking and not pushing. I was so impressed with Simone's Ob because it was then that he decided he would try to push the anterior lip back over the baby's head while Simone pushed and after 3 attempts, he finally succeeded and Simone to her sheer relief was asked to push to move her baby down her birth canal. This is when I took the gas off her so she could now focus on bearing down to push her baby through her birth canal. She was amazing!

Simone was up on the bed kneeling and leaning over the top of the bed looking at Brock and I and pushed to her heart's content and in her usual style held her baby's head on her perineum so that it could fully stretch wide open in a gentle controlled way. Her final little nudges to gently birth her baby's head were so amazingly controlled. After a short pause and one final BIG push, out swished Simone and Brocks baby's body in one final effort. This beautiful baby boy entered the world calmly at 4.37pm after what seemed like a long time but in actual real reality time was still a very quick labour. Not long after Simone's placenta came out and Madden as he was named went straight onto the breast for his first breastfeed. Everything was so smooth and peaceful in the end. We all laughed about how Simone had dilated from 4 to 8 centimetres in one hour and twenty minutes and then went to full dilation in 30 minutes and then give birth. "Wow what a woman to do that" I thought.

I feel so privileged to have been in attendance once again for you Simone and thank you from the bottom of my heart for allowing me to assist you.

With LOVE always to you and your beautiful complete family Gaby xx

The Beautiful Birth of Gala Baby No.1

When friends without children ask me if labour hurts I don't really know what to say. Childbirth is different for every woman. I have a friend who gave birth in an hour and a half and once her child was in her arms she said, 'I don't know what all the fuss is about!' I believe I could probably enlighten her. With two average-length births (approximately twelve hours) under my belt I must confess the pains of labour are excruciating. However, I must also declare that with proper education, support and physical and mental preparation, it is a pain that is bearable.

We women are made of stronger stuff than fluff. My first birth experience was in a hospital. I had decided I wanted a natural childbirth without an epidural. During pregnancy, though I kept myself physically fit, I did not participate in any pregnancy or birth-related classes. In fact I avoided them. But I chose to be in the hospital as I wasn't confident with the other options.

Having started contractions at 7 pm and arriving at the hospital at 11pm, by 5am after numerous offers from the midwife I opted for the epidural. The hospital staff all did their utmost to ensure the safe birth of my beautiful ten pound four ounce little boy, and at 7.30 a.m. he came into the world. (The obstetrician who delivered him stayed back to complete the delivery after a twenty-four-hour shift).

149

The baby was perfect and I was ready for visitors by 9 a.m. but I had a niggling feeling, which would only increase with time, that I had failed. I gave birth on my back, with my legs in stirrups, nurses pushing on my belly, in a room that looked like a dental surgery - not a homely environment. I had succumbed to the epidural and didn't have the presence of mind to ward off a huge episiotomy (leading to third-degree tearing). Though this may sound like kindergarten compared with what some women undergo, it was not how I'd imagined giving birth. In fact I didn't feel as though I'd done anything, as I felt my baby had been delivered by the swarm of medical professionals who'd surrounded me and then buzzed off never to be seen again once the baby arrived. I felt powerless.

Baby No. 2

On discovering I was pregnant for the second time I immediately started looking for antenatal fitness classes. I was only six weeks pregnant when I started Gaby's classes, but already, like those really annoying students at school who always made the class stay back after the bell had gone, I had a million questions. Second time round, I was determined to go through labour without an epidural, and feeling empowered.

We (my husband and I) opted for one of Western Australia's excellent birthing centres. I was doing antenatal aqua, antenatal yoga, antenatal meditation and active birthing classes, and had they offered antenatal nose-picking I'm sure I would've thrown myself into that as well! I decided I might need extra help, and in the third month Gaby agreed to be my doula. I already knew I had made the right choice but my husband and mother (the rest of the support team) needed convincing. My mother, a registered nurse who had studied midwifery, was sceptical about the role of the doula. She saw it as taking over the midwife's role and needed a little convincing of Gaby's function.

The four of us had three meetings before the birth and Gaby and I spoke together numerous times during and after the aquatic classes at the pool. We spoke about whatever was concerning me at the time - fear of tearing, fear of having a girl, standing up to doctors, how to have the Strep B administered, when to call her, etc.

At week thirty-nine I felt very fit and everything was ready to go. The baby's head had been down for three months, but my appointment with the midwife revealed that it had turned and was in a transverse position. The midwife started using the 'C' word and I almost broke down into tears on the spot (not that it's unusual for a heavily pregnant woman). I spoke with Gaby before my ultrasound and she assured me the baby would probably be back in the head-down position by the next day. Sure enough, at the ultrasound the bub was back head-down. It was a valuable episode as it revealed my true fears and with the help of Gaby allowed me to let go of them.

Week forty-one, the morning of 10 April, I started contractions and I knew it was all on. I called Gaby at 7 a.m. to let her know things had started but there was no hurry. Maybe it's the same with all women but I thought I was closer than I was. When Gaby arrived around nine and showed no urgency I knew I could relax. I went outside, had contractions, called my sisters, had contractions, made muffins, had contractions, my husband polished everyone's shoes, including Gaby's, and I had contractions. With every contraction Gaby or my husband came and gave me a back rub and kept my hot-pack hot.

By 11.30 a.m. all I could think of was the big bath at the birthing centre so I decided to move there. I was calling the shots. What a difference to my previous birth where I had been a slave to hospital protocol. We got to the birthing centre, only to find I had to come back into the real world for a time, to answer questions from the midwife. Then I argued with the doctor on how to administer my antibiotics for the Strep B. Though I give the doctor credit for being persistent, I won. I admit that doctors work incredibly hard, but they know about medicine and I know about me. Their knowledge must be balanced along with the understanding that a pregnant woman is not necessarily sick or stupid.

My husband, mother and son arrived just as the bath was filled. My husband and I got into the bath and time became liquid. We had music, oil and after a few suggestions from Gaby she left us to ourselves. The contractions hurt but in between I felt divine, nurtured — truly, I felt like a goddess. I'd never imagined that birthing could be this way. When my husband left, Gaby or my mum came in. They performed perfectly as a team to help me give birth in the way I chose.

When the midwife changed over at 4 p.m., the time came for an internal. I thought I was nine or ten centimetres dilated, and when I found out it was five centimetres some quick words from Gaby stopped any self-pity and helped me get on with it. At about this stage with my previous child I had taken the epidural. The two hours that remained seemed an eternity.

I was due a booster jab of antibiotics for the Strep B but at 5 p.m. I decided to pretend to start pushing so they wouldn't give it to me as I didn't really feel it was necessary to have another hit of antibiotics. Well, I did have a tiny urge to push, but at the same time I was scared to do so. This was the part where I had given my power over to the medical profession beforehand, and now I was the main player. I knew I had good support behind me to do what was needed; a great midwife, my husband, Gaby the super doula, my mum, and even my one-year-old.

The pain was like nothing I have experienced. I tore (but the tear was small) and I felt nothing but a burst of heat. And the sensation of suddenly feeling that head clunk into the pelvis was bizarre and marvellous. I am so grateful I was able to experience it. The intangible pains of contractions changed in an instant to an awareness that my baby was so close to revealing

153

itself. And when she arrived, I was exuberant, exhausted and still able to get up and walk to our room. My recovery was much faster. I had no grogginess. I had complete consciousness of my muscles and parts.

I felt empowered and strong.

My mother later commented that she saw the reason and place in having a doula — that it seemed to make everything more fluid. My husband said the support we found in her was the missing link. And as a side comment, my recovery from a drug-free birth was much quicker and I felt like I bounced back into life at home very easily.

Shannon's Powerful Journey - Birth Story No.1 – Sienna

I am so delighted to have the opportunity to share my birth story. I really believe in the wonderful work that Gaby does, and truly thank her for her contribution to Sienna's entrance to this wonderful world. I stumbled across Gaby at her antenatal aqua classes. I wanted the opportunity to meet other pregnant women whilst doing some activity at the same time. Little did I know just how valuable those classes would become.

I always knew that I would birth my baby vaginally, however that was all I knew. I was afraid to read books about those final stages of pregnancy simply because I was afraid of the inevitable. I was very naïve and happy to just cruise along and believe 'what will be, will be'.

I was shocked to hear the majority of women were either birthing at home, a birthing centre or the local Kaleeya hospital. Despite the class being in Freo – (Fremantle), the hippie Mecca of WA, the women all appeared to be normal; some who worked, some who were stay at home mothers. No presence of hippies! And what is a birthing centre? I did not know this was even an option! Attending those classes helped me learn a lot, and I was very intrigued and keen to take it all in. I left the first aqua class a little worried after finding out that the hospital I was going to had the highest intervention rate in WA! What did this mean for me...? I didn't know.

Nonetheless, I had an incredible pregnancy and was so excited about every aspect. As my estimated due date neared I felt I was gaining an incredible amount of knowledge through Gaby's Antenatal Aqua class, Couples One day workshop and the Four-week journey for women. I was like a sponge soaking it all in and growing in confidence as I became very clear about creating my idea of my ideal birth.

My partner Alan and I had to be quite firm and assertive when we showed our birth plan to our Obstetrician, yet we were forced to negotiate and give in to the doctor on certain points. We later found that a few hard conversations during my pregnancy paid off on the big day. He was very aware of my wishes and my determination to birth naturally; a wish I was not convinced he came across often as he seemed perplexed as to why I needed it to be that way. I guess he was used to compliant women who didn't often question what he said he wanted.

At almost one week post my EDD (estimated due date), on a Thursday evening in the hydro pool I got Gaby to push my pressure points during the aqua class while she floated me around. I also ran/waddled up a hill, coaxed on by Alan, and decided that evening we should follow our friend's advice and have sex a little harder than usual! To my surprise, I woke up during the night with a funny feeling. After going to the toilet and my mind racing, I stayed awake wondering, 'Is this it?'

The next morning (Friday) was the first morning I was slightly hesitant about Alan going to work (he worked an hour and a half away). However, I thought chances are there would be time for him to come home, so I sent him off while I continued on to my appointment. I was due to go to Gaby's house for a massage but was early, so I decided I might partake in a fast walk around the river to try to get things going. As I got out of the car, I felt a spurt of water, then a trickle. Was I urinating? I quickly sat back down in the driver's seat. That stopped it. I tried again to get out of the car, and it happened again. I then realised that my waters had just broken! I was so excited! Poor Alan! After just arriving at work, he received my excited phone call to turn around and come home. I then rang Gaby, informing her that I had to cancel the massage at the last minute......because my waters had broken!!! So much excitement; I was over the moon. Gaby suggested I still come for the massage to calm, and centre myself, but I was too excited and all I wanted to do was go home and celebrate.

Once Alan arrived home he wanted me to contact the hospital. I was reluctant as I knew that they would want to know when my waters broke and that would mean they would start monitoring the time. I was Strep B negative, so I wasn't in any rush, and at that stage there were no contractions. In the end, after some discussion, I rang the hospital and they asked us to go in. I made it very clear that I wanted to get into established labour at home. The nurse assured me I could go home after the initial monitoring if everything was alright. I still had no contractions at this point. I had to meet the doctor before I was allowed to leave. He said it was hospital policy that once my waters were broken, I needed to be in established labour within 12 hours. However, because I was very low risk and determined to have a natural birth, he was very happy to allow me twenty-four hours; that, I thought, would be plenty of time!

We went home and tried to focus on resting and allowing my cervix to dilate. However, it is a bit hard to relax when you know your little cherub is coming! I went for a walk around the local park and light contractions were coming about thirty minutes apart. My doctor had wanted to do another assessment to make sure bub was still happy, so by 5pm we went back to the hospital. Gaby very kindly met us at the hospital to deliver some homoeopathic remedies to bring on the contractions as they were still very mild. At that point we had decided to stay at the hospital.

Alan and I made ourselves at home and set up the birthing suite. There was a lovely big bath that I was very keen to use, a shower, a lovely big couch and a double bed. I was very impressed with the room! We set up the stations, played music, lined up all the food we had brought, watched Home and Away and just waited. Our spirits were very high. Our meal for the night came, and we watched some cricket. The midwife suggested that we get some rest for the big event, so we slowly went to sleep. Occasionally, I would get up for my contractions which had slowly increased over time before going back to sleep.

At 2 am I was woken up by my Obstetrician. He had been called in for an emergency caesarean and wouldn't be available at 8 am to induce me if I had needed it. He decided to prepare a drip to go in my arm just in case I needed it in the morning if I had still not gone into labour by then. I agreed knowing that I still had six hours up my sleeve. My contractions were five minutes apart and I had been working hard, even though I was aware they were still only warm up contractions. I always believed my body would do what it needed to, and I knew I was starting to dilate. When the doctor left, I asked him exactly, "How do you define established labour?" He said I needed to be 4-5cm dilated.

Well, 6 am came and I was woken abruptly by an older midwife who ordered me to, "get up and have a shower as you won't be able to get wet once the drip goes in". I couldn't believe it! Firstly, it was two hours earlier than expected and secondly, she automatically assumed that I had slept all night and that not much was happening on the dilation side of things! I told her! "That's assuming I need the syntocinon. I would like to think positively and that I don't need to have it". She replied by saying, "Oh yes, we all like to think positively", and then left the room. I went to the shower and just cried.

I was assessed by another midwife to find that I was only 3 cm dilated! A wave of disappointment rushed over me as I knew that meant synto was about to begin. I was no longer able to have the use of the bath I had dreamed of, and I was very aware of the cascading effects of intervention once I was induced; I wanted to avoid this from happening. I was still very determined to give birth naturally and realised the contractions were going to come on fast. I said to Alan, "I can still do this but I'm going to really need your help". All along I was convincing myself it was going to be ok.

I had already eaten the food that I had packed as it was now nearly twenty-four hours since my waters had broken back in my car! I asked for a really big feed as I knew I needed the energy. I assured the nurses that I had never thrown up and that eating always made me feel better. A huge breakfast was delivered as we changed rooms and the synto was started. I had half a bit of toast only to say, "I feel sick!"

I had a change of room and midwife, which was a blessing as I felt ready to get on with the labour! I had requested a lady called Zoe and was so pleased to have her. Then it began! The onset of labour began at 7:30am. The contractions were very frequent and at a much higher intensity; it was full on! I worked away kneeling on the bed over a belly bag (like a bean bag with a hole in the middle). In between contractions I would lay forward to rest. I had a heat pack on my back and Alan massaged me. I tried breathing through the contractions which worked well for a while. After an hour, my mind began thinking negatively and I truly believed that there was no way that I could continue at that intensity all day. As soon as my mind wasn't focused, the breathing didn't help, and I was fighting the contractions.

I finally said to Alan, "I don't think I can do this anymore. I have had enough". Of course, both Al and the midwife gave me praise, telling me how well I was doing. Deep down though, I knew I couldn't handle much more. That was it.... During the next contraction I got up off the bed and started to walk out of the door. "Where are you going Shannon?"

"I'm just going away! I want out!" I just wanted to escape and stop it all from happening.

I was redirected back to the edge of the bed. I tried the fitball, but it was not much better. Still my mind was in a very negative frame of mind despite all the positive encouragement. I thought they were 'full of shit' and not telling me the truth, because as far as I was concerned, it was too hard to do all day long and that is all I kept thinking about!

I began talking to Alan about a caesarean. After being re-directed with positive words of encouragement by both Alan and Zoe, I then demanded to have a caesarean. "I just want a Caesarean. I want to wake up and everything to be over and alright!" Luckily, I had an extremely good midwife who really believed in me and my initial wishes. Zoe reminded me of my birth plan and that I was doing really well. She encouraged me to have a natural birth. I then felt like I needed to push the issue as they were not listening! Couldn't they see that it was really hard and that I wasn't coping! Zoe then very assertively told me I was not going to have a Caesarean as there was no emergency or any need to.

At that point, Zoe very gently asked if I wanted an epidural, even though it clearly stated on my birth plan that I didn't want to be offered pain relief. I was very scared of an epidural and was always clear in my mind that I didn't want it. I tried a new position. "Sitting on the toilet often helps", she said. Well not me. I was becoming quite distressed. I began considering other pain relief options. Having gas was my only consideration. This wasn't a smart idea though because it had only been one hour, and the gas wasn't ideal to be used for the long term. I felt that was another knock back and that I was running out of options.

I went back to the bed and asked for an internal to see how far along I was. Zoe knocked me back on this as well, taking me back to my birth plan that said I did not want regular examinations. Alan had been massaging my back and then suddenly I didn't want it anymore. Then, with the next contraction, I felt this incredible urge to poo. I began making a quick getaway to the toilet. "I need to poo.... I'm pooing everywhere!" Zoe explained, "No you're not Shannon, but this is good news, and I will do that internal examination now".

In one hour and twenty minutes I had dilated from three centimetres to ten centimetres. All the uncertain thoughts and asking for a caesarean was because I was in transition. Even though I was fully aware of what transition could look like and that my actions were very typical of transition, it was a shock to all of us as it came so quickly. The sensation to push was indescribable. I liken it to a road train coming and there is nothing you can do to stop it! "I need to push!" I yelled, but my midwife had gone to ring my doctor. I knew it was important not to push until I was given the ok. I was very keen to do everything I could to preserve my perineum, but the road train was coming and that first push for me was uncontrollable. I felt my insides kind of exploding! "Z...O....E" I yelled, "Come back!" I was so dependent on my support crew. Alan made me stare into his eyes, "We are going to have our baby". It hadn't sunk in – it didn't seem real. It was only ten minutes ago that I thought I was giving up.

The next half hour was the most rewarding for me. Once I was allowed to push, I actually kind of enjoyed it. I felt in control and was able to do exactly what was asked. I did feel like I was pooing with every push; the biggest most rewarding poo that I have ever done!

I was pushing on all fours on top of the bed. I had previously had a conversation with my doctor. He had told me that once I was crowning, he wanted to have my bum on the bed in order to protect my perineum. This was a dilemma for me. I really didn't want to be in this position as I believed it would restrict the ability for my pelvis to open. I had made the decision that on the day I would refuse and make sure that I was nowhere near the bed. As it was, I was on the bed when my doctor came in! He very nicely praised me and asked for me to roll onto my back. I tried my hardest to be strong and refused his request, "No! I don't want to" I said very stubbornly. My doctor then went up a level from being nice and relaxed to assertive, saying "time to roll over Shannon."

"Ok!" I answered immediately like a little kid.

He asked me to do some practice pushes. Practice!? I don't think so! The baby was there and ready! To my doctor's surprise, as he quickly put on his gloves, he said, "oh, we're about to have a baby". I pushed Sienna Jean McLaren out in six pushes with just a slight graze and no tearing. My doctor did very well at guiding her out and yes, looking at the photos and seeing the work he did, I am very happy with the position I ended up being in.

My little girl was placed on my chest along with all the goozies. A quick wave of oxygen stimulated her first breath. Not a cry at all! She crawled straight up onto my boob for her first feed before having a skin-to-skin cuddle with her daddy. The emotions I felt at that time I cannot explain. Sienna's entrance was more than I ever expected and could ever hope for.

Thank you, Gaby, for empowering my partner and I to have the birth of our dreams!

Sienna Jean McLaren, 7lb 10oz, 23rd Feb 08.

Shannon's Birth Story - Baby No2 – Marley

It was such a delight to discover that I was pregnant again. Having said that, I had a wave of nervous feelings… how was I going to control that unstoppable train coming that I experienced with Sienna? Certainly, those feelings didn't last long as I began to plan for Marley.

As this was the second time around, I was so much more confident and clearer in my mind about what I wanted. I knew that I had no need for a private hospital and my Obstetrician.

Alan and I decided we would inquire at the birth centre. After our initial look around the centre, I felt that this was where I wanted to be.

I very much had a plan based on my experience from my first birth. I knew in my heart that I did not want to be induced. I did not want my labour to begin with my waters breaking and I had a strong desire to have a water birth.

My pregnancy flew by! I was back at work teaching and I had my daughter to keep me very occupied. I went back to Gaby's Aqua-fitness classes and did the same pregnancy yoga class that I had done previously. I felt fantastic and once again, loved the entire pregnancy. I actually didn't want the pregnancy to end.

I was very positive leading up to my EDD. I was focused on birthing my baby peacefully and relaxed. As everyday passed, I trusted more and more that my baby would come when he was ready. I knew I had at least ten days over my EDD where I wasn't under any pressure. Ten days came and went. The Birthing Centre was very aware of my strong desire to avoid induction and supported me in negotiating some more time. So, to avoid any induction (which would mean I could no longer birth at the birth centre) I needed to go into King Edward to have daily monitoring to make sure things were still going smoothly with bub. I was happy with this if it bought me time. I must admit, it was a horrible place to have to go to have the monitoring, as it was where everyone with complications presented (not the nicest place to be in when you're trying to prepare your mind for a beautiful labour!)

I was doing everything possible to get me going naturally. In the early hours of the morning (12 days over EDD) I got up and ate a big bowl of porridge as I moved through the warmup contractions. Even though I was filled with excitement, I went back to bed to be with my husband and get some rest. To my disappointment, I woke up at 8am the next morning as if it was all a dream. I was running out of time. I went to my morning appointment and my midwife suggested we did a stretch and sweep of the cervix to stimulate contractions to start again. I agreed. I had another lot of monitoring at King Edward and then went to lunch in Subiaco with my mum.

Hurray! Just in the nick of time. Lunch was interrupted with contractions. I was so excited! I had planned to labour on the boat for as long as possible (we live on a boat) so I needed to drive back to Fremantle. This was a hard decision as the contractions were increasing rapidly and I was only five minutes from the Birth Centre. I decided to go back to the boat and begin like we had outlined in our birth plan.

I arrived at the boat to be greeted by my beautiful husband who had flowers for me. He had just done a large food shop to stock the fridge. I went through the little stations I had set out, rocking and twisting my pelvis listening to Norah Jones. We were not on the boat for long. Just long enough to get organised really. Alan packed the car and I waddled out of the boat, passed the restaurant where the owners had been keeping a close eye on me over the last few days. We called out "this is it!!!"

It was an easy drive into Subiaco. It was 6pm and by that stage, peak hour traffic had finished. We dropped my little girl Sienna off with my mum who met us at the Birth Centre. Alan and I joked and played together. We set up our room and enjoyed the moment. Alan massaged me as I leant over the bed - he had improved immensely since Sienna's birth, after a little coaching from Gaby's Couples Workshop. I was quite keen to get into the tub, so at 8 pm Alan and I had a bath together, listening to our favourite tunes and adding to them with a loud, deep groan.

By 11 pm there came a point when the relaxed nature changed! I demanded Alan get out of the water as I needed my space. My loving and caring husband was snapped at quite aggressively when he touched me. Thank goodness for the caring reassuring midwife (Janet) who quietly praised Alan for his hard work.

Alan was quite aware I was in transition. I was very bossy and felt quite sick with every contraction. Every contraction went nowhere. I was nauseous, they were strong, and I definitely felt like I was in transition. But no progression! Once I realized this, my husband and midwife suggested I move to the shower to get things moving along and then I could get back into the bath. I was a little reluctant as I was scared to lose the natural pain relief that the water offered!

167

Wooow! I was right. It was very hard to go to the shower. Intensity grew which was good, but man oh man I had to breathe to get through every contraction. After only a short while, I asked Janet to examine me. This request fell on deaf ears. I was politely ignored. With my second request Janet disappeared, pretending to get everything she needed. She was gone for too long in my book. I began to get shitty!! Little did I realise; Janet was giving me more time in the hope I would progress as well as time to make sure the change in my birth plan was something I really wanted. I felt like she interviewed me! Asking me what benefit an internal examination would be. At the time, it was very annoying with what I was trying to cope with, but looking back on it, it was a technique from a very good and respectful midwife.

In Australia midwives are trained to do vaginal examinations with a woman on her back. So here I was having to lie on my back to have the internal which was just torture. It is also common practice for obstetricians to demand women give birth on their backs as well, as did mine. It was ironic that during my first birth I didn't want to be on my back and was bullied into it by my obstetrician, and now, here I was on my back (from my own request) almost being talked out of it by my support team at this beautiful natural birthing centre!

During the vaginal examination it was confirmed I was in transition and had been for the last hour! Janet was also able to feel that my waters were bulging in front of the baby's head. At that very moment I had a flashback to a comment made in Gaby's book "A Labour of Love-a guide to natural childbirth without fear". I asked Janet to break my waters for me. Again, she used the tactic of getting me to request it twice and taking her time to get the equipment she needed. Again, I was shitty! I had to get off the bed for my contractions as they were unbearable. My poor husband copped it again with me biting his shoulder. I was put in my place quickly though, as if I was a three-year-old!

I had very strongly decided that I didn't want this labour to begin like my first one with my waters breaking! Be careful what you wish for, as this time my challenge was to try to break them. They were very fibrous and tough, and Janet struggled to break them. But when she did, the release was wonderful, a huge gush of warm fluid. It felt so nice.

Then the action started immediately! Both Alan and Janet encouraged me to go back to the bath to have my waterbirth that I had so desperately wanted. Something told me to birth on the ground and use gravity. I declined the tub and began to push on all fours on a mat on the floor at the base of the bed. I had my arms on a beanbag.

Again, I was very bossy. I couldn't hear the midwife as she had a soft voice. I got aggressive and told her to speak up. I could not tolerate Alan asking questions. Alan was there to receive the baby and I didn't allow him to ask any questions!!! I had to work hard. Baby really needed big pushes! So much more than what I recalled from my previous baby. I very much needed the use of gravity. I loved the challenge of pushing. I felt in control and loved it. I pushed out my baby in ten minutes. When the baby popped his head out, I heard him puff his first breath. Alan and Janet were almost sprayed with all the goozies. Then the very big shoulders! As I pushed the shoulders through, I grazed my vagina. Alan caught our little bundle and passed him through my legs where I picked him up onto my legs.

It was the best sensation in the world! I cannot describe the moment adequately; a moment where I was rewarded for all of my hard work. To discover we had a little (or should I say BIG) boy was the most joyous moment that I had ever experienced. I snuggled him and cried out loud, "It's a boy", "It's a boy", "It's a boy", "It's a boy", "It's a boy", "It's a boy"! My baby boy, I got my boy! I fed him and he took to the breast nicely. I was covered in his first meconium poo and loved it!

I eventually sat on the birthing stool to breastfeed and my placenta came away ever so nicely with a big 'blup!' It was a very different experience to my first after-birth.

We eventually named him Marley Patrick McLaren. He was born at 1:25am on the 8th December, 2009, weighing 9lb 12oz (4.400 kg).

My family is now complete, and I am the happiest mother in the world!

Kelly Koodravsev Shares Her Stories - Birth Story- 1st Time, Round 1

Well, the lead up to the greatly awaited "Estimated Due Date" came and went... and what an anti-climax that seemed to be! Not to mention all your dearest loved one's ringing or messaging every day before, on the day and every second thereafter, just to ask whether you had popped as easy as a cheap bottle of champagne yet? And acting surprised when you kindly tell them, "No, the baby hasn't just taken the slip n slide ride through my birth canal and out of my V***** but thank you very much for asking...again". Thank goodness though, reaching deep into my natural maternal survival emotions and holding onto the things I'd learnt from other amazing, strong women that I'd been so lucky to have crossed paths within my pregnancy journey, I was able to not let these pressures of performing cloud my self-belief and the job ahead. I was entitled to birth our baby the way I wanted to and to have the strength to birth my baby at exactly the right time for us.

Throughout every pregnancy there is a journey....a story, not one is the same nor any more special than the other. Throughout the delight, for some of us, it can come with numerous hurdles to overcome. Yet, with these hurdles comes the learning of a strength that you never knew you had, making it even more of a blessing and sacred that as women, we are able to experience and give this miracle of life.

My journey was a fairly standard pregnancy, filling all the normal criteria of feeling sick up to 12 weeks, peeing constantly and consuming bag loads of Cheese Doritos amongst the healthy eating and exercising plan I'd organised. I ticked all the boxes, except for the one where I had 'Placenta Previa'. I was informed at my 20-week appointment that if my placenta did not move away from my cervix, I would not be allowed to have my waterbirth I'd so desired or have a shower in case of a haemorrhage throughout labour. Instead, I'd most likely be booked in for a C-section. My heart sank. This type of news I did not see coming as I just assumed, apart from my bungy dive into my new beloved Cheesy Chip packet, I'd been a very active, healthy, almost organic woman and assumed I wouldn't have any issues.

Nevertheless, after this appointment with the obstetrician, I started to research the topic to regain some control back. Dismally what I found was, there was nothing we could do about this issue.....hmmm, except HOPE that it shifted.

One of the most important things I learnt you can do throughout your journey is to make sure you surround yourself with great people who support, guide and help grow an empowered mind. To give you the strength to walk this path, the way you would like, and not be swayed by the numerous fears that some people will unfortunately, drag you down with. My ongoing pregnancy Aqua classes with Gaby, getting to bond with other pregnant women, holding onto lovely positive birth stories and dabbling into Hypno-birthing really was a godsend to empower my mind.

So after being told at the 37 week mark, the final say from the doctor was going to be made on how I was going to be allowed to birth….it didn't happen. My placenta had shifted a little bit, but apparently not enough so the 37-week scan showed, so my husband and I demanded another scan be done at 39 weeks…only a partial shift had happened, but it still wasn't enough to be in the clear, so we demanded another at 40 weeks and 4 days as of this point the doctor was pulling out the appointment book to schedule surgery.

Luckily for us, on the last ultrasound my placenta had shifted to exactly the margin point. This meant I could at least try for a vaginal labour but be hooked up and closely monitored throughout labour in case bleeding did occur, I would be ready for surgery. I was so relieved, and to think they were going to be happy to take me to theatre just from looking at a 37-week scan.

Though the obstetrician did end up pulling the appointment book out for induction instead, we pushed for the latest date possible to give our baby the best chance of coming naturally and when it was ready. Bittersweet, 11 days later bubs was still extremely comfortable and happy, but my husband and I agreed that 12 days over was where we felt comfortable at pushing the time factor, being our first.

Although I wasn't overly thrilled about induction, the public hospital we had chosen were happy for me to come in on the 11th day to try a gentler approach with a membrane sweep and cervix stretch, and Prostaglandin gel used in a suppository to support my desires to avoid Syntocinon the following day. Unfortunately, I didn't go into natural labour as I so dearly desired. So around 9.30am the next morning, after a very restless night, the obstetrician broke my membranes, and we started the Syntocinon drip intravenously.

It was incredible how intense the contractions shot up to a pain level of about 0-5 within 1/2hour and how consistent they were, without very much of a break in-between. At the beginning, my TENS machine was my best friend, along with my husband's hands massaging me. It was extremely hard to try and focus on breathing and being calm whilst there was no gradual lead up to the contraction's intensity. I felt overwhelmed at times, but it is amazing how you can focus on the end target, imagining your baby being born and how far this can take you.

With the strong loving support from my husband, I found a determination I never knew I had throughout the day; contraction after contraction, I kept going. Continuously standing, walking, leaning over the bench, bed or hubby all day, only to sit on the fitball on an occasion in-between contraction, in the hope gravity and good positioning would prevail us nearer to seeing my baby for the first time.

By about 3.45pm, my midwife did an internal examination and said we were in active labour, around 6cm dilated and the baby was very happy. This at least gave me hope she was pleased with our progress and we were moving forward. At around 4.30pm, the contractions were becoming quite unbearable all of a sudden, even with the help from the Nitrous oxide and pushing my TENS to its limits.

Most women are not too keen on the thought of examinations whilst in labour, but for me and being the first time, I must have needed a little reassurance that the sensations I was feeling were correct with the progress we were making. So, I asked my midwife for another examination but was denied it. She explained, "We only did one a very short time ago and we don't feel it is necessary". Being my first time, I was taken back, accepted what she said but was left questioning in my head my ability to trust and listen to my body's cues to tell me things were changing.

I started to doubt whether I could keep on going on with this new level of sensation. I wrote in my birth plan that I was absolutely against having an epidural, however I started thinking it may be my only choice to get through. I was tiring very quickly. As clearly as I could, amongst the tears, I told my husband to organise the epidural. The anaesthetist arrived shortly after. I requested the lowest dose to still give myself the options of birthing the way I felt comfortable instead of flat on my back.

He proceeded to get set up and in amongst all that, started to enjoy, what felt like a lovely conversation with my husband and midwife. I'm not quite sure if he was really going terribly slowly or it just seemed like that to me at the time. It seemed like a lifetime from the moment he arrived and told me to sit down VERY still; to the time he was actually ready to administer the epidural. I remember telling him very abruptly at one point, "You're going to have to HURRY UP as I can't even seem to sit down on my bum!"

It's crazy looking back, as this is my one and only small regret, not hanging in there and listening to my body showing me all the signs of transitioning, but I had a low energy moment. I forgot to trust it and have faith that if I surrendered completely, my body would guide the journey itself. As soon as the injection was done, but hadn't started to take effect, I began to turn completely primal. I seemed to have the guts of a bull all of a sudden and demanded another examination from the midwife instantly. Dilation was 9 cm and I was in the transition stage….that's why I couldn't sit down very comfortably, nor very still, nor very be quiet. Being things were moving very well downstairs and thank goodness I had only chosen the lighter dose of epidural; it only gave me about a 20–30-minute semi-break before my body told me to start pushing.

My most comfortable and safe position, under the circumstances of being a little off balance with the injection, was cradled over the raised bed head on all fours. So, after some

176

extremely loud, long groans and an intense burning sensation, within the next 20 minutes I was able to feel the baby's head come through for the first time. Within the next 5-10 minutes I birthed our baby boy. It was 6.05pm and he weighed in at a healthy, 3895grams. An incredible feeling after what felt like the most intense and long cross fit session at the gym I had ever taken part in, but the utmost rewarding moment of my entire life up to this date.

Nothing can come close to this feeling of pride, accomplishment and discovering a strength I never knew I had. It was truly a life changing moment for only the better. I was so delighted that under the circumstances of a low lying placenta I was able to achieve the vaginal birth I wanted, instead of caesarean - with no forceps, vacuum and no excessive bleeding.....and of course, birth the most handsome baby boy my husband and I had ever laid eyes upon.

2nd Time, Round 2

Well as per so many other people in this world, we wanted nothing more than to complete our family with a little brother or sister for our first born - it is as common as every new parent with a coffee addiction. So, as it turned out, we were heavily pregnant and doing it all over again 2 1/2years later. As I soon found out though early in the piece, not one pregnancy is ever the same. Even though it was everything we had asked for, wished for and received, my hormones decided to play havoc and left me feeling quite depressed most days until thankfully, I came out from the dark cloud by the third trimester.

I thought women only could feel that low after birth, but it turns out I was wrong. I was extremely lucky though, I was still aware that this wasn't my "normal" personality, and that kept me from falling into a hole. It was amazing when the hormones finally decided to balance out again, almost to the other extreme; I received loads of excess energy. I finally could get back into my Aqua and walking exercise eagerly without dragging my feet, and actually get excited about planning ahead for the birth; embracing the little miracle that was about to change our lives for the better once again.

Not having restrictions on possible health issues, this time I felt like I could completely focus on how I wanted to bring our baby into this world. I'll never forget how much I just wanted to welcome the contractions, as I knew that with every contraction and intense feeling, I would be closer to meeting our baby. It was nothing but absolute delight on day four past the estimated date, when I felt my first warm up sensations. Then on day seven past the EDD, a Wednesday, I started to feel the head engaging while walking up and down our stairs at home. That night I still chose to go to pregnancy Aqua class with Gaby, as I was of the belief to keep things rolling, you gotta keep moving......A small part of me was regretting that decision five minutes into the class when Gaby asked me, whilst

I was trying to balance on a noodle and kick, "What's wrong with you tonight?" Not looking at all so elegant and looking more like a drowning frog instead, I proceeded to tell her "I am fairly certain that baby's head engaged well and truly to-day"....... "Well, that would explain it!" she replied.

I now know that the feeling of buoyancy and lightness in water can only go so far...and then it stops. After having my last primal send-off chant from Gaby and the other pregnant girls I'd grown so close to throughout my journey, I said my last goodbyes and quickly headed home, straight to bed.

That night, I woke up at 1.24am startled for some reason, maybe a flush of endorphins and oxytocin? It was almost an orgasmic feeling. It was even stranger because I was sleeping alone in the spare bed. This was due to a fight for space amongst my five supporting pillows and a struggle to sleep with my dear purring husband vibrating the walls at night.

Nevertheless, I managed to get straight back to sleep, though only to re-awake at 2.45am with tightening. After con-sistently cramping throughout the rest of the night (started off at 15-minute intervals and went down to 7–10-minute inter-vals) I decided to call my Mum and Dad at 5.15am to let them know that they might need to come and look after our son for the day. I remember telling them also, "Don't rush though, as I don't want any anxiety, just relaxed feelings. Luckily, Mum and Dad didn't listen to me.

179

I was so worried about getting stressed by anyone else's emotions that it could slow my labour down. I even told my husband at 6am to go to work. Luckily, he just took one look at me and didn't listen either. So in between contractions I stuck to the normal routine of breakfast, clean-up, and washing sorted. I even snuck in a shower to wash my hair and for some strange reason, decided it was also important to look good for the day and straighten it as well. I'd like to blame the hormones for that one, but I think it was the hairdresser coming out in me instead. During the shower I had lost the mucus plug, so my baby's birthday was looking more imminent by the second.

After my parents arrived to look after our son, the bag was packed and a last belly photo was taken. I finally felt ready to hop into the car.....well I crawled by this time, hopping in fast was not an option, contractions were now 5-6 minutes apart. It was a 25-minute drive to the hospital, and I could feel in this time my whole body just starting to let go of my normal daily routine and think only about what my body was capable of doing and its job ahead. By the time we arrived at the hospital just after 9 am, contractions had now gone down to every 3-5 minutes.

We were greeted by the midwife my husband had spoken to earlier that morning on the phone. She took us promptly to an examination room where we met our lovely senior midwife Cindy, and a young girl called Charmaine who was on her first day of Prac. The two of them were absolutely lovely; they had a real peacefulness about them which was perfect. After being assessed, I was 4-5cm dilated and moving along lovely. We were taken then to our birthing suite and the midwife started setting up the bath. By around 10am, I could feel I was moving into established labour, so as soon as the bath was ready, I hopped in. I could now feel my body completely surrendering and wanting to be in a safe birthing space and for me that was submerged in lovely warm water.

Instantly there was relief in so many ways. I felt comfortable being in the same hospital that we'd had our son in. I was in the place where I had envisaged birthing my baby, listening to beautiful music, in a dimly lit room, hot water on my back, a cold flannel on my forehead, sips of coconut water and support from my husband in between. I think he was just as happy as I was that I was in the bath compared to our first time.

He will still say he suffered worse than I did, trying to deadlift my bodyweight to help me in certain birthing positions and then coming out with two crushed hands by the end of me birthing our son. This time leaning over the inflatable pool edge and squeezing his denim jeans, seemed to be sufficient enough to get through the 60-90 seconds of sensation coming and going.

Through the intensity, I focused on a very special moment I had while having an induction massage with Gaby a few weeks prior to labour. The vision was that many people from my life who had passed to the other side had all come to me standing in a line. One by one, they passed the most beautiful baby down the line. Then lastly my dear Nanna, whom I was closest to, delicately passes the baby wrapped in a pink knitted blanket to me, like it was a present. Whether it was a dream or a message from my dearest loved ones that had passed, there was nothing but love that was felt from this dream and vision and it was a delight to hold on to it for warmth and strength throughout labour. The funny thing was though, before my Nannas passing, she had knitted me a pink blanket in the hope one day I would have kids, and a girl. My mum, who had kept it in a safe place since my Nanna had left us, gave it to me a few days after having the vision.

Soon enough though the intensity was starting to make me feel I had no control over my body. I remember the feeling from my first labour, the pressure of the baby on my organs and bowels gave the strong sudden sensation of needing to go No.2 but couldn't. It was another sign bubs was close. I also automatically wanted to kind of stand up in the bath, even though I knew I needed to stay close to the ground.

At this point, I also rubbed coconut oil downstairs as I could start to feel the baby's head was beginning to crown. Cindy and my husband reminded me of the importance of short breaths, like a panting at this stage to slow the stretching down. So, with the guidance from Cindy on when I could push, I was soon able to feel the baby's whole head. Then when I felt the time was right, I pushed in the next contraction and I caught my baby in the water at 10.58am. She was a gorgeous, healthy 3520grams, with strawberry coloured red hair and a great set of lungs to match.

Her hair was an absolute delightful surprise but also a total shock to myself and my husband whom both have mousy brown hair. What was also amazing is that she was born with the membrane still intact over her head and body. Cindy had said that she saw her break out of it at the very last minute as I caught her.

Apparently, it is quite a special and rare thing to have happen. We had several other midwives come into the room, just to have a look at the membranes. The membrane almost looks like a clear rice paper sheet that you would make Vietnamese rolls out of, but so incredibly strong.

Looking back, I couldn't have been happier with how both of my journeys turned out. I wouldn't change a thing. That may sound strange as you probably gathered, my first labour tested every bit of determination and strength that I had, and then some more. The healing was longer, having received 2nd degree tearing and terrible bruising. It was truly the hardest thing my mind and body had ever had to do in my life.... but also, the most rewarding feeling I'd ever felt. It took me to a whole new place of realising the strength of the mind and how important it is to feed it well. The experience only taught and prepared me more for focusing on exactly what I knew I wanted for the next time round.

I felt it was a privilege to go into natural labour and to embrace every contraction, not fear them. Having a completely drug free birth in the water with no tearing, proved to me that somewhere inside every woman there's a natural instinct for birthing. We just have to search for the tools to learn how to trust and believe in what our bodies are built for.... birthing miracles!

A Story of a Different Kind

(Written by Gaby Targett, who was a doula for this couple.)

This couple, Sam and Ken, came to ask for support during the birth of their second child because of their traumatic first experience during childbirth. The first birth experience was truly the 'cascade of intervention' at its best. It was the usual story of induction, followed by the need to have an epidural as the contractions were just too painful, and then a long time on the bed on her back unable to move. When finally fully dilated, the baby was stuck, the mother was unable to feel the contractions or the need to push, so the baby was assisted out with forceps. In the process of having a forceps delivery, the coccyx bone was broken and a third-degree tear resulted after an initial episiotomy! Four toes (the mother's) were also broken due to the force with which this woman was asked to bear down and push doing a valsalva manoeuvre, pushing against the midwife's body.

As you can see, the first birth experience was not a pretty picture, and for obvious reasons there was a lot of fear and stress going through the second pregnancy, thinking that at the end of the road the same story could repeat itself.

When I came into the picture it was with welcome arms, and after a period of time I felt a wonderful rapport with this couple, who totally trusted and accepted what I had to say about the previous experience. Because of this trust, I was able to assist this couple to debrief and clear away the old baggage, cleaning the slate ready for the next birth experience.

After many visits to the house and lots of contact during the aqua-specific pregnancy classes, the arrival day was near. The three of us prepared the final touches to the birth plan. At the top, in really big writing, was written, 'A doula and my husband will be supporting me, to help me focus and stay really strong, as I give birth to my baby naturally with no assistance from anyone else.' This was Sam's objective.

At last the telephone call came from Sam's husband, Ken, at 11 p.m. in the night.

"Hi Gaby, it's Ken. Sam has gone into labour. I am trying to get her in the car but I am finding it really hard as she is making lots of noise and she doesn't want to move. I'll be at your house in ten minutes when I have got her in the car".

Well, thirty minutes passed by in a flash and still no car. I decided to phone just to see if Ken needed me to help out in some way, after all they only lived across our park. When I rang Ken said "I now have Sam in the car as well as our son, I'm grabbing the bag now and I'll be over in one minute". True to his word, Ken pulled up to a halt a minute later with a screech of the brakes.

I opened the door to find Sam on the back seat, half laying down, half seated with one leg in the air on the headrest and one on the floor. Sam was panting and groaning like an animal, all while her son sat happily in his car seat with big wide eyes observing in a bemused way. The first thing I suggested was for Sam to turn around and kneel on the back seat looking out the back window. At least then she could open up her knees and take the pressure off her coccyx bone and pelvis while I massaged her back. Relieved to be in a better position, we took off for the twenty-minute drive to the birthing centre.

At the halfway mark of our journey Sam started to mention the fact that she felt the urge to push a poo out and the urge was getting stronger and stronger with every contraction. Being the 'I'll do anything to support you' type of Doula, I happily suggested "Oh, just go ahead, if you have the urge to push a poo just do it, I will catch it, no problems". Well with that I lifted up Sam's dress to catch the imminent poo in my hands! Out it came before I could reach for a towel or open the window to throw it out. So now I was in a real predicament — not only did I know that what follows poo is a baby, but my hands were full of poo! Carefully I tried to rotate the window winder, to open the window enough to throw the poo out. After about two minutes of trying and thumb-cramping I was successful.

All the while Ken just cracked jokes and said "It is OK, honey, we will just tell the car-hire people we didn't smoke in the car but we accidentally got poo on the seats during the birth of our baby!" With that, I completely lost the plot laughing, not to mention Sam, who was trying to say that she could not laugh because it hurt when she laughed. It was a very serendipitous moment and one which totally shifted the energy from fear and anxiety to a calm and 'we're OK' attitude. The only difficult part of this scenario was massaging Sam with the backs of my hands as she needed pressure on her back to cope with the intensity of her pain.

Finally we arrived at the birth centre, Sam just about ready to pop the baby out, Ken feeling relieved we had arrived, their son Santi wondering what all the fuss was about, and me with residue poo all over my hands.

The midwife took one look at me and said "You had better come this way with me and wash those hands". It was a relief to be finally able to use my hands, and with that I moved into the birthing suite where Sam, Ken and Santi had been taken.

I suggested that Sam get onto a mattress on the floor to birth her baby. With that she not only went onto the floor, she lay on her side with her head completely under the bed, with her arm up and between the mattress and the base. It was here that she stayed for the remainder of her birth, which lasted all of about twenty minutes. During this time I could hear muffled sounds coming from her mouth, along with, "Gaby, help me control what I do, don't let me tear, please".

At this point I looked up to see both father and son sitting on the bed, observing quietly, in awe of Sam's strength and ability, as two midwives and myself assisted Sam to birth her baby. As Sam pushed her baby down onto her perineum her membranes exploded completely, flooding the floor around us, not to mention my pants from hip to foot! It was then that I stood up to hold Sam's leg up in the air, keeping her toes free from injury. With the help of the midwives we coached Sam's baby out through the perineum. Little by little she gently pushed and guided her baby without a tear. At last, Sam's nine and a half pound baby boy slipped gently and calmly from her body onto the floor.

Slowly, slowly, Sam moved her body out from under the bed to meet and greet her son face to face, skin to skin. Ken, Santi and the wonderful midwives and I were all laughing and crying and awash with emotion. The labour was fantastic, straightforward and wonderfully funny at times, leading to a positive birth experience. I was so privileged to have been a part of creating such a different experience from the first one, and honoured that they were open to changing their thoughts and feelings about birthing. Sam said afterwards, "I was really ready to listen and open to preparing myself this time around, I really wanted a totally different experience and I got it".

Everything that Sam had written on her birth plan (apart from the poo in my hands!) happened, and she was so thankful that she had been mentally prepared to turn her thoughts around to a more positive mindset. As for Santi, he just sat in amazement and awe of mum with her head under the bed giving birth!

Births of William and Ella - Monday 15 April 2002

No matter how many books you read or how many birthing classes you attend, nothing really adequately prepares you for your first birthing experience.

Being aware of alternative procedures prior to the birth of my baby boy, in addition to the standardised hospital procedures, gave me the confidence to arrive at the hospital armed with viable options. Having confidence is especially important to me, and going into an experience for the first time can be daunting, so having an alternative birthing plan made it less so.

I woke at 3 a.m. with some discomfort. We had open back stairs at the time and I managed to ease some of the discomfort by stretching my arms to a stair and rocking backwards and forwards on my fitball. After having some breakfast we arrived at the hospital at around 10 a.m. where I was given an immediate internal. I was only one centimetre dilated so it was a case of just trying to remain as comfortable as possible using the shower, stretching and massage.

At noon I was beginning to feel quite tired, my waters had only just broken and the contractions were steady at around five minutes apart. At 12.30 p.m. I was given another internal and was told that I was now four centimetres dilated. At this stage I was having difficulty coping with the pain and in hindsight I probably should have checked out the gas and air as a source of pain relief instead of opting for an epidural.

At 1.30 p.m. the epidural was administered and within twenty minutes all pain had gone and so all I could feel was the painless tightening with each contraction. At 4.30 p.m. my skin felt itchy all over, I'm not sure if this was a combination of the hot shower and the epidural. By 5.30 p.m. I was given a drip to help speed up my contractions. This had an immediate effect on the strength and frequency of my contractions, prompting the midwife to suggest that I lie on the bed to relieve the pressure of the contractions and to speed up the baby's heart rate as it was very slow.

At 6.30 p.m. I asked for a top-up of the epidural. I'd become used to no pain for over five hours, so as the initial epidural wore off painful contractions started to come on very quickly, becoming too much to handle, as I was by now extremely tired and feeling quite exhausted. In hindsight, once again I should have taken this opportunity to try gas and air because I'm convinced that the top-up of the epidural slowed the birth down again.

At 8.40 p.m. I was fully dilated, but I still could not experience the contractions to their full effect and had to rely on the midwife telling me when to push. On the bed I was in a half sitting, half lying position, with my knees bent and my legs held by my partner and my sister. This position does not assist the birth of a baby whatsoever, but because of the epidural and subsequent lack of sensation in my legs, it was impossible for me to get into my planned position of being on all fours and offer my baby a much better angle for delivery.

At 11.13 p.m., some twenty-odd hours after hanging from my stairs, I finally gave birth to a beautiful baby boy weighing a healthy seven pounds fifteen ounces. The euphoria was wonderful, along with the fabulous endorphins racing through my body — the whole conception of birth is an absolute miracle. New life is beyond written or spoken words. However, I can't help feeling that my miracle was only part of the true journey of childbirth because of the effect the epidural had, not only on myself, but also on my baby's first few hours.

Saturday 1 November 2003

The story continues with the birth of Ella, my second baby. During the afternoon I'd taken a long walk to try and get things started. I was far more composed with this pregnancy and I felt like I was much more in control. The fear of entering the unknown, mixed with all the horror stories that certain people feel they have to tell you, as was the case with my first birth, were not in evidence this time around. I knew that this time I would be more positive and resist the temptation of complete pain relief and give myself and my baby a far better birthing experience than before.

At around 7.30 p.m. I started to feel a little nauseous and physically tired so decided to have a warm bath and try to relax. As soon as I got into the bath, contractions started immediately. However, I was determined to stay in the bath and enjoy this experience, plus I didn't want to spend hours at the hospital again.

After ten minutes I couldn't remain lying in the bath, as things were happening very quickly and it all took me rather by surprise. My husband checked the duration and frequency of the contractions and we were both quite shocked and very excited once we discovered that they were only three minutes apart and lasting around a minute

Once my Mum arrived to look after William, we set off in the car to the hospital, which is only a twenty-minute drive away. I had to lift myself from the car seat as I could feel the baby's head bearing down. I honestly thought at this stage that I was going to give birth in the car. The time was now 9.10 p.m., and once inside the hospital and positioned on all fours on the bed, the midwife informed me that I was fully dilated. I was given the option of gas and air for my pain relief, which was fantastic. I was in complete control, managing the breathing, totally focused and being able to understand and feel my baby's journey into the world. It was an incredible experience as I felt so in touch with my baby, as we worked together in the most beautiful way possible.

Ella came into the world naturally at 10.10 p.m., with no tearing and me being on all fours just like I had imagined I would have been. This time around I felt so mentally and physically prepared and so happy. I created a much more positive birth experience for the both of us.

I can't fully explain how different the two births were. Obviously both were fantastic experiences, with a beautiful gift of life at the end. However, given the chance again, I would choose my second birthing experience over the first without doubt, as I was the one in control, yet surrendering at the same time.

Bev and Case's Stories - 1st birth of Kai

Case and I attended Gaby's 'Active Birth Workshop for Couples', which was aimed at the role of the partner as an assistant to an actively labouring woman. My husband Dr Case Sinclair, chiropractor, was really inspired by the active and factual approach Gaby used to explain the nature of labour as a process, rather than pain as we know for injury etc. I knew earlier on in my pregnancy I was looking for support to have no pain relief or unnecessary intervention during my labour and birth unless absolutely necessary, so decided to employ Gaby as our doula to oversee our experience. I attended midwifery check-ups with the hospital we chose but did not need to see any doctors throughout my pregnancy, even though I was in my late thirties.

Towards the end of the pregnancy I prepared to wait beyond week forty to have labour begin naturally, and worked with Gaby to develop visualisations, have massages on her 'big hole in the middle' table and attended exercise and relaxation aquatic classes where I enjoyed meeting other mums-to-be. Though not medically trained, I felt strongly that my body could do the job of birthing and I did a lot of reading, including some evidence-based medical summaries in relation to procedures likely to be offered to me. This gave me the confidence as a lay person to draft a detailed birth plan mapping out my preferences and any contingencies, which I wanted to convey to the

194

staff at the hospital in order to create a positive and empowered experience.

Throughout the pregnancy, Case regularly treated me (as he does with all pregnancy patients) with various chiropractic methods. He feels he helps them to achieve the maximum physical mobility so that their bodies can do as nature intended for the birth. I also followed advice from Gaby about exercises to keep the baby in a head-down anterior position using a fitball in the later weeks of pregnancy.

Gaby's Recollection of Bev and Case's Labour Journey

On Wednesday the 21st of January 2009, Bev was a couple of days from being forty-one weeks, but in no hurry to give birth - as with many couples, their home renovations were still ongoing. She came to me for a natural induction pregnancy specific massage to try to get things moving along a little. That same day in the afternoon, I was to have a chiropractic appointment with her husband to sort out my back. While I was there, I noticed Bev looked very soft in her face and blissful like she was in labour or about to begin labour. As we spoke, she mentioned to me that she had been having regular ten to fifteen minutes apart contractions for almost an hour.

She commented to me, "We weren't certain if this was it or just a warm up that could stop, so I didn't bother to contact you yet." Besides, I knew you had an appointment this afternoon with Case". I knew Bev didn't want any more delays as she wanted to go into labour without a hospital induction or having her waters broken and she was hoping this was at last happening. As it turned out, the contractions kept gently rolling along that night, and becoming a little slower the next day and the next night. By the early hours on Friday the contractions hadn't ceased; however, Bev wished at this time they would get closer together as she was getting tired having had sleepless nights and feeling a little exhausted. She was doing well resting when she felt she had to, eating good food, but couldn't sleep much between each contraction. She kept taking intermittent showers to soften the contractions. I knew that she wanted this baby to be born that day.

She called me at dawn letting me know that she was keen for my support to speed things up. Bev was doing considerably well given that at this point she had essentially been labouring two nights and a full day in between. So, I set about keeping her mind off the time, and surrendering to the sensations. I gave her ideas and helped set up various positions such as leaning over her pillows in a dark bedroom, some homoeopathic remedies and suggested she take regular showers, although she found her home shower a bit stuffy. We walked around the house and then the block using the neighbour's fences, or front wall or school fence to lean on for contractions. Bev had wanted to walk to the hospital but realised that it was going to be a hot Perth day, so keeping hydrated and needing to urinate between contractions regularly meant she had to let go of that goal. She preferred labouring in the fresh morning air and in the sunlight of their porch under a tin roof, looking out into the garden as she laboured, standing and sitting on a fitball while we watched her beautiful cat play on the grass, as hour after hour passed.

I was oblivious to the time as it just passed by without any of us giving it much consideration at all. It was however about 2.30pm when Bev decided to get going to the hospital. Upon arrival, we were informed that the hospital was very full of labouring women and unless Bev was four centimetres or more in dilation we would have to return home as they did not have a room for her to labour in! Bev wasn't enjoying the interrogation and had struggled with the whole idea of being an 'inmate' at the hospital. After much consideration, Bev agreed to a vaginal examination as she did not want to go home at this point. Fortunately, she was a good five centimetres and fully effaced with the baby's head well down. We were all relieved to hear that. We did not want to return home as we had exhausted all the labouring options there and were ready for a new fresh environment to explore.

We headed for what was to be our labouring room for the next amount of time and stage of labour. Immediately I sensed I had to try and get Bev back into good labour as all the questioning and interrogation by the midwives had snapped her out of labour. With all the kerfuffle upon admission, she had literally gone from having strong dynamic contractions to next to nothing spaced out so far we hardly noticed Bev have one contraction in ten minutes. This can often happen when women arrive at their place of birth, as there is often so much going on with midwives buzzing around, bright lights, medical procedures needing to be performed and questions asked. It is no wonder women halt their rhythm of labour as they are forced to move from the 'primal' state to one of the 'thinking rational' state where the brain is switched on in order to answer and respond to the probing questions being asked!

When we got into the room Bev jumped into the big hospital shower which she loved as it was less stuffy than the small cubical she had at home. She sat on her fitball while in the shower, and used the handrails to rock while Case and I took turns to hold the shower hose on her lower back and body. This worked so well and Bev was getting into the labour zone once again. I could see that what Bev really wanted was distraction from what was going on through using hot water, pressure, massage as she leaned forward on her arms and tried to relax her body in-between the contractions. After a while she almost fell asleep in this position. Not long after this we headed to the bath where with low light and a dripping tap, Bev felt calm enough to stay for three hours labouring beautifully. She even munched on sandwiches between crunching ice at the end of each contraction to let all the tension out of her jaw. She also used a visualisation from her days of training for team sports to treat each contraction as a dynamic sprint to a lovely big green tree and then on return slowly jogging back to the end of the contraction to rest.

We all knew things were on the move when she started to make deep noises down in her throat, which sounded very much like opening and pushing primal noises. With those new sounds, the midwife on duty came into the bathroom and asked Bev to get out of the bath just in case she began to push her baby out in the bath. This hospital had a 'no water births allowed policy' much to my and Bev's dismay.

So with that, Bev headed back to the room where she got up onto the bed kneeling and leaned over the back of the bed. It was here that she began to make the distinctive pushing and opening noises. At this point, she was working really hard and decided to try the birthing stool in which she could sit and give her legs a break as they were getting very tired. This was when the membranes broke with some meconium (baby poo) in them. Bev decided to stand, leaning on Case and showing all the signs of a woman in transition such as going up on her toes with each contraction, asking us when the baby was coming and saying she wished it would hurry up. She was restless and aggravated and moved her arms in a disparate manner, up and down.

The meconium in the waters resulted in the midwife taking the precaution to record the baby's heart rate to provide information for the obstetrician who was due to arrive soon. This meant that Bev had to stay on the bed, but showed that the baby was not at all stressed. With a vaginal exam being performed Bev was asked to stop pushing and pant until they were certain she was fully dilated. The midwife was uncertain, but the obstetrician proudly announced that Bev was fully dilated with the baby well down. With that, Bev got into her pushing with her legs up on my hip and Case's hip as she had the urge to push against something. The doctor left the room stating, "See how you go, I will be back in twenty minutes to see if you need a hand to get the baby out!" I think this was something Bev did not want and motivated her to push like hell and get this baby down and out. With such strength and great positioning, Bev worked so hard.

Ten minutes later the baby was born, with the cord around his neck which is very common and was not at all an issue. The midwife just simply released it by pulling gently on it and putting it over the baby's head. Kai was born at 10.33pm and was just over four kilograms, close to nine pounds of pure delight. Not long after, the placenta came away and the labour process was complete.

I helped Bev get Kai on to her breast after a short amount of time and he sucked for what seemed like ages. He really was a gorgeous baby boy.

Fifteen minutes later the doctor returned in disbelief that Bev had managed to birth her baby on her own, given that she had appeared to be very tired. It just goes to show you how strong women really can be, especially at the end of a very long labour. The adrenaline at the end can and will see women through, as long as there is no interference from chemical drugs on board. Bev slept very well back in the maternity ward in-between breastfeeds where her baby nestled on her chest —this was an amazing bonding experience for a tired mummy to have this little human being moving around looking to be fed between long sleeps!

I was so happy and proud of Bev and Case for creating this powerful birth experience, and getting on and just doing it as it was intended.

Anecdotally, Case feels that most of the pregnant ladies he treats, including Bev, had quite short pushing phases of their labour. Although Case had treated babies with chiropractic before he had his own baby, handling Kai with the love of a dad has really added to his confidence in working with many babies since. Parents and bub are often overtired and anxious because bub is uncomfortable, cries a lot, or has difficulty feeding or sleeping and maybe favours only one side. Babies are so supple. Case feels like he's barely touching them, he loves hearing that they did a big poo then slept like a rock or that their head shape has markedly improved after just a treatment or two. Bev sought chiropractic care quite a bit in the early days of breast-feeding as she found her shoulders needed time to adjust to various feeding positions for long periods when the baby was new-born.

Bev and Case's 2nd birth of Asta

I chose to birth at home with the CMP – Community Midwifery Program for my second baby for many reasons including:

Birth was a natural process right up until my mothers' generation, even now only 1 in 5 women should need any medical intervention – pregnancy is not an illness, unless your body shows clear signs to your health provider that you need greater care.

I did a lot of reading and it was clear that the fastest and safest birth and recovery would come from the least amount of intervention – all pain relief would prolong the birth and that was incentive enough to prepare myself for a natural birth. Ref Cochrane Report.

Women are strong, they just need to give themselves a chance to experience their ability to birth their baby without unnecessary interference.

Access to a birthing pool was the best part of my first birth (but in hospital I was asked to get out to push), so for baby number two my only choices were home or a birthing centre that allows every woman water birth by using inflatable birth pools. Hospitals with one bath may allow water birth but you compete with other labouring women on the day for access.

In an emergency I felt certain that a transfer from a home birth to hospital would be similar in time and safety to what would occur within a hospital (e.g. waiting for specialists to come to your bedside) if your birth is within reach of a backup hospital. In the hospital for my first birth, it was a busy night, I felt in the way and that I didn't need the services they offered.

Being in a home birth program has great benefits like;

- You get to know one primary midwife and a backup (secondary) midwife, so no retelling of your story over and over.

- Waiting at home for most of your pre and post birth appointments – so no travel and waiting rooms with your toddler! You just need to be flexible to reschedule if another birth is happening for another woman.

- Not being in hospital also meant we only needed one night of care for our toddler.

- Your midwife will refer you and offer to attend other related medical appointments with you if they are needed.

As is standard on the home birth program, I saw an obstetrician once late in pregnancy (30+wks) just to check that all my health indicators were appropriate for a homebirth. This took a few minutes and was the only time I saw a doctor even though I was 39.5 years old.

Patience is crucial for a natural birth. We passed the estimated due date in birth one by 7 days, and birth two by 10 days. I was very clear that I wanted spontaneous labour if possible and patience was the best way of making that happen. So I just relaxed about the day and date, and my midwife kept a close eye on me and visited me daily at my home. We booked to scan the placenta function by day 14 but the baby arrived before that so no need for concern.

I had Gaby as my Doula (non-medical birth support), onboard for my second labour again massaging my back to minimise the pain during each strong long contraction, with 5 minutes apart contractions and 2 minutes rest and recovery. I really felt I wanted to be in the water tub. I was sitting on the fitball and I had a long wheat bag on my pubic area to soothe soreness and Gaby was massaging my back. So, the race was on to get the tub full enough for me to get in and as soon as Case, Gaby and Abbey had finished filling the tub up with extra buckets of hot water from the kitchen and bathroom I was ready to step into the birth pool. What I was thinking now was that I feel really supported by the side of this tub, it is the right height for this final stage of the birth and it's easy to adjust my knee positions in the warm water. My midwife and Doula were supporting me without the need to get wet. Not long after getting in I stood up and as I did my waters broke. With that my baby dropped straight into my birth canal, and 3 contractions later and a few sort of pushes out she came. Gaby and Abbey dived their hands down between my legs to try to catch her before she went in the water head first. It was a fast experience to say the least!

None of us expected this labour to be over by now – only 1.5 hours active labour. My Baby girl Asta was born so gently and peacefully and weighed 4.025kg

3.

THREE BIRTH STORIES FROM ONE MUM

Byron's Birth - baby No 1

I really had an excellent pregnancy - my husband and I were so thrilled to find out we were expecting our first child just after we got married. I was due Jan 11th, 2007. I had no morning sickness and barely felt pregnant, except for all the beautiful kicks I got (I thought we had a little soccer player on our hands!) until I got near the end of the pregnancy and got major fluid retention and put on 30 kg by week 37. I felt like I was having a boy right from the start; I even went out and only purchased boy's things, which was confirmed at our 18 week's scan.

I was feeling really huge by week 36 and due to how much weight I had put on, a sizing scan was done which showed he weighed 3.5kg and was quite long. My obstetrician was going away for 10 days over Christmas, and with the size of the baby and because my husband works away, we decided it would be best to induce.

I was pretty calm about the birth and had done lots of research about labour until near the end where I got quite worried about his size and considered having a caesarean; I didn't want to but was really worried about tearing or being cut. The actual labour didn't bother me at all, just the end bit!

My baby was well engaged by 36 weeks, so it was just a matter of waiting till my cervix was ready. I had an appointment with my Obstetrician on 2nd January where she did an internal scan to see if my cervix was favourable. It was, so she quickly booked me in to be induced the following morning.

It all happened so quickly, and I couldn't believe we would be meeting our little boy the next day. As you can imagine, I barely slept that night just thinking about the next day.

We arrived at the hospital at 7.30am where I had my waters broken and the drip put in my arm. It was strange having my waters broken, and a ton of liquid sprayed everywhere! My husband Gareth was there from the beginning, and I also had my best friend Amy as an extra support person. I was attached to monitors but only for 20 minutes out of every hour. Unfortunately, the drip did mean that my mobility was limited but I did still get up and walk around a bit. My Obstetrician went off to work and I was left with a lovely midwife, Gareth and Amy to wait.

After the drip was put in I was having contractions instantly that were painful, but they were bearable. I had decided to try to have no pain relief earlier as I really didn't want anything to increase my chances of needing an assisted delivery which could mean more chance of an episiotomy. By 11 am my Obstetrician came back in to do another internal and found that I was only two centimetres dilated, but my cervix was thinning. This was pretty deflating news as I was hoping to be a little further along. As the drip increased every hour, it was at full dose by 12pm. This was when the contractions started to get very strong and a little more unbearable.

I continued to breathe through the contractions, mainly on the bed, and another internal was done at 2pm. I was four centimetres dilated. At this point I felt really flat as it had been such hard work for six hours and I was hoping to be a little more dilated. My Ob said that because of his size, if I hadn't progressed a lot by the next internal at 4.30pm, we would need to look at having a caesarean.

I was so utterly disappointed upon hearing this; I am almost certain it hindered my labour, but I know she needed to look at it from a medical point of view and didn't want the baby to get distressed. There was another lady who had been induced at the same time as me in the room next door, and it was at this moment that I started hearing her yelling as she was pushing and then I heard her baby cry. I felt incompetent since I wasn't already at the same stage (even though I knew everyone was different) and this, together with everything else including a change in shift of my midwife, made me really emotional. The next two hours were horrible. My husband and Amy tried to support me by rubbing my back and telling me how good I was doing. The new midwife who had taken over was very efficient at her job but unfortunately had been working for too long and had a really rough, uncaring approach. She was barely in the room with me at all for the afternoon.

Amy helped me have a shower at about 3pm, which helped with the contractions, but when I got out I felt very faint and dehydrated from the hot water. At about 4 pm I was so tired and in immense pain. It was more that it had been a long day that was making me emotional. The midwife offered me the gas to try, which I did, but I felt like I couldn't get anything from it. I found it more difficult as I wasn't able to concentrate on my breathing as much. I had been asking to get in the bath for about an hour, but my midwife seemed to keep putting it off. Finally, at about 5 pm, I asked for an VE to see where I was as I thought I may need an epidural. My Ob told me I was 9 cm dilated which was great and that she thought I should have some pain relief as I was in such an emotional, tired state

I asked for an epidural at 5 pm. At 5.30, with Amy and Gareth in the room, I felt the urge to push. It is an indescribable feeling when the head is crowning through. I am pretty sure I was yelling. I know I was crying so Amy went to get my midwife who was on the phone and told her she would come when she was ready! The midwife and the anaesthesiologist came in and I was 10 cm dilated. He got me to sit very still on the edge of the bed. This was hard as I felt like I was squashing the baby's head. I leant over Gareth who supported my weight and tried to breathe through the pain. Gareth felt really faint from the smell of the liquid put on before the needle, so Amy came and supported me. Within a minute of it being in I was on cloud nine. I was sitting in bed happily talking to Amy and Gareth and even wanted food. I could still feel my legs and walk because I only had a small dose since I was so close to pushing.

My Ob came in and said that she would be back at 6.30 in order to give the epidural time to wear off. Then I could start pushing. At 6.45 I squatted at the end of the bed with Amy holding one of my legs, and the midwife the other. We waited for a contraction to be visible on my stomach, and each time there was one I would push. After six of these the head was almost out but had got stuck. My Ob knew I didn't want an episiotomy so told me I would have to push really hard on the next one or she would have to cut me. So, I did, with all my might I pushed and his head came out screaming! It was the most amazing thing, one small push later and at 7.04 pm Byron Robert was in the world.

He was put straight on me and Gareth cut the cord. About five minutes later and a small push the placenta followed. Gareth, Amy and I all cried; it was an amazing moment to share with my husband and best friend. Unfortunately, due to my tear I lost a lot of blood over the next few minutes and passed out. While my Ob stitched me up, I was put on another drip to try to stop the bleeding. After about 45 minutes I felt a lot better and could properly take in my beautiful son. Byron was weighed and was 3890 gm, 51 cm long with a 35.5 cm head circumference. I was very sore that night and quite weak, but Gareth was fantastic and laid with Byron all night.

My tear was only 2nd degree and by the third day did not hurt much at all. I came home with my gorgeous little man on day three feeling fantastic. Giving birth is absolutely indescribable but the most amazing experience, and one look at my little angel makes everything worthwhile.

Baby No.2 - Mason - Home Waterbirth

My first birth was in a private hospital. This 2nd time around however I chose to thoroughly research my options while I was pregnant; I wanted it as calm and natural as possible. I wanted to be active and birth in a position to prevent tearing and ideally have no pain relief. What I had the 1st time around was the classic 'cascade of interventions', a labour where I was attached to the bed and monitors, threats of having not progressed far enough along and that a c-section may be necessary, pushing on my back with my legs being held and a second-degree tear. I may sound very negative about the experience, I suppose I am about it all, especially now knowing how amazing birth can and should be.

I had considered a homebirth with my first son, but in all honesty, I wasn't ready for it. I wish I was, but I still had some fear of labour, and of any possible risks. I hadn't realised yet, just how risky it can possibly be to birth in a hospital as well. I was amazed and so interested in homebirth and did lots of research about this option. I knew that when I had my next child it would be a homebirth. When I fell pregnant a year after my son was born I immediately applied to the Community Midwifery Program in Western Australia, to see if I could be approved. We are so lucky in WA that we have a program that is government funded for approved homebirths. My husband was quite hesitant. He knew I hated my first birth but was concerned about the risks of a homebirth. We discussed it thoroughly and I pointed out all the positive research and in the end, I basically said that there was no way I was birthing this baby in a hospital. Just as I had feared a homebirth with my first labour, I now feared a hospital birth, and felt home would be just as safe this time around. He agreed eventually and was over the moon when I was accepted into the program with Corrie as my midwife.

I first met Corrie at about 22 weeks and I was elated; she was calm, friendly and I felt so comfortable with her. I had a very easy pregnancy. She continued to visit my house for our lovely appointments, and I continued to grow, both physically and mentally. I was an advocate for calm birthing and was so looking forward to my upcoming labour. I kept very active during my pregnancy, and even did my daily 5km walk five hours before I gave birth. I'm sure this helped with my relatively quick labour.

My husband worked away and wasn't due back until two days before my 'official' due date. This made me a little nervous, however I was completely prepared to labour on my own if need be. Thankfully he managed to come home a week early, and as it happened, as Mason arrived the day, he would have been due back!

We spent the final week of being a family of three, preparing for the new arrival to our family and spending precious time with our first born. I was feeling slightly antsy waiting; I was so eager to meet our new baby - I'm very impatient. I'd also been experiencing 'pre-labour' for a few weeks, period pain and contractions every five minutes that would then fizzle out after an hour, so I hadn't expected to get to my due date.

The few days leading up to Tuesday I was awake for at least three hours in the early morning, feeling like labour was about to begin. Painful contractions and back ache, but it would always go away before it progressed any further. I was feeling

214

tired and knew that my husband would have to fly away again for work within ten days, so I called my midwife for a chat about what she thought. She suggested we do a stretch and sweep if I wanted it. It's not common practice for this to happen with homebirths, however I wanted it, and she didn't mind. She came by at 8.30am on the Tuesday and I was pleased to find I was 4cm dilated, could be stretched to 5cm, and 75% effaced. She thought today or tomorrow would be the day. I was ecstatic; not long till I got to meet our baby I thought.

I dropped Byron off at daycare as he went there on a Tuesday and walked around the river with our dog and a friend, just in case anything happened. Everything was ready to go at home, so I wasn't at all nervous. I had contractions about five minutes apart while walking and it was about 10.30am. I came home, and my contractions felt stronger, so being the organised freak that I am I told Gareth we were going food shopping, as I wanted chicken noodle soup for after the birth. He thought I was being ridiculous but came anyway. The contractions were about four minutes apart and getting very painful as we walked around Woolworths. I must have looked so funny leaning over the trolley every few minutes. We got home at about 12pm and unpacked the food shopping. I hopped on the computer to update friends and got through the contractions leaning over the fitball. They were very painful by about 12.30pm so I told Gareth to get organised with the birth pool, and I called our midwife to let her know that I thought I was in labour, but I was ok and would call her again soon. As it happened, she was at the office only 10 minutes away, so I felt comfortable not getting her to come yet.

We were lucky to be close with a wonderful photographer colleague Fiona Colvin and have been fortunate to have her photograph most of the special events over the last few years. She had offered to photograph the birth for me, as I had expressed interest in it and we had become good friends, so I felt completely comfortable with her being at the birth. So, I texted her and told her I thought she should come soon if she could. We were both so happy it was a daytime birth as this had been our worry; a flash through labour would not have been nice.

By about 1pm I was in lots of discomfort. I jumped in the shower as Gareth filled up the birth pool. It was 1.30pm when Corrie arrived, and I had about three strong continuous contractions leaning over the couch while she checked the baby's heart rate. At 1.50pm I was really uncomfortable, so I jumped in the pool. It was beautiful and hot and took the edge off my contractions, but gosh they still hurt. You really do block out the memory of that pain!! I was only comfortable on all fours leaning over the side of the pool and stayed like this till our baby was born. I had no idea how far along I was and thought I could potentially be 'wasting' my midwife's time. Fiona arrived at about 2.20pm and set up and tried to talk to me, but I could barely respond. The contractions were constant, and I murmured to my midwife about breaking my waters to speed things along. She said we definitely could, but I couldn't move so we didn't worry about it.

About 2.30pm I started feeling lots of bottom pressure. I thought I needed to go to the toilet, but I was pretty 'cleaned out' so didn't move. Corrie told me to go with the feeling, and push if I felt like it. The urge was so strong, and although painful, it was almost relieving. Two pushes later and I had a feel to see if I could feel a head. I felt something but wasn't sure it was a head. Another push and the head was out. It was such a strange feeling when the baby moved its head to the side. What relief I felt!! My midwife told Gareth to have a look into the water and see our baby, and he was so surprised. One more push and he would be here, but I was so thirsty and I refused to push until someone got me a drink!! Fiona ran and got it, and then one more push and he was out in the water. I pulled him up onto my front and sat back in awe of what had just happened, so quickly. It was 2.45pm on 09-09-08.

We cuddled in the pool for about 30 minutes, staring at our gorgeous new arrival. Gareth then cut the cord, and I hopped out and had a beautiful feed with our baby, while waiting for the placenta. I called my best friend Amy, who had been my support person at the birth of Byron to share the news, and she came straight over from work. She was so surprised to see me up and walking to the shower so easily after the birth. Gareth and I talked about names and we decided on Mason Parker. We chose Parker as the middle name because my maiden name was Parkes and we wanted to incorporate it in some way. The placenta was birthed easily about 30 minutes later, and I went and had a shower while Gareth and Corrie did all the checks on our baby. Gareth also went and got Byron from daycare and brought him home to meet his brother. At exactly 4.00pm we popped the champagne open, celebrating our beautiful new baby boy. Labour was 3 hours 10 minutes, including an hour for placenta birthing.

I felt incredible. I cannot put into words what an amazing experience it was for us all, and as I sit here five days later typing this, looking at my beautiful calm new baby, I cannot think of a more beautiful way for him to come into this world. My homebirth truly was incredible, and we are already looking forward to doing it again in the future!!

Baby No. 3 Indiana

As I sit here typing, with my beautiful little girl lying on my chest, I am overwhelmed by the most incredible feeling of love and contentment. I feel truly blessed and know that she was sent to us from those above who left our lives too soon.

The anticipation for our little girl began long before I found out I was having a daughter. It began years and years ago, probably when I lost my own mother at a very young age and our beautiful close mother daughter bond was gone. I am blessed with two beautiful boys who I love and treasure, so when we did find out that we were in fact expecting a little girl this time, I was completely overcome with emotion and appreciation.

My first son was born in the private system with an induction and intervention, but he was born vaginally and was perfect. I struggled with his birth though, and although I didn't realise it at the time, I can look back and say I had some birth trauma. When I found out I was pregnant with our second baby, we entered the Community Midwifery WA program, and began planning a homebirth as I wanted to avoid the cascade of intervention. I can remember the intense feeling I had that whole pregnancy – the strength and focus to have a beautiful birth this time with no intervention. I had the most wonderful birth, and it was very healing and more empowering than I ever could have imagined.

When we found out we were expecting this time, I again booked into the CMWA, and met with my midwife. She was lovely and my pregnancy continued with fortnightly visits in the comfort of our home. This pregnancy was my hardest, with all day vomiting until 17 weeks, as well as running a business and looking after my two boys, now 2 and 4. The nausea ended though and, in its place, came horrible pelvic pain and discomfort. As I neared 34 weeks, I was aware that the baby was still breech which she had been for the previous ten weeks.

My second son had been breech as well, so it didn't worry me, but I decided to book in for some acupuncture sessions.

Three sessions later and the baby was still breech, so I went for some chiropractic sessions using the Webster technique. Again, no movement. I tried being on all fours as much as possible, I had been swimming regularly all pregnancy, and I tried all other techniques to turn a breech baby. As I approached 36 weeks, I was starting to get worried. I could feel my peaceful homebirth walking out the door as the baby had to be head down to birth on the CMWA program. I started looking into private midwives that would birth breech at home just in case.

I was referred to our mainstream hospital as backup for my homebirth which was a requirement being on the Community Midwifery program. A scan confirmed the baby was still breech but on the small side, and ECV (manual turning) was suggested. I was willing to try anything at this point. I knew there was a small chance that the baby could go into distress, but if that happened, I was in the right place. Although it was uncomfortable, she was turned in a matter of minutes. I went home and did as many squats as possible to attempt to get her to engage so that she wouldn't move back to the breech position. At my midwife appointment the next day she was 2/5ths engaged and I was very happy.

As I was still working till 38 weeks, I really thought that once I photographed my last wedding, my body would be so relieved that I would go into labour quickly, and birth before my due date. How wrong I was!!

My midwife continued visits, and everything looked great. I approached 38 weeks and was so relieved to have made it through the wedding season without going into labour. My husband had been home for the last few months with our boys because it was my busiest time of the year with work. He was due to fly out on my due date and although he didn't intend to leave until I had given birth, there was pressure for him to be away on time. So at 38 weeks I had a S & S (stretch & sweep) and I was 2cm dilated; the cervix was thin and favourable. I was completely expecting to go into labour that day, as with my second son I had a S&S on his due date and he arrived six hours later. I had a bloody show that afternoon and I remember thinking "Great, we're on!" I went for a big walk, as I had been having lots of pre labour for the previous few nights.

Over the next week I continued to have contractions that would last for about 2-3 hours, completely erratic though, and then they would fizzle. They happened primarily from 2-6am, so I was getting next to no sleep. I was however getting up to date on all of my editing! I had another S&S at 39 weeks and was 2-3 cms, 75% effaced. More bloody show that night and erratic contractions. I was tired from the lack of sleep I was getting, and my body was really sore. I began to get rather desperate to get to the end of this pregnancy and birth my baby girl safely. I had been having acupuncture again to try to bring on labour, as well as a wonderful yet rather painful pregnancy induction massage, that involved having my acupressure points pushed very hard. I'd also been walking lots, bouncing on the fitball and doing squats, clary sage, evening primrose and rasp-berry leaf tea, and exhausting my husband with the awkward 'task' of having sex. At 39.5 weeks I drank the delightful 60ml of castor oil. I had heard many stories about it aiding labour, and my midwife had said that it could do the job of getting me into labour. All it resulted in was five hours glued to the toilet, and I became best friends with Sudocream in the days to follow. It was not nice, and I would never do it again!

At 40 weeks I had another S&S and I was still the same. My husband told his company that I hadn't had the baby yet, and no, I wasn't having an induction. They were quite good and extended his leave by ten days. My husband was fantastic though and assured me that if he had to walk away from this contract he would; he didn't want me to be induced or feel pressure to birth on a timeframe. I instantly felt relaxed but was losing momentum. During the days I was fine and could have stayed pregnant for a bit longer, but the nights were awful, and I spent the last week awake from 1am till daylight in tears because I was so sore and was so drained from contractions that fizzled out.

Everyday I received a new text message from someone tell-ing me, 'Today is the day, I can feel it!' I was completely over talking to people about it and was screening all calls so that I didn't snap at someone.

I can now reflect and am thankful for those last few weeks that I had, to just relax and have some me time. Work had been full on for the preceding six months, and I really did need the break to unwind, instead of launching straight into having a newborn in the house. I spent time walking; swimming and it was lovely to spend so much time as a family.

At 40weeks +6 days I had another S&S and was 4cm and thinned. I started having light bleeding that afternoon which continued all weekend. We had decided that at 41+1 (Monday), my waters would be broken at home by my midwife and hopefully labour would start. I had 12 hours to go into labour before I would have to present at the hospital for syntocinon. While this was the last thing I wanted, I was exhausted and had begun doubting my body's ability; I was wondering what it was doing with all of the stop-start labour. On Sunday night I asked my husband if we could try once more with sex, just in case it worked this time.

It was 10:30pm and I was exhausted, having not slept at all the night before, so I took two Panadol Forte that I had in preparation for the horrid after pains I was expecting after this labour and went to sleep. I was woken an hour later groggy but with a sharp contraction. Another followed two minutes later. They were painful, really painful. I lay in bed and started timing them. I stayed like that for an hour, and they continued 2-5 minutes apart. I texted my midwife telling her this might be it and I got out of bed and paced the living room. At 1am I phoned my midwife and asked her to come, still hesitant and worried that they would fizzle. She arrived at 2am and my contractions died off a bit, coming about every five minutes. However, they were still intense and on the same intensity level which I thought was about an eight out of ten. I asked for a VE just so I could know what was happening. I didn't feel as in control this time; all of the labour build up had thrown my trust in my body out the window. I was 4cms but easily stretched to 6. I continued to labour quietly over the fitball. It was a full moon, but aside from a couple of candles it was pitch black, which I loved.

Originally, I was going to have my two best friends at this birth as well as a good friend and colleague photograph this labour/birth, but instead I wanted no one around while I laboured, just my midwife. At 4am my midwife wanted to get the birth pool set up; she was worried we wouldn't end up with enough time, as my second birth was fast, about 2 hours. We got everything out, and started setting up in the dining room, with me stopping for contractions often. I remember clearly how agonising they were, they were much more intense than my last labour. With each contraction I visualised the baby moving down and my cervix opening which helped me to stay focused. At 4.30am I woke my husband and asked him to get up sooner rather than later. Thankfully, our two boys were fast asleep. My contractions were all through my back, my midwife thought that the baby had her hand up to her head. They were intensely painful. My husband came out and started applying pressure to my lower back while I leaned over the pool. At about 5am the pain was too much so I got into the birth pool.

It felt wonderful. I remember looking at the clock and thinking I had an hour until our boys would be awake, and while originally I had planned for them to be around for the whole birth, once I was in labour I wanted nothing to distract me.

I told Gareth to call Amy, my best friend, and remember hearing her in the background. I yelled that she had better hurry or she would miss it. Luckily she only lived streets away. I had three intense contractions and then felt a big movement of baby going lower. Amy walked in and then instantly I could feel her head almost there and a popping noise as my waters broke. I yelled for my underwear to be taken off, I couldn't do anything but breathe. During the next contraction I felt her head move out and I put my hand down to feel her coming, which was something I really wanted to do. The next contraction I pushed, and she was out. I pulled her into my arms, completely overwhelmed by what had just happened, my perfect baby girl, so long awaited, was in my arms.

Amy got the boys up and brought them out to see their sister. It was 5:22am. We stayed in the pool for about an hour, the placenta came out easily and the cord was clamped once it stopped pulsing. She started feeding instantly and I got to lay back in the pool taking it all in; my wonderful family, the incredible feeling of having birthed another baby peacefully at home as the sun came up. It was surreal and so beautiful. I showered while she was checked over. I had thought I would have torn, as she had come out with her hand up to her head but was pleased to have just a graze. I had time with both Byron and Mason before they got ready for school and daycare. Once we were all settled everyone left, and it was just my husband and I lying in the bed with our baby girl.

We called her Indiana Janice May. Janice was my mother's name. Born on the 16th May, 2011 at 5:22am, 8pound 14oz, 52 cm. She's beautiful and I am constantly overwhelmed with how wonderful it is to be blessed with a family.

Amy's Three Beautiful Birth Stories

I have been blessed with the joy and privilege of raising three beautiful girls. Their names are Mira, Idie and Letty. Each birth was unique, but each one out of this world, amazing and wonderful.

Here are their stories

Birth Story 1: Mira (Born 4/4/13)

We have been waiting a long time to meet this baby. Craig and I have been married 6 years now, and we both felt super excited to expand our family to 3. I had done lots of preparation through some close friends who really encouraged me to read, learn and give me information about what to expect in labour and the choices that you can make in that process. Two books that really changed my perspective and really gave me a sense of excitement and confidence in my body's ability to labour was Ina May Gaskin's A Guide to Natural Childbirth, and A Labour of Love by Gabrielle Targett.

My pregnancy was a breeze to be honest. I could have been pregnant for a few more weeks, it was that easy (people think I'm crazy for saying that). Although saying that I was pretty ready for it to happen considering I was over 40 weeks when I finally started labour, and over the abundance of people asking me "has it happened yet?" We chose not to find out the sex, we loved the element of surprise that it gave the pregnancy. My husband Craig was adamant as well that it is absolutely ludicrous to find out and he couldn't understand why people didn't just wait. Lots of my friends disagreed with him ;) We were booked to have Mira at the Family Birth Centre in Subiaco. We had a very special and enjoyable time there. My antenatal appointments all went well, we loved the staff and our team, we loved the classes, and bonded really well with others due at the same time as us. As it turned out, one of Craig's friends from his class at school and wife were in the same class as us.

I guess the story really begins on Tuesday morning on the 2nd of April. I was 5 days over my estimated date. Had my 40-week appointment and my sister Holly came with me as my husband was working. A 'stretch and sweep' was offered. My cervix was already open, which was a great sign. The midwife Jannie seemed sure it would be soon. I had slight period cramping all day, but nothing that I thought was labour. Later that night I started getting contractions of some sort quite close at like five minutes apart. I slept on the couch so Craig could get some sleep just in case this was really labour starting. I tried my best to rest but the contractions were quite consistent. I rang the Birth Centre to get some advice around 3.30am and they said to rest as much as possible and to call back in the morning unless things change. These contractions stayed through the night but didn't change.

No joke, as soon as Craig came out in the morning, they literally just stopped. Looking back this was obviously a sign of pre-labour. I was devastated that it wasn't happening for real just yet. I was also tired but tried to stay positive in my mind. My husband took the day off so he could be with me in case it started again for real. We went for a walk, watched a movie, rested, had family visit, all of it was a good distraction. I had a few strong painful cramps throughout the early evening that night. At around 11pm on Wednesday the contractions started again. This time they were a lot stronger, and they were getting stronger and stronger! I knew this was it. I had let Craig sleep earlier but needed to wake him up at 11.30pm as they were already very strong, and it was time to get the TENS machine going as contractions were about 5 minutes apart. I loved the TENS machine. It didn't take the pain away as I was experiencing this deep-down low in my pelvis type pain that was really strong. The TENS machine did help with the back pain as well as being another distraction tool. I could use the booster button when I felt the contraction coming on.

We timed each contraction, each one building in intensity and getting closer together around 3-4 minutes at this stage. I found the best way to ease the contractions was to firstly breathe! I also found I had to be up and moving about by either rocking my hips from side to side while leaning on the kitchen bench or walking around. I still felt in control by breathing and having Craig by my side. We knew it was time to call the Birth Centre soon so at 12.30am we rang them.

The midwife could hear from my voice that I was definitely in labour, but said it was up to us when we wanted to come in, that we could time them a bit longer to make sure we were getting 3 to 4 contractions every 10 minutes. I personally felt better about getting there sooner than later as I knew we had a bit of a drive ahead of us as we lived about 30 minutes from the Birth Centre. What we had been anticipating over the last 9 months was finally happening, I couldn't believe it. By the time we got ourselves all sorted and packed it was about 1.30am as we headed in. The car ride was hard, I couldn't sit down, but had to go on my knees facing the seat. I felt every turn and bump of the car, it was a relief the closer we got to the Birth Centre.

There was so much unknown being my first labour. I kept thinking "I do not want to have this baby in the car" as I had read a lot of birth stories where this had happened. Birth can be so unpredictable. We arrived around 2am. We were introduced to our midwife Debbie, who was so calm and peaceful, and Tamsin who we spoke to on the phone and was absolutely lovely. We were set up in Room 2, opposite the birthing pool. I was very keen to use the pool during labour, but I wasn't sure about the actual birthing in the water, however I was happy to go with the flow and see how my body felt at the time. Debbie let us settle into our room, we bought our own things from home – pillows, blankets and music.

I was surprised at how low I felt the pains in my pelvis, and I mentioned this to Debbie. We took each contraction one at a time, trying a few different things e.g. Fitball - which I didn't like as I found it too uncomfortable to sit on. I felt most comfortable still standing up and moving around and found this the most bearable thing to be doing. At around 3.30am Debbie came in to check on us – we both were curious as to how far along we were. Debbie never pushed this on us which I loved, and said "we don't have to have a vaginal examination as it's totally up to us". We both really wanted to have some indication where we were at, and to hopefully be encouraged. So, I went ahead with a VE. It was good news! My cervix was paper thin, and I was already 3-4cm dilated. She seemed very happy for us.

For us based on the dilation it seemed to us that we had ages to go. She said the hard work had been done, and that we would have this baby before breakfast! We were so pumped

230

and couldn't believe it was that close. A matter of hours in fact. Craig started timing contractions again at around 4am. Each contraction lasted just over a minute, so he was able to count me through them, and they were getting closer together about 1-2 minutes apart. We decided it was time to try something different as the TENS machine was kind of negligible at this point. So I opted to use the shower next. Craig and I both spent the next hour in the shower together. I stood under the shower, which Craig rubbed my back, and used the detachable shower head to help relax my back and lower pelvis area. Craig was an amazing support – he encouraged me through each contraction and kept telling me how much he loved me, gave me lots of kisses and prayed with me.

When it was time for me to get out of the shower I was getting these strong urges and lots of pressure in my bottom. I spent the next part on the toilet as I was in the transition phase of labour. This was tough as the contractions were just rolling one after another with little break in between. I remember the feeling of being in such pain, but feeling the endorphins running through me as well, it felt like I was just so focussed on the situation and breathing. At this stage Debbie popped her in to see how we were going and asked whether we wanted to try a waterbirth. I said, "yes I would" so off she went to get the bath started as it took 20 minutes to fill up. While she was gone I kept getting these massive bearing down type of feelings – like the urge to push. Next minute my waters broke (luckily, I was sitting on the toilet still!). Straight after my membranes broke my labour got extremely intense and I asked Craig to call for Debbie. The waters were all clear, which was a good sign that the baby was happy in there. I knew it was time to move, and I didn't have time to get into the bath as it wasn't ready yet.

I moved to the room on the mat on the floor that was set up with pillows and beanbags. I went on my hands and knees and found this position fairly comfortable. Soon after getting into this position, I felt this massive urge to push. It is one of those feelings you can't describe; my body just took over. It felt like the head was right there and going to come straight out. The time was around 6am. Each pushing contraction would come on and I would feel the urge to grunt and make this funny gut-wrenching sound. It was out of my control.

The breaks between contractions were so long and pain free and I remember just talking to midwives and Craig (usually apologising for the weird sounds coming out my mouth). I remember feeling a sense of being scared of the unknown and how long this was going to go on for, and feeling quite out of control with the pushing contractions as they were strong, and my body just took over. At this point, the baby wasn't moving too much, and they wanted to change my position to try and help her move through my pelvis better, whilst the midwives constantly checked our baby's heart rate. They tried to put me on my left side for a couple of contractions but I did not like this position.

Then Debbie offered me the birth stool as it would help open up my pelvis. She used a mirror to see how the baby's head was coming out. The other midwife Tamsin was in the room at this point, and she was explaining to me to listen to Debbie and to follow what she tells me to do.

The next contraction was the burning pain as the baby's head was coming out. I was trying so hard to listen to Debbie, but to be honest I didn't have a lot of control when it came to the contractions. The head was born! Debbie and Tamsin both told me to look down between my legs. It was so amazing. What a beautiful moment. The next contraction came and our baby just slid out so easily. Craig and Debbie caught her on the final push at 6.27am on Thursday morning. Debbie was right; she was born just before breakfast.

They guided the baby onto my stomach. Holding her for the first time was out of this world. All the pain just leaves you instantly, and the elation begins. Finding out it was a girl was also a massive surprise as we were expecting a boy, and Craig was extremely emotional as he wanted a little girl. It was the best best best moment. We continued with skin to skin and I had a physiological placental birth. There were no complications apart from me having some tears and some blood loss, but we were able to enjoy those first few hours with our baby girl with no interruptions and enjoying our first well deserved breakfast as a family of three. I was really proud of myself (as was Craig) that I was able to have a natural childbirth without any drugs and to be able to say that I enjoyed the experience, even though it was the hardest thing I've ever had to do in my life. We were very excited to share the news with our family and friends. We fell instantly in love with her.

Birth Story 2: Idie (Born 7/11/14)

The last few weeks of my pregnancy were really tiring and draining. We were really ready to meet this baby. Of course, the usual hopes to go into labour earlier because it's your second baby doesn't help. Again, we didn't know the sex, which made it very intriguing especially in those last weeks. We were booked in again to give birth at the Family Birth Centre after such an amazing experience with our firstborn. We loved it there, and everyone there made us feel so at home.

I had unfortunately picked up a bug on the Thursday 6th of November and I couldn't eat due to an upset stomach. That night I had the worst stomach aches and went to bed feeling pretty crappy and emotional. My due date was the Friday 7th of November and I knew labour was not far off, and I couldn't afford to be sick. About 2am I woke up with the worst diarrhoea I have ever had (sorry TMI). I was on the toilet for a good 1.5hours. I tried to drink lots of water to keep my fluids up as I couldn't eat.

Around 4am I started getting these period like tightenings and contractions. They came quite regularly but I still wasn't sure that it was as my bowel and stomach were spasming from being unwell. I tried to rest in between these cramps, as they only lasted about 20-30 seconds with about 5-10minute breaks. They were not that painful, and I woke up the next morning and they didn't seem any worse. I told my husband Craig – he didn't seem convinced it was the real thing. He was home as it was a Friday (the day he works from home) and we had our 40-week midwife appointment already booked that day at 12pm. I rang to tell them what I was experiencing but they said to just come in as usual and to monitor it throughout the morning. I tried to rest, and I tried to resume my mothering duties with my darling 19-month-old. She was really sweet and would pat my back, kiss and cuddle me.

Unfortunately, we were told that all the midwives at the Birth Centre that were rostered on for labouring duties had called in sick today. If we were in labour today it would mean we would have to be transferred to the King Edward Hospital instead. We were so devastated to hear this news. We really hoped there would be some way that we could stay at the Birth Centre. We packed our bags just in case this was the real thing and dropped Mira off at her grandparents on the way. I was feeling pretty uncomfortable by this stage though I could still talk and managed the contractions fine. Once again sitting was not the best position for me, so you can imagine the car ride wasn't the best.

We arrived at the Birth Centre at around 12.15pm and contractions were coming every 3-5 minutes for about 40 seconds. We met with the midwife Beth. She watched me throughout a contraction and checked the baby's position. Bubs was in a good anterior position (which was great news as bubs had been posterior the last few check-ups). Beth suggested that instead of doing an internal we go for a walk, have some lunch down the road and see if that gets things moving along. She said it still looks like early labour as contractions were not quite long enough yet. She suggested we don't go home though. We were worried about having to be transferred as we really did not want to be – she said to just go for a walk and we can see what we can work out. Another midwife there felt sorry for us too. We walked, had lunch (mind you this was quite hard trying to sit and eat and be comfortable). I was so hungry from not eating much the day before so ate till I was full.

We ended up setting the TENS machine up in the café disabled toilet (it was surprisingly clean and nice) as the contractions were increasing in intensity. At this point, I really wanted to get back and get settled into our room (whether that be the hospital or birth centre). It was a bit of a walk back and I found the walk very hard, having to stop at every contraction against a wall. We ended up back at the Birth Centre just after 2pm. We laboured away in the training room rocking back and forth on bean bags on my hands and knees. We waited a while until we spoke to the midwives who were so empathetic and really wanted us to stay. They suggested we do an internal to see if things had progressed. We all agreed that we would fudge it and work it out so we could stay at the Birth Centre, rather than transfer us as they knew that wasn't what we had planned or wanted. What legends!

We were moved to the birthing suite (Room 2 – same room Mira was born in) for the internal. I was 5cm dilated, and contractions had moved to over 1-minute-long and less than 2 minutes apart. We got the camera and things out of the car as it felt like things were not far away. The midwives confirmed we could stay and that was such a relief. I continued to labour standing and leaning on the bed as my main positions of choice whilst labouring and to reduce the pain. I once again had most of the pain really low down in my pelvis. Things got really intense fast where I couldn't really concentrate on anything except what I was doing. As in I couldn't really hear people talking or focus on that at all. Around 3pm I had this incredible urge to vomit.

The bath had just been put on to fill for a water birth and a shower was suggested for pain relief. I rushed to the toilet and remembered thinking that I must be in the transition phase. I again sat on the toilet, almost waiting for my waters to break again like Mira's birth. I told Beth to turn off the bath as I wasn't going to make it there. She agreed with me. Within seconds it felt like I needed to bear down. My body just seems to take over me from here. We moved from the toilet to the mat at the end of the bed on my hands and knees. The pushing contractions came with such force that it took the wind out of me! In the breaks I tried to catch my breath, but there wasn't long before the contraction came on again. My waters broke at around the 3rd pushing contraction. There was meconium in the baby's waters – due to the speed at which the baby was coming.

The midwives seemed a little stressed at this point as they needed to transfer me to King Eddie due to meconium being present, which is the Birth Centre's policy. I knew there was no way this was going to happen; I couldn't be transferred now because I could feel the baby's head right there! They decided to call the paediatric doctor down to us instead. They did a lot of monitoring of the baby's heart rate from this point and wanted me to move as they couldn't find the baby's heart rate. This did freak me out at the time, as I was feeling pretty uncertain of what was happening. So they asked me to lie on my back - my body was screaming a big fat 'no' at this point. I got onto my knees and I just felt the need to stand up. I don't remember a clear burning feeling as it was all just so intense, but the pressure between my legs was crazy at this point.

Next minute another contraction came and I remember holding onto Craig for dear life and the baby's head was born. I don't think the midwives quite expected it. I looked down and remembered asking them "is the baby okay?" They reassured me that the baby was fine. The reason they couldn't get a heartbeat at the time was because the baby was already so far down into my pelvis. They did ask me to give one last push, the next contraction came, and the rest of the baby just slipped out into the midwife's hands. They placed the baby straight onto my chest.

I must admit I was extremely relieved to be on the other side of that fast but intense experience, with the pushing stage being only eight minutes. Even the midwives were shocked at the speed of birth. We found out we were blessed with another girl born at 3.15pm on her due date! (Apparently that is pretty rare), with a full head of black hair, quite different to our other daughter. We decided again for a physiological third stage if possible. All was well post birth and I only had grazes and no tears this time. We were able to have some beautiful skin to skin and feeding time together taking the experience all in and enjoying meeting our little Idie. What an amazing experience. We have so much to be thankful for.

Birth Story 3: Letty (20/10/16)

This pregnancy was quite different in comparison to our other two girls. I carried bubs all out front and didn't crave much food this time around. The pregnancy towards the end was much tougher. By 38 weeks I was tired. Chasing two little girls around doesn't help and having the baby head down for quite a while caused a fair bit of pressure on my pelvic area, making everything feel weak down there! The best part about this pregnancy was that I got to spend lots of time with my friend Emily who was doing her postgrad studies in Midwifery. She asked to follow up and was an amazing support throughout the whole pregnancy. I really thought maybe I might go early this time around. The labour also came as a surprise for us too. Considering how fast my previous labours had progressed, I can't say I wasn't warned. My primary midwife Jannie did say that 3rd labours can throw a curveball. Let's just say this labour definitely pushed me beyond what I ever thought I could possibly handle – physically and mentally. I do love the nature of labour though and understand that everyone's different and unique in how they labour and the same can be said for each birth a woman has. You cannot compare, as there are just so many little variables in each woman's experience.

I was so excited to see how much your sisters would love you, especially your older sister Mira who was at a beautiful age.

It began on Tuesday night (18/10) when contraction type niggles began. I remember sitting at the movies with a bunch of girlfriends watching the documentary Embrace (worth watching by the way) and getting the first niggles then. Those niggles did keep me up most of that night. My due date was Wednesday 19th of October and I woke up with contractions every 10-15minutes - only lasting 20-30 seconds, and still quite bearable. It felt like this must be the day! I fancied another baby born on their due date. Craig worked from home that day, but I still had the kids to be with and to attend to. Contractions stayed all day, but the intensity did increase as the day went on. My friend Emily (who was my student midwife at the time) came over that afternoon and felt my contractions. She suggested calling the Birth Centre to let them know contractions were about 7-8minutes apart and going for at least 30-45 seconds. Jannie, my midwife, was unfortunately on leave that day but another midwife named Melody answered. We were advised to come in when my contractions were about 5 minutes apart and lasting a good 45-60 seconds long and getting to a point where I was quite uncomfortable.

We decided to pack the car and get the girls off to our parents as soon as possible, just so we could have the space and rest we needed before the baby's arrival. It was around late evening when we thought it was time to go into the Birth Centre. I allowed Craig to sleep a bit earlier as I knew I would need him later. Contractions were quite painful now and obviously after the speed of Idie's second stage I really didn't want to have this baby at home or in the car!

We arrived and we were put in Room 3 and I asked for the bath to be filled up straight away as I didn't want to miss out on using the bath this time around. Melody suggested we wait a bit. We settled into the room and then had an internal examination at about 2am – I was 3cm dilated, and she did a stretch and sweep, and seemed quite positive that I should dilate pretty quickly now. Emily was with us the whole time – doing baby's heart rate checks. It was awesome having a familiar face in the room with us. As the night went on contractions continued at about 5 minutes apart. I tried everything – walking, squatting, walking up and down stairs, walking outside. I even tried the fitball. Contractions stayed around 5 minutes apart, but the pain and strength of the contraction was long and hard.

Another internal examination was done at 6am. At this stage, I was almost falling asleep between contractions as this was my second night of no sleep. I was only 2cm and my cervix was still thick, and I hadn't progressed at all! Talk about devastating. Mentally this was hard, and so confusing for me as I was so confident from my previous labours that things would just progress. I really had to try and not let negative thoughts take over. Melody suggested we go home and try to sleep. So, she gave me a sleeping pill and panadeine forte to try to help me sleep. The Midwife reassured me that the sleeping pill would be out of my system when I was ready to give birth, however she highly recommended I take it to try to get some rest before things got really intense. We decided to stay at my folks place which was 15 minutes from the Birth Centre rather than head all the way back to Forrestdale. Our family thought it was a joke when we told them we were on our way back as they had assumed we had already had the baby based on my previous labours.

We were home and in bed by 7am. I got about 2hrs of sleep, then contractions began again every 5 minutes. I couldn't sleep so let Craig sleep while I got up and watched a movie with my sister and Mum who were home. It got pretty uncomfortable, but we still needed the contractions to get closer together. We woke Craig up at around 12 as contractions were longer and getting closer together. I remember feeling a physical drop of the baby's head – I needed some pain relief, so we decided to give the shower a go. At around 12.30pm all of a sudden contractions were just piggy backing and rolling through me one after the other. I knew we had to go in at that moment. I was pretty emotional at this point and I really had to mentally focus on what I was doing. Craig rang them to let them know we were coming back in. I couldn't even get myself dressed as I was so out of it. We rang our midwife friend Emily who lives in our suburb in Forrestdale to tell her we were heading back in and she told us she'd head there straight away.

The trip in the car was just agony – I was definitely in transition, and I was literally squeezing my legs together as I was sure this baby would come now if I let it. I really did not want to have this baby in the car! We arrived at the Birth Centre around 1.20pm. There was no parking, so we just parked right up in the driveway and I told Craig to just grab the camera, leave the car and to just come with me. We walked to Room 3 (very slowly) and had about 2-3 really long contractions and then that bearing down feeling came. I sat on the toilet for a bit, the bath wasn't ready, again! So, Sarah, our new midwife, suggested we use the shower. In the shower I found myself standing up and holding onto the rail facing the wall was the best position. I was just trying to focus to get through each intense contraction that kept rolling on and on. What felt like ages, was actually only about 10 minutes or so. I then felt this intense burn as the head was being born, it was such a strong feeling in my bottom region. You can't really describe the feeling!

Craig was amazing as usual, talking me through what was going on – telling me everything was good and that I was nearly there, only a couple more contractions. I don't remember many breaks and rest periods between contractions I had but literally within minutes I was birthing her head and with the next couple of contractions her body was born, and another beautiful (big) baby girl was welcomed into this world. She was brought up into my arms through my legs. She seemed so familiar already. I couldn't believe God had given us another beautiful gift to love and to cherish. She was a whopping 4kg, which I was a bit proud about to be honest!

After such a long labour it was all worth it and the exhaustion seemed to go instantly as this beautiful baby girl was finally here and a real sense of joy just overflowed within me. Thank you endorphins! I was overjoyed at my strength and ability to carry on. I was also able to have another physiological third stage and had no tearing or complications. Unfortunately, my friend Emily arrived 5 minutes after Letty was born, but she was able to be the first to enjoy newborn cuddles and did her first check-up. We were discharged that evening and introduced Letty to her sisters and her family, whilst enjoying a glass of sparkling to celebrate!!

Three Birth Stories

I always knew my firstborn would be a boy. In fact, I was so certain I thought I would be shocked if the ultrasound revealed a girl, not disappointed just surprised. As predicted our 20-week ultrasound revealed a boy complete with a printout of his genitals 'for his 21st'. The underwater themed nursery was completely decked out months in advance, but the baby's bathroom was still to be renovated. At the 38 weeks mark the tiling which should have taken 2-3 days was still going weeks after it had commenced. The baby had already dropped and when the tiler told me to calm down, you still have two weeks, I replied "I don't think so." It turns out I was right; I went into labour within an hour of him finishing the tiling! It was a hot day so hubby and I got into our outdoor spa to cool down.

I started getting persistent pains but just thought they were more Braxton Hicks contractions. I was still able to go to a friend's house for dinner. Curry was the main dish. The pains had been constant for a few hours but after dinner they started getting uncomfortable. I went to sit down on her couch when I heard a "pop" sound and stood up and my waters gushed down my legs. Luckily it was on the tiled area of the house. My friend was very surprised as she had elected to have caesareans, and this was all very surreal for her to see.

I calmly asked hubby to call Gaby. I laboured for quite a few hours at home, using the shower and a TENS machine for pain relief. Gaby arrived and was with me for the majority of this time. When I burst out crying Gaby saw the signs that I was in transition and we went to the hospital. I had my birth plan and a bag full of labour equipment, but I can only remember pushing and pushing. It turns out I had an anterior lip and needed an unpleasant procedure to be done by the midwife. This was trying to push back the anterior lip, as I pushed the baby's head past it. Once that was sorted the pushing went more smoothly even though I was still flat on my back (the exact position I wanted to avoid according to my birth plan). My son had his arm up near his head in a superman position, so it was quite an effort to get him out but I managed it....as the day's first sunbeams entered the room, I gave birth, and we became parents. I ended up with a small tear and had some stitches.

We were so happy to find out our second child was a girl, pigeon pair and all. She was even due to be a Taurean like my husband and I. I expected her conception to take longer as I was now in my mid 30's and the first had taken 6 months to conceive when I was just 30, but all she took was one try! The arbitrary deadline of 35 which I had set myself was met, as she was born two weeks before I turned 35. After 35 it is considered a geriatric pregnancy, how rude! As I had gestational diabetes for the second time, I was booked in for an induction at 5pm on her due date. In the lead up I had a stretch and sweep and tried all the natural methods to get things going. Nothing seemed to work, then 3 days before the due date I woke up with painful contractions. When they were 5 minutes apart, I called relatives to come look after my 3-year-old. Their arrival killed off my contractions with the comment "you don't look like you are in labour" and their decision to have a tea party in my kitchen. The night after that started the same way with contractions building this time to two minutes apart but my anxiety over when to call for babysitting put an end to it anyway.

On the last night before the induction the contractions started again. This time I already had the babysitter in the house. When the contractions ramped up, we called the hospital and they said to come in. Unfortunately, it was a busy night, and I spent the first 15 minutes kneeling on the floor in the corridor. An exam revealed that I was already fully dilated. I asked to use the toilet and could really feel pressure building. At this point they gave me a room and I went straight into the shower. I spent 5-10 minutes there on all fours alone and thirsty. When the midwife came back, she asked me to go to the bed to check on things. I just managed to walk there, rest my arms and head on the bed standing, do three pushes and out she came. While I was still standing by the bed her Dad asked the midwife "did you catch her?"

Baby N0.3

In my heart I didn't feel "done" after having my second child, although I had one of each gender and people would say you must be done if you have a boy and a girl. Despite all practicalities and the fact that having two kids already with very little support was very hard, our family was just not complete. The only thing was, the minute I convinced hubby to have a third and he said yes, my brain overrode my heart and I started to worry. We agreed that when I turn 40 that would be the end of the discussion. I was still 38 when I gagged on my eggs one morning. My 4-year-old daughter informed me there was a baby in my tummy and she was right. I am so glad our hearts won in the end. So much for being a veteran, this was my hardest pregnancy and birth. After having narrowly escaped an induction last time I was disappointed to be booked in for one a few days prior to her due date this time around. I knew that the risks of intervention would be higher, and I did not want to end up with a caesarean after two drug free natural births. As luck would have it, I was sent home and the induction was cancelled. On her estimated date due she was sitting really high in my pelvis and my cervix was not ready at all.

I decided once I got out of the hospital to go for a long beach walk. When I got home, I started bleeding heavily and the midwives said to go straight back to the hospital. I was 2 centimetres dilated when I arrived, and 4 centimetres dilated 30 minutes later. I was happy to be in labour and progressing well, but the obstetrician was concerned about the bleeding. If this was my first baby, I would have had an emergency caesarean. The compromise was to give me an hour and help things along by breaking my waters and giving me the drug to intensify the contractions. Gaby was with me as my doula at this time so I knew I would be Ok. So much for avoiding the induction, I ended up having the things I was afraid of anyway even though I was already in labour. But for me it was still better than having the Caesarean. Once the Syntocinin kicked in things were intense and quite a blur and a very short time later I had the overwhelming urge to push. Our newest baby girl was born without the Dr or Daddy making it back into the room in time! I was so glad to have Gaby with me. So, I have three very different drug free vaginal birth stories, and this is the last as Dad went for the snip when baby number 3 was 5 months old.

What a doula did for us at our birth!

With my first and second births, I felt that I really didn't have the right support around me during my labour, apart from my husband, although he was not overly excited about another birth as he didn't really want to see me go through the birth experience again. I had a friend and a non-communicative midwife present previously, both of whom offered me little to no support at all.

As a result of feeling that I had had no support or direction during both my first and second labours, I dreaded having to go through labour again. All I could remember and focus on were when the contractions started building up, the pain became unbearable, and I became very frustrated with everyone. As a result I ended up having a very negative experience that left me with bad injuries and a long recovery, in which I really felt traumatised.

When I fell pregnant with my third child I realised that I needed a professional support person, someone who could offer me emotional and continuous connection and support. A doula was the answer for me, and with little trouble I found Gaby, whom I had met during my previous pregnancies when I attended her antenatal classes at the swimming pool.

To me a doula is a guide who looks after your spiritual, emotional and physical state during the lead-up to your birth, and most importantly during your labour and the birthing of your baby. I feel that the birth of a baby is a very spiritual event, in which you are at your most vulnerable and yet connected in a way to your higher self, with the most amazing energy and inner knowing of the true forces of nature happening all at once. A doula, I felt, can nurture and protect your interests during this special time and make sure that the people around you support the type of birth you really want to have.

On the eve of my forty-week-plus-ten-days mark on the calendar, I had had enough. I was heavy, tired and fed-up. I rang Gaby to let her know that I had decided to go for an induction the very next day at 8 a.m. Gaby, knowing herself the full extent of being over the, 'dare I say', EDD, knew exactly where I was coming from. She was very supportive, but suggested I have a bonk anyway just to see if I could get things going naturally. 'You have nothing to lose by trying,' she said. With that exchange of words over the phone, I poured a glass of champagne for my husband and I, and disappeared with him into our bedroom to give it a go.

Within half an hour of doing the 'wild thing' I was in labour. Completely in labour, to the point where I needed to phone Gaby back to let her know, but I found myself struggling to get to the phone. I went from nothing to contractions three minutes apart. I decided to head over to the hospital and meet Gaby there, as things were really happening.

After ten minutes of getting settled in our room, Gaby arrived, much to the relief of my partner, who at this stage was having recurring thoughts of our last experience at this same hospital. He was looking rather white around the gills.

Gaby suggested I get into the shower as she could sense I was working really hard on the contractions. For the next hour I worked in the shower, both standing and then sitting on the fitball, as the water pounded my back. Gaby massaged my back; this combined with the water sensation felt fantastic. I also opted for some gas that they had on a portable trolley that could be brought into the bathroom, which I was especially pleased about.

After an hour I headed back to the birthing room, where I found myself wanting to get onto the floor on a mattress and lean over a bean bag with lots of pillows on top. It felt so calm and relaxing in this room as the light was soft and it was very quiet, except for the noises I was making. I stayed here to labour through to my transition stage, where I felt contraction upon contraction and again requested the gas for some relief. I also remembered throwing my head from side to side and asking, 'When is this baby coming!

After a period of time my contractions seemed to disappear, giving me a complete break from the previous intensity I had felt. I almost felt like I had stopped labour and asked Gaby and the midwife, 'Why have they stopped?' Both Gaby and the midwife reassured me that it was OK for the body to take a break so it could get into gear for the pushing part. With that I felt a huge rush of hormones and heat as the need-to-push sensation came over my body like a wave. I knew that at last I was there, I had done what my body needed to do, which was to open up, and now all I had to do was push. The pushing part is hard. It takes real focus and determination. Thank goodness for the great hormones to help. The adrenalin helps to get really primal and go within. It also aided me in making lots of noise, which is something I feel assists in getting a baby out of your body.

I suddenly remembered to start listening to the midwife and Gaby, who by this stage were suggesting that I back off a little and not push so hard. I did feel like a woman possessed, on a mission, but I decided to stay focused and do as they suggested. My female obstetrician arrived at last to find me in the throes of giving birth, and just stood back to allow Gaby and the midwife to continue doing what they were doing. Slowly, little by little, I pushed my baby into the world. All the while my husband was up my head end, giving me continuous support while Gaby and the midwife attended to my vaginal and peri needs.

My aim was to keep my perineum intact as much as possible, even though I knew I was having a big third baby. I was overjoyed and relieved when my biggest baby, a boy weighing ten pounds four ounces, came sliding into the world and was caught by Gaby.

So, my third baby came out in three hours of labour, and I am writing this story to tell you there is such a thing as a 'beautiful birth', even with having a big baby, as I am living proof of that. I am not a big woman at all, in fact I am very small and petite, and yet I birthed a whopper baby. It truly is amazing what women can do when they are given the right mental preparation and emotional support during labour, and, above all else, the belief that they can birth their baby.

Gabrielle Targett's Birth Stories

(Excerpt taken from A Labour of Love – a guide to child-birth without fear) written by Gabrielle Targett

The day before the estimated date of arrival of my first baby I desperately wanted to drive down to Bunbury three hours south of Perth, Western Australia, to have a swim with my friends the dolphins. Since returning from Japan I was a regular swimmer in the waters of Bunbury with my flippered pals, thanks to my good friend Rowena, whom I met in Bunbury. Rowena became my constant swimming companion with the dolphins. Over the years since my return from Japan, we had experienced some awesome and unforgettable interactions that we hold in our memories and hearts forever. Some dolphins I befriended, particularly females in the pods, who would always come and show me their babies. When I was pregnant I'd had a strong sense that they knew I was carrying a baby, as their interaction times increased, and they seemed to intensify their visits with me whenever I entered the water.

On that day in April 1995, I got into the water and had the most amazing interaction with the dolphins. They were all around myself and Jerome. I frolicked and dived and did som-ersaults for hours with them. At times, I just floated and they cruised slowly under me while I relaxed and caught my breath; being heavily pregnant the dolphins' pace and excitement tired me out quickly. I was at peace, feeling content and reassured by their presence. At one stage they jumped out of the water over Jerome and I as if to express their pure delight and excitement for the interaction and experience. I really think the dolphins sensed that I was very close to birthing the baby I was carrying.

I arrived home from our outing to Bunbury feeling up-lifted, energised and physically tired. I rang my midwife, Mary, to tell her that I was back in one piece from our amazing adventure and that I was so glad to have gone down to the dol-phins, because now I felt ready to give birth. On that note she suggested I go to bed early to get some sleep.

At 4 a.m. in the morning I was woken by a trickle of water coming out of my body. I sat up, saying to Jerome "I think my waters have just broken". I stood up and with that the biggest gush of water left my body. I walked to the bathroom to get a towel to clean up the liquid on the floor. I went back to bed unfazed about my waters breaking and tried to get some sleep. I found sleeping impossible, as I knew I was going to be having a baby that day and I was so excited.

I rang Mary about 7 a.m. to tell her my waters had broken. She explained that she couldn't get to me till 1 p.m. so she would send around a backup midwife, Bronwyn Key, to check on me. At 11 a.m. Bronwyn came over to check my progress and to have a cup of tea. All was well, and I just plodded around the house with the period cramping I was feeling, which was getting stronger and stronger by the hour. I had at the back of my mind that I had to wait for Mary to arrive before I could go into proper labour — whatever proper labour was! I guess to some degree I was holding back from actually allowing myself to really get into the swing of strong contractions as I wanted Mary to be there. I was not complaining, however, as I had a lovely warm-up which helped prepare me physically and mentally for the labour that was to follow.

On the dot, Mary arrived with her big hug and reassuring smile. It was a relief to see her, because at long last I could let go and allow myself to go into proper labour, and I did. Like clockwork the contractions started to intensify and hold me up from walking freely around the room. At 2.30 p.m. Mary suggested I get into our normal oval-shaped bath for a little natural pain relief. For all of ten minutes I stayed in the bath, as I found that sitting on my bottom with my legs out straight was agony. I could not cope at all with the contractions and I told Mary so in no uncertain terms.

Women in labour need not worry about what they say to others in their labour state, and need to be forgiven for the way in which they speak and for what they actually say. This is the given right of a labouring woman.

I moved from the bathroom to the papasan chair in the bedroom. At last I felt comfortable! At about 4 p.m. I remember saying "Mary, I really need to poo!" She replied in her very casual manner, "That's OK, I have my poo-catcher here, I will just catch it". But at that point Mary called for Jerome. I noticed a little quiver in her voice which suggested this was urgent

— she told Jerome to quickly go to Woodside Hospital and set up the proper birthing tub as I was going to need it very soon.

I was heading to Woodside, our local maternity hospital, as I have a blood disorder called Von Willebrand's Disease, which means my blood has problems clotting. In my case, the specialists weren't sure if I was going to bleed abnormally or have a haemorrhage. Just in case we had planned to go to the hospital towards the end of my labour, to experience my water birth, where they had clotting factors waiting for me in case I needed it. (As it turned out I didn't, and all was fine).

So, I watched Jerome take off in the car to go and set up the tub. I realised that my friend (another Gabrielle!), who was to be my birth support person, was still down the street in my car with the screws and bolts to put the birth tub together! There was nothing I could do but pray that somehow she would be back in time for the birth. In the meantime, I was getting louder and louder in my noises and Mary suggested we also get to the hospital in her car.

I can tell you that it was easier said than done! Heading down the stairs I was trying to put on a dress and have a contraction at the same time! I can remember that the journey down those stairs seemed to take forever. When I finally arrived at the bottom step I burst out of the house and onto the front lawn for all the neighbours to see, my ass in the air, and me yelling, "Mary, just leave me here, I want to have the baby here!" With that she picked me up and got me into the car for the quickest drive around the neighbourhood I had ever experienced. Suddenly, like a miracle, we arrived at Woodside's back door.

I again flung myself out of the car and onto the lawn. I presume this is a regular occurrence for the locals who live across the road from this maternity hospital — a woman in labour, on all fours, yelling something obscene to the driver of the car!

Yet again Mary lifted me up and told me that under no circumstances was a baby going to be born on the lawn outside the hospital. She marched me inside telling me to pant. Inside I saw Jerome and Gabrielle madly trying to get the tub ready while I laboured on the bed. Gabrielle wanted to show me the dolphin photos from the day before, thinking I would find this calming and relaxing. At this point I have to say all I wanted was to get into the tub and push. Looking at dolphin photos lasted about thirty seconds and then the need to really push became so overwhelming that all I could think about was the tub, water and the birth.

I learned a very important lesson during this birth, and that is just how important it is that you are clear with your support people and tell them exactly what you expect from them and what is appropriate or not appropriate at any given time.

At about 4.20pm I got into the tub, which was wonderful. At that moment I felt calm, relaxed and again able to surrender to what was happening to my body. I had about four contractions where I pushed really hard and my baby pushed out to her ears. At this point all I could feel was the 'Chinese burn' sensation in my perineum as it stretched. Mary supported the baby's head, which allowed my perineum to expand and give. I then had another really intense contraction where I made the most amazing noise like a primal animal. It bellowed out of me from deep within and seemed to echo through the room and down the corridor. With that sound, I pushed Jaeosha out of my body in one push, and she slipped through the water over to the other side of the tub as if swimming.

It was 4.32pm when Jaeosha rocketed out of my body. Mary had to move over to the other side of the tub to pick her up and she placed her gently on my chest. I remember saying "look, it's a baby. I can't believe I have had a baby". I am not sure what I thought the outcome would be!

With Jaeosha on my chest we sat for what seemed like an eternity, just looking at each other, looking deep into each other's eyes. The weight of her body, the warmth, smell and softness of her skin were beautiful and uplifting. At last we had met face to face, skin to skin.

Our journey together was just beginning, and I felt we had got off to a great start with the most amazingly fast, positive and beautiful birth experience.

I got out of the tub to deliver the placenta, which I have to say felt like a big wet jellyfish sliding out! Having had Jaeosha so quickly I had little trouble in expelling the placenta. The only downside to a really fast birth is occasionally the body goes into shock, and this is what happened with me. I had a really high temperature and was sweating profusely, and my blood pressure was high, all symptoms which are not unusual after a quick birth.

Something I hadn't counted on was having very strong afterbirth contractions, which really blew me away. Every time I went to breastfeed Jaeosha the contractions became so intense that I had to breathe slowly just to get through them, just like I had done during the labour. For a while I really thought that maybe, just maybe, I was having twins and I had forgotten about the other one! These afterbirth pains went on for about three days, all of which is considered normal with very quick births, but is more likely to occur with second and third births than the first.

Although my first experience was fast, I have to say it was indeed a positive birth and one I will always remember clearly. The first time any woman births the experience is so new that every sensation is observed and analysed with your conscious mind. And often lots of questioning goes on internally. Is this supposed to happen? Is that OK? And so on. These thoughts and feelings are all very normal and to a certain degree teach and prepare us for the next experience. If there is a next experience. In my case I knew there was going to be.

During their second labour women often relax a little more, knowing they have a fair idea of just what to expect and that there is light at the end of the tunnel. After all the hard work, the birth of a baby is the end result. Sometimes women actually forget that this is the true purpose of labour, as I seemed to during Jaeosha's birth. Despite this fact, having had a positive first experience does prepare women to look forward to the next with great anticipation, as I did.

My second birth journey

The second of my births started like my first with the 4 a.m. wake-up call. However, this time it was a very strong contraction that woke me. I waddled to the toilet in readiness for my waters breaking, but to my dismay this didn't happen. I had looked forward to this unusual sensation and wanted this to be the real thing as I was ten days over my supposed due date and getting very heavy and tired. I went back to bed having mild period-pain-type contractions that kept me in a half-sleep and half-conscious state, my brain mulling over the fact that today I was going to have a baby. The excitement once again set in and I found it hard to get any more rest.

At about 7 a.m. I rang Mary, the same midwife I had had for Jaeosha's birth, to tell her of my contractions. Mary had in

261

the back of her mind that I would be having a pretty fast labour, and said she would be straight over as soon as she showered. I then took to walking the streets block by block to try to get things moving along. Walking the streets in early labour always reminds me of a friend who lived in Alice Springs who walked through the labours of her four children and as a consequence had very quick, easy births. This inspired me to do the same and off I headed. I always wondered what people thought of a big, heavy pregnant woman walking the streets with a towel slung over her shoulder.

What, you may ask, is the towel for? Just in case the waters break! Stopping to have contractions leaning on people's fences can be very entertaining, especially if noises are coming out from deep within your throat as you puff and pant through a contraction. This always draws people out from their houses to discover what is going on!

I walked and walked till I felt it was time to move my labouring body back to the house for Mary to check my baby's heart rate and have a feel of the baby's head from the outside, to see how far down it was into the pelvis. All was going well, and I wandered around the house going to the toilet as often as I could to relieve my bladder, which was being squashed flat like a pancake by the baby's head pushing down.

In my anxiousness to go into labour I had set up the timber frame of the birthing tub the day before, in readiness for the birth and to try to spur it on both physically and subconsciously.

We were having this baby at home. As I wandered about the house having the odd strong contraction, I started to get anxious about getting the soft foam and liners into the tub's frame, ready for the water. Oh the water! How I dreamed, leading up to this birth, about wallowing around and really enjoying the sensation of the water for a much longer time. In hindsight, we really do have to watch what we ask for, as I got just that, a much longer time!

After many trips to the toilet to check on the show (mucus plug or bloody show as it is often referred to) in my undies, many games of UNO — a great card game — and a really funny laughing session looking at Gary Larson's Far Side calendar, I finally went into proper labour. Proper labour is known as established labour, and you really have to concentrate on each and every contraction - usually by closing your eyes and burying your face. After a substantial period of time in established labour Mary felt I was far enough along to get into the birthing tub. By hopping into the tub too early I could have slowed down or even stopped the contractions. This is always a possibility as water is so relaxing that the body sometimes responds by relaxing a little too much.

I stripped off as fast as I could and dived in. Well, I would have dived in had my belly allowed me that privilege! Once in the water I felt at peace with my body and relieved to have the weight off my feet, legs, pubic bone and pelvis. At last I could float totally suspended if I wanted to. The best part about being in the water was that when the contractions really started to get tough I could surrender and work with my body, not against it.

Once in the water I felt like the edge of the pain in each contraction was being taken off so I could work with my body and not fight these natural, rhythmical waves of openings that were flooding through me.

Once in the tub, that is where I stayed - from 2 p.m. in the afternoon until my baby arrived into the world a little over four hours later. Apart from wanting a longer birth and more time in the tub (and I certainly got that!), this time I distinctly re-member going through the transition stage of labour.

It has been noted in many textbooks that transition can be a time when a labouring woman snarls, swears or becomes abu-sive to anyone around her and for a short period of time acts totally out of character!

For me, transition was marked by sharply telling Susan Jane, Mary's apprentice homebirth midwife at the time, to stop massaging me. I remember snarling "Don't touch me, just leave me alone". With that I went and sat myself in the middle of the tub where no one could reach me. I then said to Mary "I just want this baby out of me now, get it out, I have had enough".

Mary looked at Susan Jane in a knowing sort of way and both said 'transition' in unison. Afterwards I apologised, as I felt incredibly rude — Susan Jane had been massaging me for about four hours continuously before I reached transition and I had found it incredibly calming, not to mention wonderful having the pressure on my lower back and pelvis.

Just after the end of my transitional stage it was as if a miracle had happened. The intensity had shifted in my body from deep within my pelvis, cervix and vagina to my bottom, where once again I felt the need to do a poo. Oh, the poo sensation, how I longed to feel this again. It was a welcome sensation, as I knew at this point, with the urge to push, I was nearly at the end of my marathon and had about two kilometres to go to get to the finish line. The only problem was I was hitting the wall fast. I knew I just had to keep going, so on I worked, and pushed, vocalising rather loudly! The raw energy and adrenalin of birth once again supported me and saw me through. At last I was having a moment of 'runner's high', and it was great!

The pushing sensation took over my whole body and, as in my first labour, not pushing was impossible once the urge came on. I felt this was a big baby and Mary was coaching me, sensitive to the fact that I was getting pretty close to pushing this baby out. We had previously discussed that when the time came and the head was pushing through my perineum I would take it easy and pant and resist pushing, and really listen to what Mary was saying, if I could. This would prevent my perineum from tearing badly. Mindful of tearing I made the effort to pant like an animal in the wild giving birth! Then, without any consideration or thought on my behalf my waters broke. This sounded like the cork on a champagne bottle flying off, for all in the room to hear. The celebration of birth had begun, and I was overjoyed that soon I could be drinking real champagne to celebrate.

At last the 'Chinese burn' came and lasted for what seemed like an eternity, but as requested by Mary, I panted through the next contraction so the perineum could retract and slide back over the baby on its own. With the next contraction, as with Jaeosha's birth, I expected my baby's body to fly out of me. Well, not with this baby! I had to work him out on every contraction, to the point where he was hanging out of my body, totally stuck with my perineum around his stomach, as he was so large around his midriff. I ended up saying "Mary, can you please just pull the baby out, I've had enough". With that he slipped out calmly and peacefully into the water at 6.16 p.m. on the 16th day of May in 1997.

I attempted to turn around, so I could hold my baby, but I kept getting caught up in his very long umbilical cord. I actually had to lift my leg high into the air to get up and over it, so I could at last sit down and cuddle him. We were finally able to meet face to face and skin to skin. Words cannot even describe this moment. All I can say is that when you look into your baby's eyes for the first time it is the most wonderful moment a mother can experience, making the bond and connection very strong on every level possible.

I looked with Jerome and Jaeosha who had both been amazing birth support to see what sex this baby was. I had guessed by looking at my baby that he was a boy. He had 'boy' written all over him. By gee he was a boy. He had huge testicles and a penis that would make any man proud! The large size, due to swelling and hormones, is quite normal Mary told me after his birth. The reason the boys look so well-endowed is because of the amount of blood that flows to the genitals during the birth. Boys' genitals do go down after the birth, to be more in proportion with the rest of their body.

Benjamin, as we named him, was a good eight and a half pounds of muscle; he was solid but chubby as well. Best of all he was so healthy and happy-looking that I just wanted to eat him all up. Your own baby always looks so scrumptious and has the most incredible baby smell. Yummy.

Finally, I got out of the tub to deliver the placenta, as I had done before, and to be monitored for blood loss. Right on cue the placenta slipped out like a big jellyfish, all soft and squishy! It was a delight to have finished the process of giving birth and have Jerome finally cut the cord. This, to me, symbolised all the work I had done and the journey I was to start, as mother, provider of food, protector and nurturer for the years to come. To me, birth represents the beginning of the process of life together as mother and child. "Wow, a boy. My baby boy, Ben".

My third birth journey

Once again, the sharp pains of contractions at 4 a.m. in the morning disturbed my sleep. I don't know what it is about 4 a.m. in the morning and going into labour, but that is how and when my labours all started. I got up on this very cold morning in June and decided to light the fire, so I set about chopping wood and getting the kindling alight in the open fireplace. I imagined that this is how it must have been for women in early Australian settlers' times - lighting the fire and doing the odd job, knowing that a baby was going to be born on that day.

I did some exercises and yoga in front of the fire to try to get things going. I was eight days 'overdue' and really BIG. This time I wanted a birth that was not as long as Benjamin's, as that felt like it had been a little too long! In my head I was requesting a three-hour birth. This I knew I could do. After some time in front of the fire I decided to go back to bed as I again felt tired and thought maybe I should get some rest before the big event.

At 6 a.m. the contractions were starting to feel really intense when I was lying down, so I got out of bed. The intensity surprised me as I thought that I would have more of the period type of pain as a warm-up before I got to this point. I decided at this stage that I had better phone Mary. Once again, Mary Murphy was supporting me with her excellent midwifery skills. I think she felt this was going to be a fast labour, as she said "I'll jump in the shower and be right over in twenty minutes!" This amused me as she lived about thirty-five to forty minutes away. I had visions of a speeding midwife on the freeway zooming through all the cars that slowed her down, waving her hand and yelling, "Get out of my way!" All in the name of birth!

This birth was another planned homebirth, with both Jaeosha (now four) and Ben (now two) with us at home. In the time it took Mary to arrive I proceeded to really start to labour. My only problem was that Benjamin was really driving me crazy. With each contraction he saw, he wanted to be picked up and cuddled by me. Some two-year-old's do not understand what is happening to Mummy when they see her in labour and can get very needy at this time. This was happening to Ben. As soon as I could muster up the energy I blurted out to Jerome "Phone the neighbours to come and get Ben, right now please".

When I finally saw Ben walk down the driveway holding my neighbour's hand, I could at last let go of trying to hold myself together.

This was another lesson I learned about women in labour. They should never have to hold back and not do what their body wants to do as this is not surrendering to the natural process of birth and will ultimately interfere with progress.

Pam England and Rob Horowitz refer to this in their book Birthing from Within as 'Performance Anxiety'. They suggest that external factors, such as being watched while in labour, can slow a woman down, due to the subconscious mind telling your body that you are not feeling very comfortable about your situation. This is exactly how I felt with Ben being in close proximity to me. I knew the only way to stop this was to get him out of the house.

I walked back into the house and headed for the bathroom to take up my favourite position of burying my face into the towels on the towel rack while groaning and grunting. I asked to get into the tub, however the tub wasn't quite ready. Also, a needle in the bum had to happen first. I was dreading this more than anything, and in fact felt I could handle contractions any day over 100 millilitres of antibiotic in the backside while in labour!

I will digress here to explain the reason I had to have the antibiotic. I'd had group Strep B detected with a swab in my vagina. No one is sure how you get it, but it is known as a flora of the body. If detected in large quantities of the bacteria in your vagina around birth time there is a small risk the baby may pick it up. I'd had it three times previously throughout this pregnancy, so it was not a shock when on my estimated due date after having yet another internal swab, I had it again.

Group Strep B bacteria can pass from the mother's fluids into the baby's mouth, nose or eyes during birth and they can become very sick. At the time of this birth, the protocol to manage Strep B included; immediately post birth the contents of the baby's stomach being sucked out and sent off to the lab and tested, with strong antibiotics to be given to both the mother and baby by injection. This can be enough to stop the baby from getting sick, and in my case it was, as my baby ended up testing negative.

Boy, did I squeal like a pig when the dreaded injection went in. I think it was because I was so close to transition and my entire body of nerve endings was on alert due to the intensity of the contractions. I have to say I also hate needles! With the jab over and done with, I bolted from the bed and into the tub. That was the pay-off for having the injection and being brave. Once again I slid into the tub and felt at home. A sensation of peace and tranquillity swept over my body as my great friend Sue put her warm and loving hands onto my back and started massaging. Sue massaged me till the end of my labour, and for this I am eternally grateful.

The labour intensified even more when I got into the tub. The edge was taken off the top of each contraction due to being immersed in the water and being massaged, however they were still pretty intense and occurring very rapidly with lots of piggyback contractions. These are contractions that are very strong and come one after the other consecutively, with no rest in between. It was at this stage I remember saying "Fuuuuuuuuck", drawing out the sound as long and hard as I could. What I was trying to do was find a sound I could identify with and use to help me get this baby out.

Jerome suggested that I try another word, as he was concerned that with Jaeosha present at the birth, she might start to

271

imitate that sound and word after the birth! Mary suggested that it didn't even sound like the actual word and to keep going as it was helping me to open up incredibly. I remember at one stage looking over at Jaeosha as she whispered in my ear, "It's OK, Mummy, you are going to have the baby soon". With that she placed a cold towel on my forehead and kissed me. It was one of the most moving parts of the whole labour. Incredible to think that a four-year-old could acknowledge what was going on and totally support me in every conceivable way. This I will always remember.

Before long I was pushing and working really hard. This puzzled me, as my contractions were five minutes apart. I remember asking, "Mary, how can I be pushing? My contractions are still five minutes apart". As always Mary reassured me that it was totally possible, and my body needed the time in between contractions to rest and recuperate before the next one came.

With this change in stages, it was time to call my attending doctor who was needed to oversee the actual birth and the procedure that the baby had to undergo for the Strep B. The urge to push became stronger and stronger and before I knew it my baby's head was pushing on my perineum. Just as with Ben's birth my waters broke again, sending a loud popping sound out into the room for all to hear. My children loved coming into this world with a pop!

Mary supported me once again by reminding me to pant as my perineum stretched as I worked at taking it easy, so as not to push too quickly or forcefully. Having a midwife coach you through this stage can really help avoid a big tear and keep the perineum in great condition. My eyes remained totally closed for this part of the birth as I felt I just had to focus all my thoughts and feelings inwardly and really concentrate on the business at hand. I squeezed Jerome's hand so hard that his rings actually cut into his skin, which I figure is a small price for a father to pay during childbirth!

Within five minutes and with two really strong pushes I had birthed my baby into the water at 9.30am. Once agai, I turned slowly around to feel his warm soft skin as he was placed on my body, which assisted with melting away the memory of the intensity of contractions that I had experienced only minutes before. All was forgotten in an instant, and all I could do was look at this incredibly beautiful angel-like figure on my chest. I was in love.

Together we sat in the tub just looking at each other. Jaeosha kissed and kissed his tiny little head. Someone suggested that Jerome and I look at the genitals to see what the sex of the baby was, so we did. At first I said "Oh, it's a girl", then someone suggested that I look again. To my surprise (I actually thought I was having a girl) this baby was actually a boy! He looked so small and perfect with amazingly beautiful eyes that seemed to follow me everywhere. I felt totally connected with him on a very deep level.

I turned and asked Jerome if I could have some lunch, as I was starving. "Lunch? Don't you mean breakfast?" said Mary. "It is only 9.30 a.m. in the morning". I was really surprised with this reply as I thought that I had laboured for a lot longer than I had. I was totally oblivious to any sense of time, and had no clocks or watches around me. I have always done this with my births, because I believe time has no relevance where birth is concerned.

It was finally time to hop out of the tub and onto the floor, where I then delivered the placenta. The cord was clamped and cut by Jerome when it had stopped pulsating. Jarrad, as we named him, was bundled up in towels, beanie and booties, ready for the tube down his throat and suction of his stomach. The downside to this was I didn't get to breastfeed him immediately, as I had done with Jaeosha and Ben. This first suckle can really help with the bonding that a mother and newborn share immediately after birth, as well as beginning to establish breastfeeding. To me, this first feed is always a special memory and moment. But in this case I had to put it on hold temporarily.

I couldn't watch the procedure take place. I was in the room though. The thought of not being able to see him or hear him made me aware of just how painful it must be for parents to have their newborn baby taken away for tests or to another room immediately after birth. The feeling of loss must be incredible.

Jarrad was finally passed back to me, where Mary had set me up with lots of pillows, nice and snuggly on the couch in front of the fire. It was here he had his first feed and I dressed him in his new suit, which was pink! I had honestly thought I was having a girl and was a little shocked when I had looked again, to see that he was in fact a boy!

After the birth I felt fantastic. This was due to the cocktail of natural opiates my body was producing during the final stages of labour. After a couple of hours rest I decided to take a shower, in which I felt even better than I had with Jae's and Ben's births. I didn't even feel sore through my perineum and there was absolutely no stinging from a graze or anything. I ended up walking around for a little bit doing the odd job around the house, in disbelief that I had just given birth to an eight-and-a-half-pound baby.

I thought to myself, if only all women could experience how great they can feel after natural childbirth, the fear aspect would be completely gone forever. I was high from birth and high on life, overjoyed and content that my last birth experience could finish on a positive and empowering note!

4.

FOUR MAKES A
FABULOUS FAMILY

The Barrett Boys

In Bali, Ferg and I conceived our first baby. I knew straight away as I felt really strange. Whilst in Bali we thought we would pop back to England to get married; I would then apply for residency to Australia, and we could live happily ever after... On returning to England (whilst having a night out with some girlfriends) I found out that my friend was pregnant too! I called Ferg in the early hours of the morning, to let him know the good news about my friend!

I was having a night out with my girlfriends enjoying her hen's night when the next thing I knew I was feeling fully nauseous and unable to enjoy the hen's night. I could no longer drink champagne at all, bugger! There I was, hitched and then alone (as Ferg had returned to Australia) waiting for my

Australian residency to come through...... time was running out... then at seven months pregnant, I was granted residency and at last I could fly to Australia. The last time I'd seen my husband I was (though never skinny) a whole lot smaller than when I waddled through the arrival gate in Perth, Western Australia ready to start a whole new chapter of my life!!!!

Having spent a lot of time reading and checking out pictures showing the growth of babies during those first nine months, knowing what it may be able to hear, thinking about what I should eat, doing some swimming, taking up yoga, playing beautiful music, I had really only skimmed through the birth bit. Yes, I had been wonderfully informed on natural birth etc. but somehow assumed it would come naturally!

At 8 ½ months pregnant I had been a support for my sister during her caesarean (her son was breech). I ended up watching through the glass doors of the theatre rather than holding her hand supporting; I think it was due to the high risk of getting in the way!!! They may have been right!

Ten days over my official due date I had a hearty breakfast at a local café feeling horribly nervous at the prospect of being induced, that was what the doctor ordered, and like a lamb to the slaughter I went. After being examined, I was told by the doctor what drugs would be administered and that an epidural would be a good idea because of the intensity of being induced! A nurse popped her head in afterwards and said "You know you don't have to have an epidural. You can do what you want".

However, since I had been told by the doctor that the drugs are what I should do, I thought it must have been the right thing to do, and I did what I was told!

Fifteen hours later I was still lying on the hospital bed. Eventually I had stopped being able to walk around, my body was apparently contracting but not getting far (I could not feel a thing) ... my husband had popped out for a pizza and was given a little bed in the room (at least that stopped him filming me and playing with the bed controls). The epidural started wearing off and I called the midwives a few times, not used to the pain that was creeping in. I felt like I was just desperate for a poo! This, according to what I had read indicated to me that I was close to the pushing time. The midwife passed me a bed-pan! I threw up on her. I was then examined again, twice! This had gone on during the whole labour as a student midwife was present and was also required to examine me. I felt like I was going nowhere.

Eventually the doctor appeared and again I was examined, apparently - he then drew a little diagram on how I would be cut for a caesarean (only my rather shocked husband was able to see this!) Before a caesarean was done the doctor used forceps on me but they didn't work, and then the vacuum! This too didn't work. Time for a Caesarean, more drugs and off I went. I have to say that having just watched my sister have a C-section now it was my time and I knew exactly what was going to happen. I was completely exhausted from the hours gone by. I was a bit of a wreck; I was shaking all over yet they set to work. I remember lying there trying to visualise a beautiful field full of poppies whilst my body was pushed and pulled, my little baby was stuck in the birth canal and he had to be pushed back up so he could be pulled out, during this my toes started to wiggle, I think the drugs were wearing off! By the time I had my baby handed to me, I was so wasted that I couldn't hold him. I was scared I would drop him since I was shaking too much, and my mind was all over the place. This was not the picture I had seen for the birth of my first son, Finn. Not because I had any feelings about being let down personally regarding the birthing process, but more about how my son had been born while I was drugged up to the eyeballs.

When I found out I was pregnant again, I wondered if this could have been avoided and I went about making a plan...to inform myself and avoid that scenario happening again.

With a bit of informative reading and of course a wonderful aqua pregnancy class, I worked out my next move (this was not without obstacles). First, I had to find a doctor who would let me birth vaginally after having had a caesarean – bingo, I found Him but said, I would have to have a IV bung in my hand during the birth in case I needed to be attached to a drip of some kind. I agreed as I felt I could cope with that; I am not a huge risk-taking kind of gal and that seemed like a good compromise. Second, I roped in a friend, who was also a physiotherapist. This meant having great support and great massage during labour (quite useful thought!). Her main role was to speak for me when I was unable to.

So with plenty of reading leading up to my estimated birth day/night, and an amended birth plan, I was ready to go...... however ten days passed (I should have known!). On the day our home was opened for people to view as we were selling it, I started having contractions, which helped address the 'keep active' line on the birth plan.

Eventually I had to leave the home open which was a relief as I was with my 'beloved' nearly 2-year-old who was running everywhere. So we headed off in the VW Kombi van. First stop, my friend's house, as she would be coming to the birth with me. She was however still at work, but her hubby kindly made us a cup of tea and sat there cringing as I was having ever increasing contractions. We left so as not to make him feel any more uncomfortable and went to the hospital for a check-up. Labour was progressing well, but I still had some time to go. I was invited to stay but decided I would rather keep away from this hospital and stay active. Off we went again in that bloody bumpy old VW Kombi van, down by the river.

We did a drive through the takeaway food place (can't remember if I ate) ... bumpety bump, ooooooh, right oh, NOW it was time to go back. My friend left work and turned up with wonderful timing at the hospital. I kept moving and using good active labour positions around the room. I had wonderful back rubs and kept focused within. The only pain I remember now is the pain of the IV bung sticking out of my hand, as I moved, and the tube jabbed into my hand…. "OUCH". Eventually, against my plan, I still somehow ended up on my back! But then my baby came, another beautiful baby boy. We named him Gus. I slept the rest of the night in the hospital and eventually had the IV bung removed (I think that was the most blood loss that I had!) and off I went back to my family home.

Having avoided the hospital for so much of the last labour (purely so I didn't get persuaded into pain relief), I decided to opt for a home birth for my 3rd birth. I was in the hands of the most beautiful midwife who was so understanding and with me for the whole pregnancy. If I had a worry she helped me and soothed my thoughts; she was a source of great information and calming words. A waterbirth seemed so perfect and with a little more research I found an accommodating doctor who would assist or be of assistance if required! As it was, it all went swimmingly! As suspected though, I went ten days over my estimated date again! The tub was in place and the other boys were at their Aunt's house for tea. We phoned her and she held onto them a bit longer because conveniently, I went into labour whilst they were over there at her house.

I had soft music and warm water, the ultimate in pain relief; such a beautiful labour, and there was Magnus, my third son born into the water with ease and grace. As I sat up after giving birth, my other two sons were brought home and carried through to my bedroom. They enjoyed meeting their baby brother, it was so beautiful. I woke up the next morning with my baby Magnus in my arms and my two other boys looking at him adoringly.

A few years later with three beautiful sons I felt quite complete (but hadn't thought about how to keep it that way!) We headed off to England for a holiday and were quite excited that I had no breast-feeding babies and wasn't pregnant, and with family to baby-sit this could be our chance for a few nights out. The first night away from Perth we stopped in Mauritius. Cocktails on the balcony overlooking the beach aaaah… ooops, pregnant!

An unusual pregnancy, I was quite worried about the prospect of another baby, wasn't our life crazy enough with three boys? It took a while to get my head around it. The last birth had been so perfect, so I didn't think twice about making the same arrangements, but I had some underlying worry all along. I explained this to the midwife who just kept everything so calm and outlined that all options were available; if I felt I wanted to go to hospital then that was always available and if I wanted to stay at home that was fine too. It was the perfect situation, but still I had a strange feeling which had been with me all the way through the pregnancy!

I think it was 14 days over my estimate when I eventually had to have my waters broken. However, I returned home to slip slowly into contractions, much slower than I was expecting. The boys were out of the house and we were completely wallowing in having the house to ourselves, although also waiting for the appearance of our 4th baby…. Slowly but surely things started picking up and we filled the tub. My midwife was at another birth which made me slightly nervous, but I got into the water and everything slowed down a little. My 'backup' midwife arrived, and I felt reassured.

I felt like I was drier, and it was harder for my baby to move, and at the end, just as my midwife arrived I was almost forcing pushes which felt wrong but necessary. I was just ready for this to all be over when out came my baby, another boy, looking a little bit chilly. I held him to me rubbing him to get his little body warmed up, I think a bit vigorously, I remember someone saying, "I think that will do!" Poor little thing was getting 6-year-old rubs instead of newborn rubs!

I climbed out, I was bleeding quite heavily, and it was hard to tell in the water how much it was so it was better for me to get out. It took a while to pass the placenta and I was also passing plenty of large clots. I went to lie down and whoosh, the world went spinning round. It was then off to the hospital. I lost quite a lot of blood. The next day I had a small bit of placenta removed surgically that was a little stubborn and refused to come out. After that it was all fine, but I was pretty drained for some time. I will never know whether I had some kind of intuition about the birth, or whether my negative thoughts had brought this on, but I was happy to be on the other side of it. So thankful for the wonderful midwives and convenience of the local hospital nearby!

I am now blessed with four beautiful sons, Finn, Gus, Magnus and Iggy. I will not be birthing any more babies, but should someone give me another I would be happy to receive!! It has been a wonderful life experience to have experienced so many different births and this has opened my eyes up to so much. I can appreciate the wonder and ease of natural births, the amazing effect of water and birth but also the wonderful job of midwives. How lucky am I. Thank goodness I did get pregnant again or I wouldn't have ended up with Iggy, the missing piece!

Lisa

Two Hospitals, a Car Park and an Unplanned Home Birth

On my 30th birthday I stopped taking the pill and we started trying to fall pregnant. After 12 months of trying I remember looking at myself in my bathroom mirror and saying "no-one will ever call me Mum". I am now 38 and the mother of 4 beautiful boys and have 4 amazing birth stories to share. It also feels like someone is calling me 'mum' every minute of my day ☺!

I finally fell pregnant with my first son Jackson after 14 months of trying. We were elated and then shortly after the morning sickness started. I vomited for 23 weeks but didn't care because I was having a baby! Now I needed to decide where to have this baby. My husband is a Chiropractor and is very open to natural birthing practises (his father and 3 siblings are all Chiropractors!). His sister Sonya had already given birth to her four children at home with a midwife present and my other sister-in-law had also had a home birth. This was a very new concept to me and whilst I could see the merits, I just couldn't bring myself to have one so booked in for a hospital birth under the care of an obstetrician. In hindsight, I think I am very fortunate to have had such a positive outcome under the hospital system, particularly given it was a first birth and my lack of knowledge on the subject.

There were a couple of key decisions which I believe contributed to my overall positive experience:

- While pregnant I attended an active birthing class through the Community Midwifery Program.

- I had regular chiropractic adjustments throughout my pregnancy to align my pelvis correctly and give the baby the best chance of facing the right way for birthing.

- My obstetrician was generally happy to go along with what I wanted (e.g., minimal scans) as long as my and my baby's safety were not put at risk.

- My husband and sister-in-law's presence at the hospital during my labour – I will elaborate on this later.

- My decision prior to the birth that I would not have any pain relief drugs. The main reason for this was because I was worried they would interfere with the natural stages of labour and as a result, increase my chances of having an emergency caesarean.

A couple of weeks before the birth my sister-in-law, Sonya (who had the experience of 4 homebirths), offered to be present at the labour. While I thought it would be nice to have her experience on hand, I politely declined as the thought of her seeing me half naked was mortifying ☺.

10 days before my estimated due date my waters broke in the early hours of the morning while I was sleeping. The contractions didn't start straight away so I had time to have a nice shower and finish packing my hospital bag. We then tried to remember what we had learnt at the active birthing class and laboured at home with me moving between the shower for pain relief on my lower back and the toilet because the water just kept on coming! At one point I tried to eat some toast but vomited it up. The contractions were quite close now, but I was slow in getting to the car because water kept trickling down my

legs even though I had a maternity pad on (I learnt for subsequent labours to use a nappy!) I had already soaked through several by now.

On arrival at the hospital, I burst into tears from nerves. I was so scared about what it was going to feel like to push this baby out but the midwife who greeted me was very reassuring. Upon entering the birthing suite, I had to lie on my back for a very uncomfortable internal examination. I was suddenly bombarded with questions about pain relief and felt pressure to select something. I said I didn't want anything but felt very vulnerable and turned to my husband and asked him to call Sonya to come after all. Luckily she was not far away (she was holidaying several hours drive away but had jumped in the car when Adam told her my waters had broken on the off chance, I needed her!) and was only 10 minutes away when Adam called her. I felt more at ease to have the strength of two advocates with both my husband and Sonya present.

I was told to lie on the bed for the baby monitor to be fitted but I literally couldn't lie down, and I remember Sonya firmly saying to the midwife "she can't lie down!" The midwife still wanted me to wear the baby monitor while I was standing up and I tried for a short while, but I felt very constricted and didn't want it on me. When I expressed this, I was told that it was hospital policy, and I had no choice. This is where my advocates were able to back me up and reiterate to hospital staff my wishes. As a result, the midwife phoned my obstetrician, and he gave "permission" for me to not wear it. I was able to labour standing up, leaning over the hospital bed with my husband and Sonya coaching me through contractions and supporting me with heat packs on my lower back, sips of water through a drink bottle with a straw and placing my jumper on and off my shoulders as I swapped from being hot and cold between contractions.

As I was nearing the final stages of labour, Sonya suggested that I start thinking about moving across to the mat on the floor so that I wouldn't get too tired. I moved onto my knees and leaned onto a fitball for the final contractions. My obstetrician was now present and suggested I change my 'groaning/breathing' to deeper sounds for these final contractions. After several big pushes and 5 hours from when my waters had broken, I gave birth to my 9-pound baby boy, Jackson. He was immediately placed onto my chest and I realised for the first time that I was a mother. Everything had gone well, my baby was perfect, but I had a 2nd degree tear, possibly from pushing him out too quickly, and collapsed briefly afterwards in the shower from so much blood loss. I felt quite drained over the next 24 hours and was sore when going to the toilet. (I didn't tear in my subsequent labours and was amazed at how great I felt afterwards). Interestingly, the hospital midwives were encouraging me to have a home birth next time now that I knew that I could give birth drug free!

When I fell pregnant with my 2nd baby, Lucas, I considered having a home birth but decided to stick with the same winning formula as last time - my husband, Sonya and the same obstetrician. A girlfriend had dropped a book off on my doorstep the morning that I was in labour with Jackson called A Labour of Love, by Gabrielle Targett. Jackson had arrived early, so I missed reading it in time, but read it leading up to Lucas' birth. Reflecting on Jackson's birth while reading the book I could now clearly see all the places where things could have gone wrong and felt confident that I could have a natural birth in a hospital again if I was well informed and had the right support team.

My waters broke in the early hours of the morning again, but this time I was 1 week past my estimated date. I had refused an induction because I was worried it would interfere with the natural order of the labour process and had turned to chiropractic and acupuncture to help bring the labour on naturally. This time the contractions started straight away and came on thick and fast! I had hired a tens machine to try this time, but I think my labour was progressing too quickly as when I tried to use it, it seemed like the contractions had already built up too fast and it was uncomfortable. I again moved between the shower and toilet and was on the toilet when I could suddenly feel the baby's head pushing down! I said to Adam that we have to go to the hospital NOW! I was still upstairs in our house and couldn't walk down our stairs because the baby's head was pushing down. Adam had to carry me with my big pregnant belly - it would have been quite a sight!

I knelt on my knees on the front passenger seat of our car, hugging the headrest, butt facing the windscreen, for the less than 10-minute drive to the hospital. About halfway there I could feel more pressure from the baby's head and then realised I could feel the head with my fingers! I told my husband and he said "no you can't be feeling the head yet", and for some reason I believed him....so then I started thinking "what is that then, my liver, the placenta?

Adam phoned the hospital to inform them that we were on the way and they needed to be out front waiting because this baby is coming NOW! I think they must have thought it was just another panicked husband calling because no-one was out front when we got there. We parked at the door, Adam opened my car door and then started ringing the afterhours bell. It was then that I felt the urge to push. Adam stopped ringing the bell and turned around just in time to catch baby Lucas. He placed Lucas down on the car seat between my legs and went back to ringing the bell! I was in such shock, I just stayed still with poor Lucas underneath me. The hospital staff came running out and whisked him into the hospital while I was put into a wheelchair moments later. It wasn't too long before I got to hold him in my arms. I only had superficial tearing this time, no stitches. Lucas was born 1 hr 20mins after my waters had broken and weighed a hefty 11 pounds!

Needless to say, when my waters broke again in the middle of the night one day before my estimated date with my 3rd child, I made a mad dash for the car before my husband stopped me and calmly asked "do you have any contractions?".......and I didn't. I think this is my favourite labour because there was time to calmly go through each stage. With Lucas' labour in mind, we gathered everything we needed and went downstairs, packed the car and Adam even drove it out of the garage, ready in case of the need for a quick exit. My sons were picked up by relatives and then the contractions started to build up. It was a balmy summer's night in January, so we spent a lot of time on our front porch working through contractions and going for walks up and down the street, chatting between contractions.

When my contractions were about three minutes apart, we drove to the hospital and Sonya met us there. In the birthing suite we kept the lights dimmed and played Christian music from my phone which calmed me. With my husband and Sonya obviously taking on very active roles, attending to me with heat packs and sips of water, the midwives left us to manage on our own, just checking in from time to time. Similar to with Jackson, I laboured mostly standing up and leaning on the bed with my arms and moved to a mat on the floor for the final stage, upper body draped over a fitball. The midwife came in for the birthing stage and did a wonderful job of coaching me through breathing and pushing the baby out and I had no tearing. Nate was born 3 hours after my waters broke and was to be our 2nd smallest baby weighing in at 10 pounds.

My 4th pregnancy was definitely the hardest physically. I had the same morning sickness as with the others, lasting until week 23, but in addition I had terrible varicose veins on my left leg and developed an awful skin irritation on the veined area which kept me up at night because it was so itchy. Some nights I would sleep with an ice pack between my knees to try to dull the itch. My baby belly also seemed huge! From as early as 30 weeks I would be stopped by strangers asking when I was due and was I having twins. My obstetrician thought that my belly was large, but I didn't have gestational diabetes and we both just assumed that I was having another big baby (and that my belly had been stretched before so perhaps not much tightness left to hold everything in.

As with my other pregnancies I only had one scan at 20 weeks. As we got closer to my estimated date my obstetrician was debating the merits of a scan for baby size but then we decided that I had had big babies before, and it probably wouldn't change our approach to the labour so therefore not worthwhile. In hindsight I am so glad that I didn't have this scan as I think it could have changed events for the worse given the large size of this baby.

In the month before the birth, I struggled physically to care for my 3 little boys (aged 5, 3, and almost 2). I was physically exhausted from carrying around so much extra weight (I weighed 20kg over my pre-pregnancy weight) and had enormous pressure pushing down on my pelvis which made it difficult to walk sometimes. I found chiropractic adjustments helped enormously at this time with easing the pressure. Amazingly, I did not have any backache.

At my 37-week obstetric appointment I had the routine Strep B test. I had forgotten all about this and hadn't had a lavender bath beforehand (as recommended by Gaby) and unfortunately came up positive. I was devastated as I didn't want to be encumbered by an intravenous drip during labour so read my 'A Labour of Love' book as soon as I got home to refresh my memory on my options. Gaby outlined the options including asking for the antibiotics to be administered through injection in my thigh or bottom rather than the drip. This would mean four hourly injections during labour which were a much-preferred option, particularly given that it was unlikely that I would be in labour long enough for a 2nd injection based on my history! My obstetrician agreed to this request with no reservations.

Even with my positive labour history I felt very nervous leading up to my due date. I feel like a ticking time bomb, going to bed each night wondering if this is the night that my waters will break (because that's what has happened every other time). When I woke up each morning and nothing had happened in the night, I would go about my day as usual waiting for the next night.

I prepared for the labour spiritually, mentally and physically. I prayed a lot leading up to the birth, handing over control to God and to the body he has given me to birth this child. I know my body is capable and I reminded myself that it can be trusted to respond naturally better than if it is altered by drug intervention etc. I prepared mentally by reading the 'A Labour of Love' book and reminding myself of the stages of labour and things that have helped in previous labours. I love Gaby's advice on thinking of each contraction as only 40 seconds long, breathing in through the nose for 4 seconds and out the mouth for 6 seconds and knowing that you will only have to do this 4 times and it will be over. I also found Gaby's chapter on 'avoiding the fear-tension-pain syndrome' very useful. Getting my husband to refresh his memory by reading the chapter on 'choosing and educating your birth support people' was also essential. And physically I prepared by having regular chiropractic adjustments to ensure my pelvis was aligned optimally for birth. Once I had done all these things I felt as ready as I could be....and just waited.......

I woke up the morning of Australia day, three days before my estimated date, and decided that today was not the day because my waters hadn't broken in the night. But I was wrong. Around 9am my waters broke! We quickly organised for my sister-in-law Sonya to pick up our three sons. She dropped them off at her house just around the corner and then returned to check on us. I was having contractions, but it still felt like the early stages of labour and I was enjoying sitting on the toilet. Suddenly I felt a lot of pressure. Sonya offered to take a look and I hesitantly agreed. She informed me that there's still a little way to go. She walked away and literally returned two minutes later when I exclaimed that the baby is coming now, and we need to go to hospital, she took another look and said, "you have a choice of either having the baby in the car or at home!" I decided that home was the preferred option.

Adam swung into action grabbing the yoga mat we had ready to take to hospital and placed it on the floor of our foyer. I remember saying that I needed a fitball to lean over so they grabbed the closest chair and a cushion as a substitute. Sonya called the paramedics and kept them updated on my progress. Adam supported me as he had with my other labours, saying encouraging words over and over, stroking my back, informing me how much of the baby he can see. Once the baby's forehead was out, he seemed to be stuck. Sonya and Adam were telling me to push, and I was replying that I'm exhausted and can't push anymore. I heard Sonya go into the next room, in an attempt to be out of ear shot, saying to the paramedics that the baby is very blue. I am glad that I overheard this as I think it gave me the incentive to keep going.

The paramedics suggested that I change positions to laying on my back to get the baby moving again but Adam remembered that this position hadn't worked for me in other labours so instead got me to sit a bit more upright. Suddenly there was a shift, perhaps in gravity in my favour, and the pushing got easier. Much like he had seen the midwife do with Nate's labour, Adam coached me through pushing the baby out and he was born into his arms moments later. We waited breathlessly for a sign of life. I can clearly hear the relief in Sonya's voice when she tells the paramedics that he is breathing.

The paramedics arrived two minutes later, perfectly timed to cut the umbilical cord because with an unplanned homebirth we have no expertise to take care of things from here. We decide that I can birth the placenta at the hospital and the ambulance officers assist me in walking to the ambulance. Much to my surprise, the placenta births itself and comes crashing out onto our garage floor! I remember looking down at it, glad that it just missed the kid's hats and shoes ☺!

The ambulance drive to the hospital was really enjoyable, cradling my newborn bub and taking stock of the eventful morning. We later obtained a copy of the ambulance phone call recording and discovered that the last stage of labour was only seven minutes long (my waters breaking to birth had taken 1 hour and 10 minutes in total!). All my worries with the positive Strep B test were now obsolete.

My obstetrician was at the hospital on my arrival. He checked me over and gave me the all clear with no tearing. He commented that the placenta looked very healthy and very large. The midwife checked our healthy-looking baby boy, and it wasn't until he was weighed that we realised how big he was; 5.95 kg (13 pounds, 2 ounces), and 60cm long. He was too big for the newborn sized nappies! I think if I had known how big he was beforehand I may have thought he was too big to push out. That might explain why his forehead seemed stuck.

I feel very blessed to have had four natural labours and even more so, to have four healthy beautiful children. I am so very grateful to God, Adam, Sonya (and Gaby, for what I learnt through reading her book) to have supported me on the four most important days of my life and know that I could not have done it without them.

☺☺! Just one more thought, I want to share with women that are reading this. I'm not big in size – I am about 166cm tall and weighed 58kg before I started having babies and my new norm is now around 68kg....but my main point is that I was able to birth big babies. I share this with you as I feel many women are potentially robbed of having the opportunity to attempt natural labour because they are told that they have to be induced or have a caesarean because their baby is too big, and their pelvis is likely to be too small! I would like to inspire women to not get caught up on size (half the time the size scans are way off anyway!). I've had a lot of people comment when they've met me that they expected me to be a much larger size. Anyway, just a thought that I would share with you the reader with that additional information ☺. Gabrielle and I both think this has become an issue for birthing women when it should not be. The bottom line is to TRUST and have faith in you and your body that you can and will birth your baby vaginally and naturally if that is your wish and desire.

Thanks again and all the best to you, Nina July 2017

5.

ACCIDENTAL
HOMEBIRTHS

Belinda and Nick's Birth of Alexia

On the day of Tuesday 30th August 2017, I was sent a text by my friends Nick and Belinda to say it looked as if Bel was in what looked like imminent labour.

The text read, "Some early contractions? No bloody show yet and some tightening and downward pressure". I wrote back, "How often are the contractions happening?" To which the response was "every three minutes from the end of one to the start of the next – like clockwork". I then asked about the intensity level, to which Nick texted, "she can talk through them, but she says they are pretty intense, and by the way, the lift here is broken in our building so Bel is going to have to navigate six flights of stairs at some point to get down to the car!!!"

I thought "oh shit, that is going to be interesting" and ran around getting my doula bag ready along with some food and drinks.

I arrived to be greeted by Nick after climbing the six flights of stairs and then walking the length of the building to get to their apartment. To say it required some effort would be an understatement and I did think "how are we going to get Bel to do this in labour and get her down to the car?"

Upon being welcomed into the apartment I put my gear down and went to find Belinda who was sitting on the loo. I waited for her contraction to be over and then I said "hello" and asked a few poignant questions like, "Are you going O.K?" "Are you feeling like you are in established labour?" "Have you got lots of pressure in your bottom?

To which she answered "Yes" to all, so I suggested we wait a little while, gather up all the belongings and bags we needed and take it all down to the car and then make a move to go to the hospital. Taking the gear to the car was also problematic in that it would require going down all the flights of steps and Bel wanted Nick and I to both stay with her. Nick decided to leave it and to focus on supporting Bel with me.

At this point Emelia had gone to Nan and Pop's home to be taken care of. Emelia is Nick and Belinda's beautiful two-year-old daughter who was a known breech to all of us but was born via caesarean after she decided to put one foot down making it difficult for Belinda to birth even though she was 10 centimetres dilated. Belinda had done an amazing job during that labour (with me as her doula) and nearly got to experience a breech vaginal birth. It would have happened had Emelia not dropped one foot down and despite the doctor's best efforts to release the other foot.

So here we were, Bel now in the full swing of labour receiving what seemed like contraction after contraction one on top of the other. I suggested we get to the hospital, to which Bel replied, "There is no way I can walk. I think I have to have the baby here!" And with that she slumped forward off the toilet and crawled onto the floor and said, "Gaby, my legs just won't work, I can't make them work". I knew that Bel was experiencing the same thing she had during her previous labour where her legs just would not cooperate. It is like the blood just flows out of them rendering them useless.

So, with that statement she went onto her hands and knees on the floor, and I asked Nick to go and get some pillows and some towels so we could pad Belinda's body up against the hard tiles on the bathroom floor. It was here she was for what seemed like next to no time at all, and then she began to push.

It was then the reality had hit that Belinda was going to be birthing this baby right here at the apartment at this moment in time. So I said to Nick and Belinda "O.K, so I need to say to you both out loud you have three options here and you need to tell me what you want to do. The first is, we stay and you give birth here. The second is we try to get down to the car and make it to the hospital. The third is, we call an ambulance to take you to the hospital probably after the baby is born as this is happening really fast now".

They both instantly agreed to stay and that we would call for assistance from the paramedics. So with that Bel continued to push, on her side with her leg in the air, on her hands and knees face buried into Nick's lap, on her side with one leg up on the shower screen. I was so impressed by Belinda's flexibility at this time as she intuitively moved into positions that she felt would assist her baby down and out.

The final position was a hands and knees position, and as the baby's head crowned I was confused for a moment as to why I wasn't seeing the baby's face looking up at me. I was thinking well it's not a bottom, so it is not breech, so what am I looking at? To my astonishment I realised I was looking at the back of the baby's head which means Belinda was birthing a direct Posterior facing baby. At that point I was so amazed that she was able to do this as she was so calm and quiet and just listened to me suggesting when to nudge her baby down and when to back off. Belinda showed extreme control; I was so impressed and as a result she did not tear at all.

One final push was given and out shot the baby in one go. I attempted to receive this very slippery, wet gorgeous baby but she slipped through my hands and thankfully landed on the towels on the floor in a puddle of amniotic fluid. WOW, I could not believe Belinda had just naturally, calmly and gently birthed this posterior baby. Her dream of having a successful VBAC had been achieved, little did she know it would be a HBAC – Homebirth After Caesarean! I was so proud of her and what she had just done. I cried tears with Nick as I do at all the births I attend. It is such a magical moment, and I was so honoured to have been in attendance at this time.

Still kneeling on the floor, Belinda looked down and Nick and I assisted Bel to pick up their baby onto her chest where she let out a noise as if to say hello! Bubs was pink, breathing and with eyes wide open looking around. She did have a pressure mark on her head where she had been trying to come through the cervix at an interesting angle! Other than that, she was looking so healthy and a really good size.

In fact, beautiful Alexia was 8 Pounds (3.635kgs). I could not believe it as Belinda is such a lean woman and really had a very normal sized pregnant belly.

Not long after the commotion of the baby being born, I looked up to Nick and said "you had better go downstairs and let the paramedical guys up and into the building". In next to no time he appeared back at the bathroom door with two male paramedics who had some idea of birth, were happy and jovial, and went about congratulating Belinda who was still sitting on the floor on towels with her beautiful baby girl now breastfeeding happily.

Now it was time to figure a way to get Belinda out of the apartment block as the lift was still out of order. After we clamped the cord, Nick cut the cord and I took some photos, we got Belinda up off the floor and I ran around looking for some clothes to put on her while Nick held the baby. I also assisted Belinda to put on disposable pull-up undies for adults (these are the best things in the world when you still have a placenta inside and you have some blood loss and have to travel!) Next, I took the baby to the nursery to dress the baby as we were heading outside for the ambulance ride to the hospital and I didn't want the baby to get cold. More skin to skin would have to happen again once at the hospital.

Finally, we headed out the door with Belinda being wheeled in some random makeshift wheelchair the paramedics brought up the stairs. I asked the obvious question "So how does it go down the stairs?" To which one of the guys replied "We have to carry it down the stairs, so Belinda will have to walk down." "Oh my god" I thought to myself, not only has she just given birth to a baby, she has a placenta still inside her body and she has some blood loss, she is shaky and not 100% with her low blood pressure and now she is going to have to navigate getting down the stairs to get out of this building. I looked at Nick and said, "This is going to be fun!" As usual, Nick just smiled his beautiful smile and laughed as did I. Belinda had just given birth so I knew she could do anything she put her mind to, after all she was high on adrenaline, and this was a walk in the park for her after giving birth.

So, there we all were at the top of the stairs, Nick with all the bags and supporting Bel, myself with the precious cargo - the baby, and the paramedics with all their gear and the wheelchair! I was so impressed with Belinda who walked down two flights of stairs and sat on the chair to take a rest for a few minutes as she was feeling a little dizzy. We took our time, and I was so pleased the ambulance guys were so patient, so we really felt there was no stress or pressure. We chatted and it all seemed very surreal to me, and I am sure to Nick and Belinda, as everything before this moment had gone so fast.

Belinda, Nick and the baby ended up going to another hospital closer to home as it seemed pointless to travel now to the original hospital where they intended to go. They and I were well received and surprised to hear that the baby was born in a direct posterior facing position and Belinda having a VBAC as well. Everything went well post birth except for Belinda fainting when she was sitting on the toilet peeing, when we were at the hospital. Thankfully, I caught her as she slumped her whole-body weight onto mine as I called for help from the midwives.

It was decided that Bel would stay that night in the hospital as the lift in the building was not going to be operating until the next day. So with that being decided I headed back to the apartment to assist Nick to clean up the mess on the floor in the bathroom so that when Belinda arrived back home it was clean.

I feel this is such a brilliant story as it just shows you the power and strength of the female body and the possibilities of what the body can do when birthing. All credit to Belinda who was strong and empowered, and never once complained or said a thing about it all being too much. She just put her head down and did it. You were amazing Belinda and I thank you for trusting in me to assist your baby to come into the world in such a calm, peaceful and relatively uneventful way. Nick, you too were as solid as a rock for Belinda and incredible support to me - thank you both. This birth will forever be etched into my mind and one I will remember fondly forever more.

Baby Alexia was born on Tuesday 30th August at 11.32 am

Kristy and Stu's Birth

Wow what can I say except to state that this was the first birth that I have ever done with this particular outcome which was incredibly positive and powerful but not one I had intentions of being a part of at all.

I received a call at approximately 6.15am and was woken from a deep sleep thinking that I had been dreaming about my phone ringing! Well it actually was I missed the call and immediately called back as I had a sense this was birth related.

It was Stu on the phone explaining to me how Kristy's membranes had just broken and that she was doing OK, but felt she needed me right now. I could hear her in the background making lots of noises and thought to myself "She sounds like she is giving birth right now". With that she screamed out "The baby is coming, tell Gaby to hurry." With that I tell Stu I am on my way and ask him to call me back in ten minutes. That way I can tell him what to do over the hands free speaker in the car.

Sure enough, he calls me back as I do 140 kilometres down the freeway in my car towards Fremantle. The first thing I say to Stu is "tell Kristy to get out of the shower and onto the floor and put her head down and bum in the air to slow things down." Kristy of course says "What? Gaby wants me to get out of the shower and what?" I say to Stu, "tell her I said, NOW and I really mean it." He repeats what I say.

She begrudgingly does as I suggest, thankfully.

Next, I say "It sounds like the baby is coming down the birth canal, so you have three choices. Do you want to call for an Ambulance, travel in the car or stay at home and give birth?" I also add that at this point "I think the baby is going to be born in the car on the way to the birth centre, so if you don't want this to happen stay put as I am now five minutes away". Without hesitation Stu says they will stay put. I then tell Stu to get Kristy to breathe slowly and in a calm way and tell her not to push at all, and just pant and breathe through the urge to push. She says she can't….. And I relay through Stu, "Look, I know this is tough but tell her she has got to try". He relays my message. I then ask him if he can see the baby's head and he says "No, but it is all puffy down there". I smile to myself as that is exactly what it can look like prior to the baby's head coming out. "Good answer" I think to myself.

I ask Stu to listen carefully and in the break between contractions I begin to tell him how to assist with the baby should I not make it in time. With this he goes very silent. Thank goodness I was pulling into their street at this point, flying past the neighbours and into their driveway. I am never one to speed so this is really a first for me but well warranted I felt at the time.

I run inside and assess the situation. I take a deep breath and begin to talk to Kristy in a slow deep voice which instantly reassures and calms her. Next I send Stu to get me some clean towels, a face flannel with hot water on it, heat bags and then the camera ready to film and take stills. Remarkably he is so compliant and calm, and fantastic support for both Kristy and I.

In the next few contractions, the baby comes onto the perineum and slides back in playing peekaboo. This I explain to Kristy is for the very reason of completely stretching up the perineum and with this sensation I apply a hot compress/face flannel and Kristy instantly says "Oh, I love that feeling".

After about four pushes and peekaboo appearances the head finally makes an appearance on the perineum and I suggest to Kristy to just pant and nudge the baby out of her body, trying to resist a big push. She does this so incredibly well and listens to everything I suggest. Finally, the head gently glides on out of Kristy's body, and I put my finger past the perineum and along the baby's neck to feel for the cord, but instead I feel two little hands in a fist shape waiting to be born.

With the next contraction I tell Kristy her baby's body is being born, and to assist by giving a really big push. With this effort, the baby slides on out all soft and wet and slippery into my hands. I gently lower the baby onto the towel below and check her over observing her breathing, pulse and colour. She is perfect and happy. I slowly pass her through Kristy's legs and place her on the towel in front of Kristy. As I had seen before, women take their own time to realise their baby is there in front of them and pick up the baby, and Kristy was no exception. She was crying tears of joy and happiness, leaning back on Stu and hugging bubs. It was truly a beautiful moment, and then out of the blue she say, "Oh my baby, my beautiful baby," and scoops her up onto her chest and hugs her tight. I grab the camera and take photos of the three of them.

After we had all looked her over we wrapped her up, I was faced with the prospect of assisting the placenta to come out. I began to make suggestions about how to go about this. Firstly, I felt it was probably better for the placenta to come out if her bladder was empty. I suggested Kristy hold the baby and go to the toilet, being that they were still attached together. In the meantime, I asked Stu to go and get some shoelaces from a pair of shoes to tie off the umbilical cord. He said he always knew his new Dunlop volleys with new shoelaces would come in handy one day. We all laughed.

Just before Kristy went to sit on the toilet I said to Stu "can you bring a bowl from the kitchen to catch the placenta please?" With that he brought back a tiny little bowl, bless him. I kindly suggested I think we are going to need something a lot bigger than that. As he passed me the new bowl I was telling Kristy to hold on sitting down on the loo while I put the bowl in the bottom of the toilet to catch the placenta, but before I could get it in place 'PLOP' goes the placenta into the toilet with a huge splash. Yes, I then had to put my bare hands in the toilet and fish it out, and all I could think to say is, "well I guess you won't be eating any of that then?" With that we all rolled around laughing. We had such a laugh, it was brilliant.

With the placenta birthed, Stu cut the cord and I got Kristy dressed in some warm clothes and got her to rest on her bed and feed her baby. Like a natural she fed beautifully straight away. While Kristy breast fed the baby, I made her Milo and Stu fed her some toast while I cleaned up the bathroom floor and toilet.

Finally, it was time to ring the birth centre where Stu began talking to Fran, my friend and birth centre midwife. After a time he handed the phone to me so I could tell her what had happened. Fran was so supportive and happy that they were all doing so well and told me what I needed to do and be aware of with both Kristy and the baby. She also suggested that the choice was really theirs to make as to if they wanted to go to the birth centre or not. We all agreed it probably was the best thing to have the baby weighed and measured and for all the visitors to come to the birth centre that day rather than to their home.

All in all, it worked out perfectly. In the pouring torrential rain we ventured on our 20-minute drive to the birth centre where we were greeted well. Kristy and Stu's baby girl came into the world weighing 8 pounds and was named Isla.

At our debrief session a few days later Kristy had told me that during our hypnosis sessions prior to the birth she had been unable to see herself birthing at the birth centre and no matter how hard she tried she could not see herself giving birth there. I wonder whether she herself knew subconsciously she was going to birth at home being that it would be so fast. I certainly knew that she was very clear and open to the birth energy and suggested to Kristy at the time that I would not be surprised if her labour was going to be very fast and she smiled and said, "Yes I hope so". Our thoughts really do create our reality, for sure.

Thank you, Kristy and Stu, for trusting me enough to be there for you when you needed it most. Words cannot express how privileged and honoured I feel to have been a part of this wonderful (fast) journey of birth accidentally at home. Thank you xx

My Beautiful, Accidental Home Waterbirth

My whole life I had been terrified of birth because of all the horror stories women tell each other and what I had heard. I always said that when it comes my time I will use all the drugs available and have a C-section.

But once I fell pregnant I dived into research and read a lot of books on natural birth. It seemed so normal that women were built to birth naturally without intervention.

I was particularly drawn to waterbirth, but we ruled this out as we lived in the outback town of Karratha in WA and the local hospital didn't have the facilities. We decided the best option for a natural birth was to labour at home for as long as possible and then drive to hospital which was barely 1km away.

I resigned from my job four months early to prepare myself for my birth. I read as many books as I could on gentle and natural birth and watched videos on home, water and hospital births to help prepare my mind. We flew down to Perth to have birth preparation training with birth educator, Gabrielle Targett. I walked every day until I became too uncomfortable and then did laps in the local pool instead. I had acupuncture and aromatherapy treatments to help relax myself and tried to say affirmations every day and visualise my positive birth experience. I was lucky to find a Doula, Fran in Karratha who was able to help us.

Two days before my due date, we decided to go on a two hour drive out to a remote swimming hole called Python Pool. The local midwives told us bumpy roads can often bring on labour. That night I awoke at 1.30am with mild stomach cramps that felt like period pain. I assumed it was the hot curry my husband had cooked for me.

The stomach cramps continued with a pattern of twenty minutes apart and I spent time on the toilet with diarrhoea. I felt this was my body's way of getting ready for birth. I knew that this was it!

I was so excited and happy that our little baby had chosen today to meet us.

I moved to the lounge room to let my husband Grant sleep. I didn't tell him I was in labour as I assumed being my first baby that I could be in labour for well over 24 hours.

I took a necklace of beads and trinkets that my girlfriends had sent me to symbolised their wishes for us during labour. I wore a beautiful charm bracelet given to me by a dear friend. It had St Gerard - the Saint of health and safety in childbirth - and I wore this bracelet for weeks after birth.

I lay down on the couch with a doona and lots of cushions and listened to the 'A Labour of Love' hypnosis for birth scripts my friend had lent me. I slept in-between my contractions. I focused on the light of a rose quartz lamp and gently breathed the pain out through my toes.

I used my 'Labour of Love' heat pack on my tummy and sometimes moved to the kitchen to lean over the bench and breathe.

At 5.30am I had blood tinged, egg-white mucus. I told myself this was normal, and my body was opening up. It was such an exciting feeling knowing my baby was really on the way now. It began to get light outside and it felt like the last five and half hours were only one hour.

My husband woke at 6.00am to find me at the kitchen bench breathing through a contraction. I told him I'd been labouring since 1.30am. He broke into the widest smile and said how excited he was that our little baby was on the way. Plus, he was proud as punch that his curry had started labour (so he thought!). He was amazed at how well I was coping. We both thought there were hours to go. Grant announced he was going to wash the car seeing as I was doing so well. I told him he had heaps of time. So, he had a shower and cooked himself a full breakfast and paid some bills online. Grant kept checking on me in between chores, bringing me ice cubes to suck on or Gatorade drinks for energy.

By 7.30am I could feel my contractions coming closer together and picking up with intensity. I walked around labouring upright and rolling on the fitball as I now felt safe to speed up the labour because Grant was awake. I called my Mum, who lived in Victoria, and Grant booked flights and buses for her to fly over to meet the first grandchild in our family.

I called my Doula Fran - she said she could come over anytime I wanted. I said I'd call her again when the pain got scary. I lay down again to conserve my energy.

By 9am I was getting nervous and called the midwives at the hospital. They told me it would probably be a long labour, to have some breakfast and rest as much as possible. I was finding the contractions tougher but managed to eat some toast my husband had prepared for me.

By 9.30am I felt like I was in a land far away. I called Fran to come over and told Grant to fill the birth pool.

Our doula lent us a blow-up birth pool to use for pain management. It was nice and deep with a little seat at one end and grip handles around the outside for support. Grant filled the pool to 37 degrees while I was struggling with the contractions. I was kneeling next to the couch and yelling out the pain as I banged my hands on the couch. I needed Grant to rub my lower back and count out loud until the contractions passed.

Fran arrived at 10am and breezed through our front door with a huge smile and announced "what a beautiful day to have a baby!"

She sat with me and quietly told me I would wear myself out using all my energy, and encouraged me to breathe slowly, breathing in with the count of four and breathing out with the count of six. She put my hypnosis scripts on and breathed with me for the rest of my labour.

I looked in her eyes and breathed with her and felt my body relax and all panic disappear. Miraculously, the pain seemed to melt away as I stayed in the moment and concentrated on each calming breath. I trusted her. She had given birth to four children and birthed her son at home in Karratha five months earlier; a 10lbs 13oz baby boy in the same birth pool we were using. I knew I would be OK. I knew it would all work out if I kept concentrating on breathing with Fran. By now my contractions were 60 seconds long and three minutes apart.

At about 11am I decided to get into the pool. I'd read that water was a great pain management tool and I waited to use it as a last resort.

I stepped into the pool and my whole body went soft and floppy. It felt like I had just been given pain relieving drugs. It was actually fun to experience my contractions as I floated in the water and my husband joined me and rubbed my lower back. Fran stayed near me and kept breathing with me.

I remember chatting and laughing between contractions. They were two minutes apart and 80 seconds long. Concentrating on the breathing got me through.

I winced on three contractions - they were quite intense, and then I suddenly felt a massive push sensation as my waters broke. Fran told Grant to get out of the pool and call the hospital to tell them that we were on our way.

Suddenly my body wanted to push, and I felt it shudder violently. Fran asked me if I wanted to stay there or transfer to the hospital. I could think of nothing worse than getting out of that water and risking birthing on the side of the road or in the hospital hallway in front of everyone. So we decided to stay at home.

Fran told me not to fight my body and to relax with each pushing contraction. I felt the baby fall through my cervix with such force that it felt like my insides had blown out through my vagina. I became scared. Fran held my hands and breathed with me. I was on my knees and leaning on the side of the pool gripping the handles and looking at a collage I had made of how I wanted the birth to go. I kept saying out loud, "I can do this. I can give birth to my baby. It's natural. There are thousands of women birthing with me all around the world. It's safe. I'm safe. It is safe, little baby; you can come down".

There were incredible relaxing periods in-between the contractions with no pain at all. I hung there over the side of the pool smiling and saying "I'm alright, this is actually OK". Then I could feel the wave of another contraction starting deep within my body as I mentally prepared myself for the next onslaught of power.

317

At some stage Fran ended up in the pool with us to help. I was so glad she did because I gripped her thigh and took in her powerful, divine, feminine energy to help me push down our baby.

It took four contractions for the crowing stage, and I felt like I was going to split in half. Most of the pressure was on my clitoris and I was so scared that I was going to tear there! I kept yelling out,

"Ring of fire! Ring of fire! It's the ring of fire!"

Fran helped me to breathe and told me not to push until she said so. It felt like I was hanging there in limbo, half alive, half dead, and reaching across into another dimension to bring forth new life.

I felt my baby's head with my hand, and it felt like a beak as the bones had crossed over to make the passage. I was frightened and didn't want to touch it again. But later I did, and I could feel my baby's beautiful hair swaying gently in the water.

The baby's head retracted back inside me and I yelled out "It's gone back in! It's gone back in!"

Fran explained that it is nature's way of stretching the perineum and that it's all ok. Fran helped me to slowly breathe my baby's head out. She checked there was no cord around the neck and told me to give the biggest push that I had ever given in my whole life. Like I was doing the biggest poo ever, the size of a watermelon.

Fran helped me steady myself and kneel more upright. She helped me grip the handles so I could push as hard as I could. It was the best feeling in the world feeling my baby's body slip out from me. My husband Grant caught our baby and passed him/her to me through my legs.

I blew gently on our baby's face and watched as our baby took its first breath. I sat back and marvelled at our beautiful bundle of joy in my arms. My husband sat next to me in the water with a single tear rolling down his cheek.

I'm not sure how long we were like that in our own little world before we lifted the towel to discover we had created a little boy! We later called him Liam Jackson Cucel.

Grant held our son while Fran helped me out of the pool and onto a chair. The placenta cord was very short, and I could feel it tugging as I negotiated stepping over the side of the pool. Once I sat down I asked about the placenta and two minutes later I could feel it on its way. Fran helped me to squat on a bucket and I watched in amazement as my placenta slid out of me to plop neatly in our cleaning bucket.

What a feeling! It was all over! I achieved it and gave birth to our son!

Grant and Fran helped me into our family car lined with garbage bags and towels. I was in a dressing gown and held our son against my bare chest. We pulled up at the Emergency Department and a midwife happened to be walking right past our car. Fran opened the car door to reveal me sitting there with a newborn on my chest and his umbilical cord still connected to the placenta in a bucket between my legs!

The midwife took my baby and the bucket while someone else helped me into a wheelchair. It felt surreal being wheeled through the hospital with people staring at us.

Grant went with the staff to get our son checked over while I was whisked away to room ten to be checked over. I was ecstatic to learn that I didn't need any stitches! I had a slight graze internally on my perineum. I was even more surprised when Grant brought our son to me and announced that he weighed 8lbs 12oz! Wow! I really did it! It was the most amazing feeling of accomplishment. Our son was the picture of perfect health as he attached and began breastfeeding.

I was on a birth high for many days afterward. I was so proud of my accidental achievement. It was the most empowering, beautiful, divine experience. It was a gentle, unobtrusive birth. Whenever we hear Johnny Cash's song, 'Ring of Fire' we crack up laughing.

Baby Liam Jackson Cucel-8lbs 12oz 52cm long

My birth story of Amber by Rachel

Born Monday 25th January 2010 at 12.23pm

After the traumatic birth of my first baby where I was ill prepared, in denial and well and truly stuck in the fear-tension-pain cycle, I had gone to the hospital at the very first sign of labour which is what they advise when your membranes rupture. It was a fairly long and painful labour that I tried to manage with TENS. I tried the bath, but I was very uncomfortable and eventually ended up having an epidural, gave birth lying on my back (the worst position to be in to allow your pelvis to open) with the help of an episiotomy and a 3rd degree tear with a large amount of blood loss and emotional scarring to boot.

When I discovered I was pregnant with my second baby I was keen to educate myself and do whatever I could to ensure I had a better and more empowered experience. I had heard a little of Gaby and her classes from mothers' group friends and people I'd known who had done her workshop. I had intended to go along to the classes during my first pregnancy but did not prioritise it and never got around to it.

This time round I started going to Gaby's aqua classes when I was 11 weeks pregnant. Gaby often joked that I had been going since conception! I loved them and I only missed one week when I was away. Once I finished work, I started going twice a week for the last eight or so weeks of my pregnancy. I also did some research about doulas (having previously thought, "what would you need one of them for?!") and read Gaby's two books. After reading her books including all the wonderful birth stories and going to her classes, the healing process had well and truly begun. I understood where I went wrong last time in my lack of preparation. I decided to ask Gaby if she would be my doula and when she said yes, I felt a great weight had been lifted. I really felt I could do this with her supporting me.

My husband Pete agreed also as I think my first birth was quite traumatic for him as well. I did quite a bit of preparation with Gaby, including a hypnosis session. I also listened to her hypnosis scripts most days towards the end of my pregnancy. I bought an 'Epi-no' and used it to stretch my perineum for the last two weeks as I was concerned about another tear or need for episiotomy. I believe that as well as the physical preparation that it gave me, it also added to the psychological preparation by giving me that sensation of the perineum stretching.

So, when the time came I was relaxed and ready to give birth. It was about 5pm and I began to get quite strong cramping every 3-5 minutes. I carried on having dinner with my husband and two-year-old daughter Holly, and gathered the last-minute items I needed for the hospital. The cramping continued over the next hour, so I phoned Gaby to let her know what was happening. She reminded me it could just be a warm-up, but I was pretty sure it was the real deal. We got Holly ready to take to our friends who had agreed to look after her for the night and Pete took her over. I felt she knew something was happening as she was uncharacteristically cuddly and wanted to hold my hand.

Pete returned at about 7.30pm and at this stage I was well into established labour having between 4-5 contractions every 10 minutes. I was very keen not to call Gaby too early or rush to the hospital as I felt it could be a long night. I felt comfortable labouring at home at this stage. I was in the zone breathing through the contractions and kneeling on cushions over the couch. I still felt like this could go on for hours. I remembered Gaby advising me to try and sleep through the small stuff, so at about 8.30pm both Pete and I decided to try and get some rest even though I didn't really think that what I was experiencing was "small stuff." I thought I should try anyway but I still wasn't sure I was coping a lot better than with my first labour. This was probably a combination of my mindset and the fact that my membranes were still intact, so I still had the benefit of that cushioning.

Anyway, I only lasted one contraction…it was much too intense and in hindsight, it was crazy to think I would be able to sleep through that! I got Pete up and told him to call Gaby as I really felt I needed her here with me. I was also burning up (later Gaby told me that this was a sign of transition) and wanted the air conditioning on and buried my head in a cold pack.

At this point I was sitting on a fitball that Gaby had loaned me and leaning over the dining room table, all the while trying to tell myself to relax and surrender. I was trying to listen to Gaby's hypnosis on my iPod, but the contractions were too intense and I needed quiet. I hadn't even thought of my TENS machine or using the shower which was all set up with a fitball. I wanted to delay all that until I really needed it. The only pain relief I used was a heat pack and Pete massaging my lower back.

Gaby arrived at about 9.30pm. I think she could tell that I was in transition, but I still had no clue as to how close I was! I felt pressure in my bottom and needed to go to the toilet (this should have been a clue, but I felt this for much of my first labour due to the membranes having ruptured). Gaby helped me up from the fitball and to the toilet. With the first step, my membranes ruptured with a big gush. At the toilet I was too uncomfortable to sit down - the pressure was immense - but I still didn't realise that birth was imminent. At around this point, which was only five minutes or so since Gaby had arrived, she said "I don't think we're going to make it to the hospital, I think this baby wants to be born at home. I think if we try to make it, you will end up having the baby in the car". Gaby suggested Pete call an Ambulance as a backup as she could sense this was happening right no.

For a moment I was horrified, but I was more horrified about the prospect of giving birth in the car or in a Bunnings car park! Anyway, I quickly regained composure and was totally reassured that Gaby was there and I just had no doubt that everything would be fine. Gaby said, "do you trust me?" and I said "yes". I just decided I didn't really have any choice in the matter and remembered everything that I'd learned from Gaby, and just focussed on my breathing and Gaby's words as she guided me through the pushing stage of the birth. The sensation was intense but so much easier than my first experience, my 'Epi-no' use had paid off and I only had a very small tear that did not require stitching. I was aware of the ambulance officers asking lots of questions, but I didn't let it distract me.

My beautiful baby, Amber, was born at 10.06pm and I can honestly say it was one of the most amazing experiences of my life. It was so much more relaxed and calmer than my previous experience. I was amazed and overjoyed that I had just birthed my baby at home on my living room floor and I had so much energy left. After thinking I was in for the long haul, I felt as if I could have run a marathon!

After Amber and I had lots of skin-to-skin contact (I actually had the strength to keep her in my arms, unlike Holly's birth where I felt so weak from the epidural and the blood loss) and the cord had stopped pulsating, the cord was clamped, and Pete cut it. I was totally in love with my warm little bundle who had entered the world in such a surprising way. I gave her a breastfeed and after a little while we made our way to the hospital where my obstetrician was waiting for me. I thought he seemed a little miffed that I had done it all without his help! The placenta eventually came away naturally without the help of syntocinon. I don't plan on having any other babies, but if I did, I would definitely be looking at a planned home birth. My perception of birth has been totally changed by this remarkable experience with the expert help of one special lady.

Rachel and Pete's birth of Amber

I met Rachel soon after she had discovered she was pregnant with baby number two, but she could hardly talk about her pregnancy due to having so much trauma associated with her previous labour. That to me spoke 'alarm bells' as I knew she had a lot of work to do to clear herself of her previous labour journey so that she could create a new fantastic experience in her future with the baby she was pregnant with. At that time I really hoped and prayed that she would seek me out to assist her to get to where she needed to be mentally, physically and emotionally to birth in an empowered way. You see, I knew she could change and heal but only if she was prepared to take full responsibility to do so.

Thankfully Rachel started coming to my Aqua–fitness classes where she started to listen to me talking about just how positive birth could be. Little did she know she was coming to my classes for childbirth education rather than the exercise! All the same, it became the highlight of Rachel's week and as the weeks went by, I could see Rachel's energy and enthusiasm change around the way she was thinking and feeling about her imminent journey.

By the time Rachel got to her 25th week she decided to ask me to be her doula which I was excited about as I knew now I could really get into Rachel's head, and find out exactly what was going on in her psyche. During the next ten weeks we set about doing a three-hour intensive hypnosis session, childbirth education sessions and we spoke for a few hours at a time. For our very last session we had a coffee in a coffee shop as I wanted to look Rachel in the eye and really see where she was at mentally, physically, emotionally and energetically. I can honestly say that she was in such a clear and open place with no hang-ups or baggage at all. She was totally free of the past labour journey and I knew from the bottom of my heart that Rachel was truly ready to give birth in the most amazing and open way.

About two weeks prior to Rachel's estimated due date I went to her home to meet with Pete, her husband, and ask if he had any questions. The subject of homebirth came up and the usual question of "what if we have the baby at home?" To which I responded, "if a baby comes into the world that quickly I can assure you there is nothing going wrong with you, your labour or with the baby". That said, I reassured them that the likelihood was there, that it could happen, however there was usually enough time to get to hospital in time so there was no need to worry or focus on that.

So as the next two weeks went by and I kept intuitively thinking that Rachel was going to have a homebirth, but I did not want to share this news as I knew it would potentially 'freak' both Rachel and Pete out so I kept this very strong premonition to myself. However the funniest thing happened. About a week out from Rachel's actual birthday she runs up to me in the pool during the middle of my class and asks me "so how many accidental home births have you done?" I glanced at Rachel trying not to give too much away in my facial expressions and said "about 6 or 7, I will talk to you later about it", and proceeded to move off into the middle of the pool and change the subject. Later, after the birth, we laughed about my lack of commitment to get into any type of discussion going that night, due to me trying not to 'spill the beans' over the fact that I already had a strong feeling she was going to be home birthing. Rachel said that she just thought it was odd the way I responded and then swiftly changed the subject, which was not at all like me!

So during the afternoon of the day of our last session (our lunch-time coffee date) Rachel went into labour, which incidentally was the day I had forecast Rachel was going to have her baby. So as we sat there drinking our coffee and it rained outside Rachel said to me "I thought I was supposed to have the baby today according to you and your psychic ability?" I smiled and said "today is not over till midnight Rachel – you still have plenty of time!" We finished our meeting and I said "ok, I will see you later on today" and we joked around smiling, hugging and then said goodbye; off we went our separate ways.

That evening, whilst out walking my dogs, Rachel called at 6pm to tell me something was going on that felt very different. She could feel her body was moving into action but did not want me to come over at that point but was giving me the heads up that something was going on. We talked about this potentially being a 'warm up' and not the real deal, but I put myself on standby anyway. So with that I walked the dogs home, prepared the family dinner and mentally prepared myself to be going to a labour.

At about 8pm I had not heard any more from Rachel, so I jumped into bed thinking that maybe Rachel had a long way to go. At about 8.30pm however, I was awoken by Pete who requested I come straight away as Rachel suddenly really needed me. I immediately jumped out of bed, literally threw my clothes on and drove over to their home as fast as I could because I had a very strong sense that now this baby really did want to be born at home.

Upon my arrival at their home I found Rachel sitting on my fitball that I had left for her a few days earlier, listening to my hypnosis for birth script whilst burying her face into pillows and a cold pack leaning on her dining room table. As soon as I touched her arm and she saw me, she looked up and pulled her earphones out and said "I am so over listening to this, thank god you are here. I have so much pressure in my bottom!" So, with all of that information I asked Rachel when she last went to the toilet as I felt she should go to try to relieve some of the pressure. In my mind I knew perfectly well that she looked like she was transitioning due to her grumpy demeanour, and if the baby was really sitting inside her birth canal, I knew that she would start pushing once on the loo.

It took a few more contractions, a bit more convincing and a few more grumpy words from Rachel before she finally was ready to go to the loo. As Rachel went to stand up though her membranes broke all over the fitball and the floor. I said "oh that's wonderful, well done, things are really on the move now. Come on let's get you to the toilet while we clean up". So as Rachel sat on the loo, I could hear her starting to puff and pant and then push, whereby she said "Gaby I need to push". I thought she might as the breaking of the membranes often means the head is just sitting in the birth canal and the pushing stage of labour is about to begin. Sure enough, contraction af-ter contraction, Rachel began to push. I suggested we move to the lounge room but before we did, we needed to quickly dis-cuss a plan of action. I said "I don't think we are going to get to the hospital, this baby wants to be born at home. I think if we try to get there you will end up having the baby in the car!" The plan of action was to ask both Pete and Rachel if they gave their full consent to birth at home right there and then in which they said "Yes". Secondly, I had to ask them if they wanted to call an ambulance as a back-up to have some extra hands avail-able if I needed, to which they also said "Yes".

With that I walked Rachel to the lounge room with Pete and then he proceeded to call the ambulance. He was then on the phone talking with someone who was asking 100 questions while I asked him to go and get towels, baby wraps, baby wipes and tissues. Poor Pete, he was having to multitask to the 100th degree. Then he watched and gave the woman on the other end of the phone a running commentary on what he was seeing. Rachel, this whole time, was so calm and listened to my every word. I had a little bit of time to give her some water, calming remedy and apply some perineum balm to her perineum to assist it to stretch as I was determined to help Rachel stretch wide open this time around and not tear. To Rachel's credit, she stretched beautifully thanks to using an Epi-no and with the assistance of my coaching.

I was so proud of Rachel as she was amazingly calm, centred and totally in the moment. She also listened intently as to when to push, when to back off, when to breathe slowly and when to nudge her baby down. Her biggest distraction was the ambulance guy wanting to ask a heap of questions of me about Rachel's history as I tried to focus on suggesting to Rachel what she needed to be doing. As a result of Rachel's inner focus and awareness she birthed her beautiful baby girl into the world at 10.06pm on the 20th November 2014, in the most calm and peaceful way, with Pete by her side and all three of us on our knees on the lounge room floor.

After a few minutes had passed and we all shed tears of joy and relief, Pete and Rachel looked to confirm that indeed they had a baby girl who was divine, pink, alert and beautiful. Due to the placenta not coming out after feeding Amber (as she was later named) for approximately 20 minutes, it was off to the hospital in the ambulance for the birth of the placenta there. Not long after our arrival it decided to slide on out and into this world having done a brilliant job over the last nine months.

It was then that Rachel got up and had a shower, fed Amber some more and bounced off the walls due to such a fantastic labour journey. She looked absolutely amazing, fresh and so happy and content with her labour journey. She kept saying to me "Gaby, I just can't believe it, I just had a homebirth" smiling from ear to ear.

I truly am so happy to have been of assistance to help Rachel and Pete to create this wonderful experience; a journey that has helped the both of them heal and a story that can and will empower other women who read this to trust and know that they too can turn their beliefs and thinking around to create an amazing journey. Rachel is proof of that for sure.

Inge's Rapid, Amazing, Unplanned Home-birth

Sunday, at 11 am, I was cutting bread we'd bought on the market that morning. My husband and toddler were visiting some neighbours. I was making the most of having a quiet moment to myself while feeling what felt like more of my "warm up" tightening which I'd had for weeks. I was cutting the bread feeling quite relaxed being 41+1 that day, when I realised I'd had about three sensations in about half an hour. I got very excited and took my phone to download a contraction app.

I had been anticipating a moment like this for weeks, yet I was still caught by surprise. I had been pressured to be induced from 39 weeks due to my age, by a hospital doctor. I could, initially, also only birth at the Birth Centre until 40 weeks for the same reason, based on age and statistics etc. I had seen a doctor every week and had ultrasound appointments at the main hospital in the last few weeks, jumping through all of their hoops. After advocating fervently for myself and my baby in the last weeks, I got an extension to 41 and then to 42 weeks, when eventually I was heard and seen for my good health. This healthy pregnancy and my previous natural birth that took place at 41+6 at the age of almost 41. So finally, I could relax and let go.

As I figured, the real deal had started and when my family came home, I started to sit on the fitball, not saying anything yet. I was thrilled inside about what was starting to happen. I had put on some special music and soon after I showed my husband the app. Soon after my little daughter sat on the elevated area where I had my fitball and rubbed my hand with every tightening. My husband called Gaby at around 12.30pm to give her a heads up, saying we didn't need her yet. My daughter excitedly packed her suitcase for her first sleepover. She got so excited about the sleepover that she started to drive me nuts. I needed more rest and quiet, so my husband took her to friends around the corner. He called Gaby at 2pm who said she would be there in half an hour.

He was only away for a maximum of 15 minutes but in the meantime, I had to go to the toilet.

Somehow, I still thought I was quite a few hours away from anything happening but when I came off the toilet, I couldn't move more than 3 metres during the rest between the contractions. When my husband came back, I was still stuck trying to get around my bed on my way back to the fitball in the living room. I was getting cold when my husband found me there and I found that he put the worst socks on my feet that he could find, too slippery, which made me panic and express that I wasn't sure if I could actually do it this time.

He had quickly grabbed our beautiful birthing bowl that friends lent us and started playing. The next break he helped me to quickly get back to my "rescue spot" - my fit ball. There he started to play the bowl again which we had practised before, and I remember thinking "let's visualise the baby getting through the cervix" which I did, and which then totally happened! I could exactly feel it happening and thought subsequently "oh no what did I just do?!!". I yelled to my husband

"Gaby has to come NOW!", my body knew what happened although my mind didn't catch up yet.

My husband had called the Birth Centre to talk with them about what was happening. In the mean-time, Gaby arrived and came straight over to me. I was so relieved. Soon I had a contraction coming whereby I said "I can't sit on this ball any-more", not knowing what to do then and not realising why. Gaby said "well get up then", which I did and I felt I had to push against the whole world's gravity to just get up and straighten my legs. At the same time Gaby asked if she could pull my tracksuit pants down and have a look at what was going on! She then ordered my husband to get clean towels, hot water etc. etc. They both got really busy while I felt and said out loud, "Gaby don't leave my side anymore!" My husband called the Birth Centre again saying we wouldn't make it. We were asked if we wanted an ambulance, but we decided confidently to do this together and we knew we could call an ambulance if we needed it.

Gaby came back from washing her hands and asked me if I could climb up onto this lounge area we have built in the wall. Funny enough, I said "I want to give birth in the bath!" think-ing of the wonderful bath and my first experience in the bath of the Birth Centre which I had planned to go to. Well, that wasn't happening; I climbed up and the baby came. Gabrielle applied really hot towels on me and heaps of oil to help my perineum stretch wide open, because it was going so fast. From the moment I had got up from the ball, I felt such strong pushing urges which Gaby had asked about. I had replied I could not resist pushing which was a new sensation for me, so I allowed things to open, stretch gently and carefully. With Gaby's guidance I felt I could surrender, trusting her completely. I then realised my precious girl was being born because I felt the perineum stretch, with no break in the burning sensation. That's when my head realised that I was giving birth NOW, and it was really happening.

My baby had done a fresh green poo inside so came out with her face covered which was all at once wiped off by Gaby. When only her head was out, waiting for her body to be birthed, my husband got nervous not seeing her breathe yet but when Gaby told him to take pictures, he got that all was good and how it's supposed to be. Once her body came out on the next contraction she cried and pinked up pretty quickly and took her first breath. Gaby just held her face down to drain all the fluid out of her mouth and lungs before I turned around to receive her on my chest skin to skin.

At 3.38pm our beautiful baby girl Sterre, arrived and so much joy and relief went through me, having this quick wonderful homebirth that I wouldn't have dared dreamed of. I stayed with this beautiful baby girl on my chest while Gaby and my husband looked on laughing and smiling at what had just happened. I was just thrilled with how my girl decided to come, with all that just happened. I was in shock a little due to the speed at which she came, and Gaby and my husband began to feed me some food which helped as I started to shake from all the adrenaline I had onboard. Gaby asked if my husband could find a clean shoelace in which to tie off the umbilical cord as she didn't have any clips on her. He came back with a new clean one which Gaby tied in two places and my husband cut between the two with some sharp scissors. Finally, I could bring my baby onto my chest skin to skin as the cord was quite short. After a little while our beautiful little girl began to breastfeed beautifully.

After half an hour Gaby suggested that I go to the toilet to do a wee to see if the placenta would release itself from within me naturally. As I sat on the toilet, I held onto the umbilical cord and within a second it had plopped out of me straight into the toilet. I screamed out to Gaby who was running to go and get a bowl for the placenta. Too late... it landed in the loo.

I decided to take a shower at this time while my husband did the skin on skin. Gaby assisted me, dried me and helped me get dressed. After feeding Sterre, we got into the car very relaxed and in awe and headed to the hospital. It was just for a check-up to see if I had a tear, however they wanted me to stay so they could watch my baby for the next 24 hours due to her doing the fresh baby poo in her amniotic fluid. I did in the end need a few stitches inside as well but not on my perineum which I was pleased about.

All in all, I could not have been happier with this amazing labour journey. My Birth centre midwife was away and as it turned out they were full and would have asked me to go to the main hospital anyway, so it was just perfect the way it all turned out.

6.

EMPOWERED POSITIVE
SECOND BIRTHS

A Powerful Second Birth

My first child was born after 34 hours of hard labour. I remember always being afraid of having to give birth but even through the pregnancy I never dealt with my fear. I knew it would be amazing to be a mum and I kept thinking of how lovely it would be to have a family but throughout the pregnancy that fear was like a little black cloud. I never talked about it much with anyone, there didn't seem to be much point - I knew the baby would have to come out inexorably. So when my daughter was born after an ambulance ride, an epidural gone wrong and being pulled out with forceps, I swore I would never go through it again.

But I did do it again - four years later when I gave birth to a little boy and his birth was the most amazing experience.

When we decided to have another child the memories of my first birth had not really faded but I had talked to a lot of women that had had a positive birth experience, so I was determined to conquer my fears and find an option that suited me. I remember one of the only positives with my daughter's birth (except of course the fact that she was born happy and healthy!) was resting in the shower and having a bath. Being in water calmed me down and eased the pain. I did a bit of research on birthing alternatives and when I found out I could have a waterbirth I knew it was for me. That decision, along with some positive affirmations and the support of a great midwife, made me confident I could do it.

So when the day of the labour came, I felt excited and prepared. We stayed at home and had a late lunch with friends and waited for our babysitter then got in the car and drove to the birth centre. I remember how different I felt and how much more in control. I was surprised at how manageable the contractions were, but I believe that feeling so much fear in my first labour made them feel worse. This time I kept thinking about how each contraction was something positive that would bring me closer to having my baby.

At the birth centre we were greeted by our midwife who had set up the pool. It was perfect. Just seeing it there set up in the room made me feel relaxed. I wanted to use it only when the contractions intensified so I strolled around outside a lot, focusing on my breathing and rested on the bed in between.

When the contractions were very close my midwife asked if I wanted to get into the pool, so I did. As anticipated, being in the water made me feel light. It truly felt like the pain subsided. I remember I was surprised when my midwife gently told me that I was ready to push, it seemed to be too good to be true. Even while I was pushing I kept thinking that it really wasn't too bad at all.

Our beautiful baby boy was born into the water in his caul. This meant my waters never broke and he was still in his membranous sack. My midwife came to the end of the pool and gently opened it with her fingers and then I picked him up from the water and held him for the first time. He was perfect.

Then of course came the nappy changes and sleepless nights, but I didn't mind. Our daughter had a baby brother who she loved. Instantly I was really proud to have turned my fears into a beautiful experience. A waterbirth might not be for everyone, but it is finding out what makes you feel relaxed and safe to have the best birth possible.

Annelie Hansen

Crystal's Quick Birth Entrance

I had my first contraction at about 10.30pm that night. It was strong and I remember thinking to myself - here we go again - I'm in labour!

I waited anxiously for the next one to come but it didn't happen. Disappointed, I showered and went to bed, only to wake up about four hours later with another two contractions, 15 minutes apart. I phoned my mum to come and collect my daughter, as she was going to look after her during the birth. We had chosen, once again, to give birth at home and I felt my daughter was too young to stay and she wouldn't understand what was happening. I also needed to just focus on myself and the baby. My mum arrived and waited for the next contraction to come but it didn't come for over an hour. So Mum took Giselle and I went back to bed. In the morning I got up and had breakfast but was starting to feel quite frustrated as this was so different to my last labour - things weren't progressing! I continued to have the occasional contraction but there didn't seem to be any rhythm or regularity with them.

By about 11am I was beginning to feel a bit over it all and quite upset, teary and frustrated. I decided that it was perhaps time to try taking some homoeopathic remedies to help get things going. My partner called a family friend of ours who is a homoeopath and described what was happening and how I was feeling, and she suggested I take Pulsatilla. She said that this should help to regulate the contractions, generally help labour to progress and help me to refocus. Matt was asked to give me one dose each hour for a couple of hours. About 20 minutes after the first dose my contractions kicked in at 15-minute intervals. Just after the second dose Matt said he was going to call the midwives, but I tried to protest this as I was feeling so much calmer and in control compared with my daughter's birth. He called them anyway!

In hindsight that was probably a good thing as one and a half hours later we welcomed our beautiful son Maddox into the world. My waters didn't break at all - his head was birthed while still in the sac. This is considered lucky and is celebrated in many cultures. It is called 'bearer born with veil'. They say babies born this way bring luck and protect the family.

I definitely believe that having homoeopathic remedies really helped me during my labour. I had taken the remedy at a point where I was starting to feel frustrated about my labour not progressing.

It assisted me to overcome those feelings of hopelessness and at the same time completely regulate the contractions. The remedy therefore helped me on both an emotional and physical level. It was a completely different experience to my first labour where I had felt so overwhelmed, almost as if I couldn't manage it, and even feared death. With Maddox's birth I was calm, focused and felt empowered.

By Crystal Johnson

Emma's Beautiful Experience

I just thought that I would write and share my experience with a Labour of Love.

My first childbirth experience was so harrowing, that when I found out that 'Baby Number Two' was on the way I knew I had to try a different approach.

My son was born in a hospital and I had little knowledge of what to expect. We went into the labour ward after several hours of mild contractions and settled into the birth suite in time for the heavy contractions to start. Immediately I freaked out at the amount of pain I was in and started screaming out for drugs!! The midwife quickly gave me a shot of pethidine and laid me on my back on a hospital bed. Things got worse from there on as I seemed to not handle the effect the pethidine had on me, but it was too late – the drug had been given. My son's heart rate started dipping with each contraction. As it was not coming up again, I ended up having a foetal scalp monitor attached to the baby's head and remained on my back in a bed for the remaining labour. My son was born blue and whisked away before I could even see him; I was petrified at what might have happened. My son is now 5 and healthy, but his stressful entry into the world certainly reflects the early troubled infancy that we experienced with him.

When my son was two, my husband and I decided that it was time for number two and so we started trying. We were quite surprised to fall pregnant immediately, so we started talking about the pregnancy and birth ahead. I knew that there had to be more to the fact that many women had said that pregnancy and childbirth were beautiful experiences. So I got online and 'googled' beautiful childbirth or something to that effect.

I came across A Labour of Love and contacted Gabrielle. I bought everything Gabrielle recommended and waited for it to arrive. The moment the parcel arrived I was a changed person. My pregnancy from there on was beautiful and I discovered a newfound respect for my pregnant body. I found myself even looking forward to my imminent birth ahead.

So, after around 20 weeks of regular massage, affirmations, birth planning, meditations and guided visualisations – I was ready to give birth.

Once we arrived at the hospital, I politely asked the midwife to leave my husband and I alone in the room and that we would call her when I was ready to give birth. I also explained that I would not be needing any pain relief and that I would be using a combination of music, meditation and herbal remedies to gently aid me through the labour.

I can honestly say that giving birth to my daughter Lauren was the most beautiful experience of my life. It hurt – a lot but using my body for the purpose of creating and birthing a baby and feeling so present in the moment made it the beautiful experience that women talk about. My daughter is now almost three and is a beautiful, calm little girl and has very few fears.

So, thank you Gabrielle. Thank you for your program, thank you for empowering all women to take charge of our own child birthing experiences, and thank you for helping me through the birth of my daughter.

Emma Newman

A Positive Second Birth

It was a year ago today that my second baby girl, Eve Summer, was born. I was woken at 7am by my first daughter, Maia Rose (22 months old at the time). My partner, Phil, was already at work, and Maia came toddling into my bed to have her habitual morning snuggle and "susu" (our code word for breast milk). I had never found the appropriate moment to wean Maia with the amount of movement in our lives leading up to Eve's birth.

After Maia finished her feed I needed to run to the toilet, and for the next hour I was running to the toilet every ten to fifteen minutes, clearing my bowels. At first, I thought that it may have been part of the awful flu that I had for the previous two weeks. It was a really hard and very expensive flu to shake. It was expensive, as I was determined to clear it as naturally as possible. I spent quite a sum of money between naturopath and acupuncturist visits, not to mention herbs and homoeopathic remedies. It was not until the day before the birth that I gave in to the infection and went on antibiotics. Thank goodness that I did as the next day, when I gave birth, I felt ten times better.

After various trips to the toilet, I realised the visits were just a little too regular. I rang my midwife and she decided to cancel her bookings for the day. I called Phil around 8.30am and he made his way home from work. It just so happened that I had a cleaning lady organised for the morning who arrived at 9am. I pottered around with her for the next three hours, organising and 'nesting' in preparation, all the while having mild contractions every 7-8 minutes. Phil arrived home during this period and hung a swing for Maia in the backyard.

The cleaning lady left just before midday, and I made a fruit platter for the three of us to enjoy outside. I had been keeping my midwife updated on my contractions via text. At 12.30pm I lay down with Maia and gave her some susu to put her to sleep. When she fell asleep, the contractions suddenly picked up pace. Phil was lying down in bed to have a rest and he asked me to lie down with him. I declined and asked him to fill the pool for the waterbirth. He then suggested that he skip off to the markets, to pick up some sushi for later. I did not think that was a good idea, and once again asked him to fill the pool. He then suggested picking up a few things from the supermarket (which was 50m down the road). I replied, with much agitation in my voice, "no! Phil! Fill the pool now!" Phil finally got the picture that the baby was coming and filled the pool.

I started to cut up some veggies to prepare for dinner. The contractions quickened to every five minutes and I texted my midwife. Five minutes later, I could hear the front gate open. I went to the gate to greet her, and as I waved my hand and said hello, my waters broke on the front doorstep. Amazing timing! My midwife came in and took my blood pressure, and I then continued cutting carrots. However, dinner preparation did not last much longer as the contractions became too intense. I walked around the house to focus more. After being asked whether I was ready to get in the pool, I certainly did not need to think twice about it.

The warm pool offered welcomed relief. I spent the next 45 minutes on my knees with my head resting on the edge of the pool. I sipped on a solution of honey and black salt dissolved in water to keep my electrolytes up. Phil massaged my sacrum in circles, from which I refused to let him have a break. I gave deep earthly grunts as I welcomed each contraction on, knowing they were temporary. I considered each one a blessing when they passed as it meant the birth of my baby was closer.

A substitute midwife turned up whilst I was in the pool, whom I met briefly between contractions. Maia woke just as the baby's head was crowning. Maia came into the lounge, entering a very still and quiet space. A couple more contractions and the baby was born, very gently, in the warm water of the pool. Phil was a very proud father whilst he caught the baby underwater. Our baby was a girl, born at 2:36pm.

My midwife suddenly noticed some excessive blood in the water and took over. It seems that the cord broke as she passed through my legs. She acted quickly and clamped the cord to stop any more blood loss. I sat back and gently pulled her out of the water and on to my chest. It seems that the cord was very short. I stepped out of the pool with my baby so that the blood loss could be monitored better. We got comfy on a small mattress on the floor and breastfed the baby for the first time.

Of course, seeing me breastfeed our new little baby made Maia very upset. We immediately called my mother who arrived within 10 minutes to pick up Maia. My mum later told me how amazed she was at the peaceful and loving energy in the room. There were no disturbances from various hospital noises and disruptions, or fluorescent lighting. There was just gentle, dim, natural lighting, quiet voices and the fresh scent of a perfect summer's day, not too hot and not too cool. My mum took Maia home with her and Maia spent her first night away from us.

We rested and snuggled with our new baby girl whom we named (three weeks later) Eve Summer. Our midwife helped clean up and left us for an afternoon nap. As the sun was getting close to setting, I was back in the kitchen chopping veggies, preparing our dinner.

I say now, that after experiencing the birth of my daughter Eve Summer (even though I am not planning on having any more children) I would really love to experience a birth like that again. What a phenomenal day!

Jody's Positive Birth Stories

My name is Jody and I have two little boys – Kyle, 3 and a half, and Logan, 4 months. I had both my boys at the Family Birthing centre at King Edward Memorial hospital because I didn't want any intervention at all unless absolutely necessary.

My births were completely different, both physically and mentally; so different I could never have imagined they could be that way.

My pregnancy with Kyle was uneventful. I only had a small amount of nausea which disappeared within 12 weeks. I walked approximately 10 kilometres every day and worked until I was 38 weeks pregnant. It was a wonderful time and pregnancy.

The labour itself was fast and furious and all over and done within five and half hours which on one hand sounds great. Unbeknown to me, I was five and a half centimetres dilated without even having one single contraction and then there I was suddenly holding my son. I hardly remembered anything about the birth except the pain and fear I was feeling. I could not believe I had survived it and thought that I definitely could not go through that experience ever again. I guess you could say I was traumatised due to the speed in which my body laboured and expelled my baby out into this world!

I know lots of women who would love this type of experience, but it does come at a cost sometimes.

This was a huge dilemma for me as I had always wanted at least two children. In my head I felt very fearful and trapped and agonised over whether I should try to have another child or not. I knew in my heart that if I fell pregnant again, I wanted to have a completely natural experience with no medical interventions or drugs. However, at the same time I was frightened about doing the whole natural labour process again.

Finally, I came to terms with the fact that I was going to have another baby. I fell pregnant and realised I had to find someone who could help me through this dilemma and the fear I had brewing within me. This is when Gaby came into my life. I had read her book A Labour of Love - an Australian guide to natural childbirth (everyone should read this book!) and felt very strongly that she was the one person who was going to be able to help me get through this labour and birth naturally, in a positive and calm way, this time around.

Lucky for me Gaby lived in the same state as me and not too far away so I knew there would be this opportunity to work with her. When I felt the time was right, I rang Gaby, and we organised a three-hour hypnosis session. At last I felt like I was moving in the right direction so that I could gain some perspective on my past labour experience and move forward in a positive way. Well I can tell you, I could not believe the results!

When I finally came to sit on Gaby's couch, she asked me to describe my first experience. I told her that previously when I had talked about it I had had panic attacks and felt very uncomfortable. I truly was in a bad way. However, Gaby reassured me that by talking about it I was debriefing myself and looking at this experience as a past event that is over and done with. My biggest problem was every time I went back to that experience in my head, I became terrified about my imminent experience just around the corner.

By the end of the three hours, I walked out of the session with a completely different outlook on my first experience and felt so excited about my impending labour. Who would believe that!

During this second pregnancy I had nausea and vomiting constantly for twenty-five weeks, which was just so debilitating as it would go on for 24 hours each and every day. However, the hypnosis completely alleviated this. Whenever I felt unwell, I would do my deep breathing techniques and listen to Gaby's hypnosis scripts and I would feel so much better and re-energised. I really don't know how I would have coped if I had not learnt these skills.

Finally, after going over my estimated due date by thirteen days, my waters broke at 9pm on a Thursday night. I don't think I have ever been so grateful. People were starting to whisper in my ear about inducing me and I was trying to stay positive and not buy into this panic and pressure. The cut off day for my birthing at the birth centre was 14 days over so I knew I was cutting it very fine with my pregnancy gestation.

My labour was a lot longer than the first, which was exactly what I wanted; however, the contractions would start and stop, go to 2 to 3 minutes apart then disappear. I was not perturbed by this, as I just listened to Gaby's voice on the hypnosis scripts and felt calm and relaxed. I also used the TENS machine which helped me immensely to stay relaxed and positive. I felt so empowered, strong and in control (to a degree!) of what was going on this time around. I know Gaby says, being in control is the wrong way to go about labour and that it is about surrender, and staying out of your head and just allowing the process to take its course. I definitely was doing this during labour thanks to learning relaxation skills, how to breathe through the contractions and how to 'let go' through using hypnosis from Gaby.

As I look back and write this story, I can honestly say that this was the most beautiful, amazing birth experience. I ended up water birthing in a calm and relaxed way, with no interventions or drugs.

If I never have any more children, it would be perfectly OK, as I feel I have reached the pinnacle of what natural birth is all about. I birthed with no fear, instead feeling strong, confident and excited.

Preparation is everything and I highly recommend that all pregnant women listen and use Gaby's techniques and hypnosis scripts before giving birth; it will change the way you think and feel about labour.

Jody Blake 2008

Lincoln's Birth Story

"I'll see you after the birth, then?" I said with a smile. My obstetrician – such a lovely man – smiled sweetly at me, as I walked out of his rooms for the last time. I could tell by the look on his face that he didn't actually believe me, but God bless him, he nodded and wished me luck. Crazy pregnant woman, he was probably thinking. Even though my EDD was actually a few weeks off, I knew this would be the last time I would see him before the birth.

You see, in the politest way possible, I had told my doctor that I didn't want him at my birth. A funny request really, considering I was giving birth in a private hospital, under the care of my chosen obstetrician...but my choice all the same. My obstetrician knew that I wanted a natural, non-intervention birth. He knew I wanted to be left alone to labour how I wanted and for as long as I wanted. He knew I wanted to stay at home to labour for as long as possible. He knew that I felt that my obstetrician for my first birth didn't honour all my wishes. He also knew that I was confident in how I wanted to birth this time and that I had complete faith in the midwives at the hospital to assist in my birth. And he respected that – for which I will be eternally grateful.

I was birthing at Galliers, the private wing of the Armadale Health Service, which is located in the foothills of Perth, Western Australia. It is also what I consider to be the best maternity hospital in WA. Filled with wonderful nurturing midwives, all supportive of natural birth and non-intervention, I had complete confidence that my midwives would provide me with the best possible care both throughout my pregnancy and birth. After all, that is what they are trained to do!

I have always been blessed with ailment-free pregnancies, and apart from the frustrating 25kg weight gain I always endure, my pregnancies are always a time of great enjoyment and reflection. For this pregnancy, I had totally indulged myself with my preparation. I had regular naturopathic appointments (to ensure my vitamin and mineral supplementation intake was perfect), acupuncture sessions and homoeopathic appointments. I had regular sessions with my kinesiologist who ensured that I was balanced mentally, emotionally and spiritually…and how I savoured those appointments! She would talk

355

to my baby and I loved the little tit-bits she would share with me about my baby. "Oh, this baby is a talker!" she told me during one session. I took comfort in knowing that my baby was being well-nurtured in my belly and that he/she had many precious angels around, looking out for us both.

I also took Bach flower essences as well as constitutional homoeopathic tissue salts throughout my pregnancy and participated in Pregnancy Yoga classes. But the activity I enjoyed the most was the Pregnancy Specific Aquatic exercises classes with Gaby at Fremantle Leisure Centre. These weekly sessions were for me, a turning point in my birthing journey. I have always followed a natural pregnancy, birth and parenting model and had at times felt quite alone in my way of thinking. But to meet Gaby and be around so many other like-minded mums was just wonderful. Our hour of ante-natal swimming exercise became about the networking and discussion with the other mums more than the exercise. My husband fondly referred to the class as "exercise of the mouth" because we would all be talking non-stop the whole class. The 50-minute drive down to Fremantle each week was never an issue as I looked forward to my class more than anything else in the week.

Through Gaby I also participated in an Active Birth workshop with my husband as well as a 4-week journey workshop (which was just for the girls!!). For me, these workshops were exactly what I needed – and had been searching for. And yes, even though I had already experienced a vaginal birth two years earlier and knew what to expect, I still felt that there was more knowledge and wisdom to be learned.

Gaby filled my head with confidence. She went through scenarios with us, helped us focus on what we wanted to achieve and best of all; she helped us to see that as intelligent, independent birthing women, we do have rights! These workshops, coupled with my extensive reading throughout my pregnancy, certainly allowed me to be in the right headspace for my forthcoming birth. I had prepared my body diligently with exercises and stretches, to ensure my baby was in the optimal position for birth and I had spent hours listening to Gaby's hypnotherapy preparation. I had a clear birth plan, I was armed with knowledge, brimming with confidence... and now, ready to give birth!

40 weeks came and went, with still no sign of my little cherub. As this was my second pregnancy, I was sure I would have gone into labour early, but apparently, my little baby was quite content in my tum. My lovely midwives monitored me weekly and reassured me that everything was on track. Having undertaken months of preconception care and planning for this pregnancy, I knew my dates were correct and that I was in the best state of health and mind for this birth. I was ready...and 6 days after my EDD, my little darling too was ready.

My first contractions started about 8pm – very mild and about 10 minutes apart. I hopped in the bath at home to try and relax and just see if what I was feeling were in fact contractions. The deep tightening feeling inside continued, and I hopped out of the bath in excitement. I quietly played with my 2 ½ year old son Lennon on the big mattress on the lounge room floor, trying hard to disguise the mild contractions I was experiencing. The night continued, as did my contraction, and soon my son went to bed. I kissed him goodnight knowing in my heart, that this would be the last night with just him to consume my life. A small wave of sadness came over me as I contemplated the end of one very special chapter of my life. But this was very soon replaced with a twinge of excitement, as I knew our new baby would be here with us soon.

My husband Chad and I watched the end of a movie, with my viewing being interrupted every ten minutes or so with my very mild but manageable contractions. I sent my husband Chad to bed knowing that it was going to be a long night – and one of us might as well get some sleep! I too tried to lie down and sleep between my contractions but by now the contractions were getting pretty consuming. I started my first doses of my homoeopathic remedy Arnica at this stage - and continued to take this regularly throughout my labour. With no bloody show or evidence of ruptured membranes, I still felt my baby was a long way off. At about 12.30am I got up, finished off my last bit of packing, brushed my teeth, and I think I might have even got my hair straightener out! It was at this time that my husband got up and together we made our way out to the family room, and the double sized mattress which we had out on the floor in preparation for this time.

From there began one of the most special nights of my life.

Together as planned, Chad and I laboured in our family room. I was on my knees on the mattress for most of this time, with Chad gently massaging my back with each contraction. As rehearsed, we had my kit of homoeopathic remedies out and he administered these as they were required. Arnica and Rescue Remedy were used frequently, and I occasionally sucked on some Rescue Remedy pastilles. The pain relief side of my labour was something I knew I just wouldn't have to think about. Chad, being a confident user of homoeopathic remedies, knew one of his roles for my labour was to give me remedies as I needed them. I am so proud of the way he calmly did this throughout the night, and not once did I question him.

For most of the early hours of the night my contractions were between 5-7 minutes apart; very strong, but still very manageable. During this time I was amazed at the rhythmical sound of humming and the deep, monotone sounds that were spilling out of my mouth. Different sounds to my first birth too, I now recall. I laboured on a chair, on my fitball, on my hands and knees – wherever I felt relief. I was confident in how I was feeling, and I knew instinctively that there was still no need to make my way to the hospital yet.

Looking back, if I had been able to write a script for my ideal birth, it really couldn't have been any better. The universe handed to us the perfect scenario for my labour. By labouring throughout the night, I didn't have to worry about my 2 ½ year old son and was able to concentrate wholly on my baby and forthcoming birth. And so we laboured peacefully, in the dark of the house, in the comfort of our home, with no other distractions or interruptions. One of my friends described this scene as "sounding very romantic". And in a way it really was. How much more intimate and special can you get, but to share a beautiful night together, preparing for the imminent arrival of your precious baby?

At one point during the night I remember we could hear Lennon in his room, calling out restlessly. I went into his room and knelt down beside him. He was tossing and turning and calling out deliriously "Baby... Baby!" It was as if on some unconscious level he knew that I was in labour. How precious! And how precious to know that our dear little boy was about to become a big brother!

At 3.30am we rang the hospital to let them know I was in labour. "Please don't ring the doctor, I'm fine", I told the night-shift midwife. I said to the midwife that I would like to try and wait a few more hours before I came down to the hospital (so I could wait till my son woke up in the morning). I also sent a text to my dear friend Claire to let her know that I was pretty certain this was it! Claire, a trainee doula, was desperately hoping to get to our birth. I had sent my mum a text a few hours earlier to let her know that things were happening, and she arrived about 4 am with my very excited dad.

I continued to labour for a few more hours, and despite the many suggestions that we head to the hospital I knew that I still had plenty of time. However after a few contractions only a couple of minutes apart my dad put his foot down. "You are going to the hospital... RIGHT NOW!" he insisted. So reluctantly I made my way to the car – but not before I defiantly announced that if I wasn't a good way dilated I was coming straight home again! Chad and my mum accompanied me to the hospital around 5.30am – my dad staying at our house to wait for Lennon to wake.

On arrival at the hospital I again reminded Danielle, the midwife on duty, that I still didn't need the doctor. I had already decided that I wanted to find out how dilated I was – and was pleasantly surprised to find that I was already 6 cm dilated! That was the only time throughout my labour that I had an internal. I had planned for a very active birth and so I can assure you, that lying on a bed finding out how many centimetres I had or hadn't dilated was not something I planned on doing! "I'll have my baby by 10.30am" I called out, as they started to run hot water into the bath.

At 7.00am the staff changed over, and I was greeted with the familiar faces of Barbara and Leone, two midwives that I knew very well. At 7.15am Claire, my doula arrived and from there, like a well-rehearsed dance recital, she and Chad nurtured and supported me whilst I laboured. In the bath, Claire massaged my legs and knees, whilst I clung onto Chad. When

I started to get the shakes, Chad gave me my homoeopathic remedy Gelsemium and when the water started to get cold I hopped out of the bath.

Instinctively, Claire and Chad grabbed the mattress off the sofa lounge in the birthing suite and placed it on the ground. After they covered it with a sheet I knelt down gratefully for my next round of contractions. All I was aware of was Claire massaging me and Chad holding my hands and shoulders. I knew my mum was coming in frequently, and I knew the midwives were there, but they really were in the background. I spoke very little throughout this time. When I felt like a drink, it was there in my hand before I needed to ask. When I felt that a flannel would provide relief on my face, it magically appeared. It was as if my two-support people knew exactly what I needed before I did. Despite the continuous low rumbling sounds pouring from my mouth, it really was a very quiet and peaceful labour.

For me, having a doula was just such a wonderfully positive experience. She was there, providing words of encouragement, support, and love - whilst at the same time massaging and soothing me. And my darling husband did not leave my side for the entire labour. He held me, squeezed me, and coached me. I needed to see him the whole time and needed to be able to hang on to him with each contraction. For me, I loved having that beautiful feminine energy of my doula supporting me throughout the labour. But I also desperately needed my husband. I needed to be able to feel his strength and hear his words of encouragement. When I felt too tired to go on, I needed him to remind me of just how close we were. I needed to be able to squeeze him and know that he would not pull away. I needed to feel his unconditional love. It really was a magical combination – and one which worked so harmoniously together. Although it was never discussed, both Claire and Chad knew their very different roles and what they needed to do. They worked together beautifully.

And so it came time to start pushing. I didn't want to hop back in the water, although we had of course discussed the possibility of birthing in the water. For me, at the time, it felt right kneeling on the mattress. Rocking and swaying on my knees with my head resting on the bed. It was at this point that Chad grabbed hold of me and said "honey, this is it. You are going to start pushing now – would you like me to see if your mum would like to watch the baby being born?" For this I am eternally grateful to my husband. To be honest, I hadn't been aware of Mum not being there. I was so focused on my own body, my breathing – that I was quite oblivious to everything going on around me. I guess you can call this being 'in the zone.

And so mum ecstatically appeared as the final part of my labour journey began. I remember my dear midwife Leone asking me "now, you sure you don't want me to call the doctor?" But she already knew the answer to that. With Claire filming, Chad holding me and my mum watching by my side, my midwife coached me through the breathing and panting of each contraction. I could feel my baby descend and I knew I was almost there. My body was bulging, stinging, stretching... "One more push, Kristy" my midwife cried excitedly. And with an ecstatic "THERE'S YOUR PUSH!" and a loud sigh, I birthed my beautiful baby into the awaiting arms of my midwife.

The next ten minutes were the most wonderful, special ten minutes of my life. My midwife followed my birth plan perfectly. My baby was placed straight on the mattress in front of me – and it literally took a second or two for me to register...my baby was here! I reached down and picked up my beautiful little boy for the first time and held him against my skin. He then opened his eyes and looked up at me. A mother never forgets the first time her baby looks into her eyes, and for me it was as if we were the only two people in the whole world. We sat there staring at each other – a look of joy and familiarity mirrored on both our faces. Finally, we were here together. My precious boy still had not made a sound and Leone, my midwife, knelt down beside me to make him give his first little cry. It was as if he was too consumed with the enormity of the moment to even think about crying! We instantly fell in love with our little boy – and named him Lincoln.

We sat together there on the bloodied mattress and I brought him straight to my breast. He suckled sleepily and nestled into my chest. Chad stroked him gently and we sat there so happy and content for about ten minutes. Chad then picked up my beautiful umbilical cord (so lovely and white) and announced that it had stopped pulsing. Leone brought over the instruments and with all the last nutrients having passed through to our baby, Chad clamped Lincoln's cord. As he was no longer attached to the cord, I then gently stood up. My midwives knew that I wanted the placenta to come away naturally and whilst Chad cuddled our baby, I gave a small push and out slipped my placenta. As simple as that!

Beaming, I hopped up onto the bed. We had always said that we wanted big brother Lennon to be the first one in to see our new baby – and so we called out for my Dad to bring him in. In bounced our very excited 2 ½ year old – and he ran straight over to us and hopped onto the bed with me. "This is your baby brother, Lincoln" we told him. Lennon instantly put his arms around to cuddle him. "Oh Mummy, can we take him home?" he asked so seriously. "Of course, darling" I replied, with tears welling in my eyes. We were a real family now, I thought. I had beside me my wonderful husband and my two beautiful boys. Life doesn't get any better than this!

As I had anticipated, Lincoln was born before 10.30am - 10.22am to be exact! Somewhere in all the excitement of our birth, my doctor had been rung and appeared around 11.15am to congratulate us and check over our baby. This was the first time Lincoln left my side. The midwives weighed and measured him (a lovely 7lb 8oz) and then performed all the obligatory tests and checks over him at this time. I am so grateful that the midwives allowed me to have that precious time with Lincoln before they did all their checks. For me, that time after the birth was the best part of my whole birth experience.

I can honestly look back now and say that my birth was a wonderful, wonderful experience. Every moment is still so vivid and fresh in my mind. I felt so empowered and in control the whole time. I listened to my body and trusted the beautiful, miraculous process that is birth! I am eternally grateful to all the people that made my birth the beautiful experience it was – because without their support and assistance, it may not have turned out the way it did.

Births happen every day, to thousands of women around the world. We need to honour and cherish our birthing mothers. We need to encourage and support them throughout their pregnancy and give every woman the opportunity to birth how she desires. It might only take one person to share a positive, empowering birth experience with a pregnant woman for her to start thinking - "YES! I can do that! That is the birth I want!".

And wouldn't it be wonderful if every mother had a positive birthing story to share?

Lincoln Grant Brookes was born on 21st October, 2007

Greg and Natasha's Birth of Tahlia

The night before giving birth to our daughter I stayed up with my Mum and husband Greg watching "Memoirs of a Geisha", interestingly about the plight of under- privileged girls in Japan. I couldn't help but think how lucky our soon-to-be-born daughter was to be born in Australia at this time. We stayed up until 11 pm, despite saying to them, " I'll be cross with you if I go into labour tonight, you've kept me up!", and I felt compelled to replace a few final things in my labour and hospital bags, so eventually I got to bed at 12 midnight.

I was woken up after a good six hours sleep to a familiar sensation - it was the same as the start of my birth with Abi, our first born who was now 4 years old. Too excited to stay in bed, I got up and got dressed, and pottered around the house. By 7 am I had two more contractions and felt it was time to wake Greg. He was physically out of bed before he quite knew where he was – the excitement was contagious. I wanted to go for a walk to keep things moving so I woke Mum and let her know what we were doing and where we were going.

We slowly wandered down Beaufort Street, a busy well-known road in Perth, about 1.5 kms to the only café open early on a Saturday morning. The whole experience was a bit surreal, and I had to answer the inevitable question by an inquisitive café worker who asked "when are you due?" I answered "I'm in labour now, so sometime today I hope!". It was very

367

entertaining watching and hearing the other patron's sitting around us as they reacted and stared.

I managed to eat half a piece of toast casually while Greg calmly drank his coffee and read the paper. I had just sa "It seems to have slowed down," when all of a sudden there I was clutching the table and breathing as quietly as I possibly could from a rather intense sensation, for the sake of not scaring off the other patrons! With that we decided to head back up Beaufort Street, only this time the journey back was a lot slower that's for sure. One thing I knew at the back of my mind was that Greg promised to run home and get the car if I really needed to be driven. As it turned out I managed really well, holding onto Greg for a couple of the stronger contractions I had on the way back.

At one point I remember him asking how I was feeling, saying "because if I were you right now, I'd be sh…ing myself!!" I wasn't at all feeling this way. I really felt empowered to face what was to come and most of all I was really ready to meet our little girl. Nearer to home, we saw that some neighbours had a mature tree for sale which we organised to buy and made arrangements to have them drop it off in the next week - a birth present for our daughter Tahlia! The things people do when in labour!

We arrived home to find our cleaning lady had arrived, so I had a full house! It was time for Abi to go to Greg's mum but before she arrived to pick her up, it was lovely to spend a bit of time with her and talk to her about what was happening. She was quietly overwhelmed by the whole thing I think, but certainly didn't make a fuss leaving which I was relieved about. We decided it was time to call our doula, Gaby, to let her know what was happening and we arranged for her to come over in a few hours time.

We watched a baby settling DVD that had been given to us the day before, and as I watched I made sure I bounced and rocked around on the fitball to keep moving and active to keep everything moving along! Gaby arrived about midday which was perfect timing as the contractions had been 15-20 minutes apart and lasting for one minute or so. We talked for a while and made lunch for everyone present and just relaxed. The first contraction Gaby observed she got me to relax my shoulders and stop locking my knees out as I stood leaning forward slightly. This helped immensely as the next contraction was a lot easier to say the least.

An hour later the contractions still hadn't begun to get any closer, so Gaby suggested I take two homoeopathic remedies every 15 minutes to encourage the contractions to be a little more regular. It worked!! Half an hour later they were three minutes apart and Gaby recommended I hop into the shower for some natural relief. Again, a great suggestion as I really got into a rhythm (at first I knelt down in the bath with Abi's bath books under each knee and then Gaby came up with the idea of leaning over the fitball in front of me which was just bliss). The hot water hitting my lower back felt wonderful.

Gaby kept reminding me to surrender to the contractions and as I did I started to make groaning noises with each one. Meanwhil, Mum was cooking in the kitchen while Greg was asleep on the couch!! Gaby let me be, apparently fielding a few questions from Mum as to when I would be going to hospital - understandably she was a bit nervous but could tell from my groaning when the contractions came that I was getting into good established labour. After a while Gaby came in to give me water, a cool flannel for my face and offered gentle words of encouragement which made all the difference. I felt safe surrendering to the whole process because I knew that she would guide me through this next stage of my labour.

After a while I started to feel my ankles and feet swell from kneeling and sitting on them for an hour and a half (which had felt like 30 minutes!) Gaby helped me out of the bath, and I sat on the toilet for a couple of contractions. I wasn't finding it easy to manage at all after having the wonderful hot water on me which seemed to help me cope. Gaby suggested we head for the hospital so I could use the big bath at the hospital on the labour ward, so I got dressed and started to get some bags together. Greg was woken up with little fuss and felt refreshed having gotten some sleep. He then assisted us to get all the bags in the car. I was helped into the back of Gaby's Tarago where I was on all fours so I could carry on labouring. I remember smiling, waving and blowing a kiss to Mum as she waved back from the front lawn. I wanted her to know I was alright - because I was, I really was.

I remember feeling a little anxious as Greg was driving ahead of Gaby in his own car and the route to hospital seemed to take forever, especially when finding there was nowhere to park as the curb on one whole side of the street was being re-done!! Regardless, we parked on the side of the road. When I got out of the car I stopped to experience one intense and noisy contraction on the footpath, and then managed to get up the steps and into the lift to the second floor. As the doors rolled open I had another contraction at the reception (I'm just glad it wasn't the day for AnteNatal tours!!). Finally, we arrived at our room. The first thing we did was ask if the tub was available, and to my sheer relief it was.

After I organised my bags it was time for the dreaded internal check up by the midwife. "I don't want to know if it is under 6cm!" I said as I attempted to lie on my back. I found the internal examination very painful, probably mostly from being a little uptight and worrying about being in a new environment which I hadn't felt completely settled in at this point in time. The hospital setting is not like the comfort of your own home and took some adjustment. The midwife performing the vaginal examination said she couldn't really get a good idea of what was going on in terms of dilation and was happy to leave it at that. However I wanted to know how dilated I was so agreed for a second try. This time she was happy with her assessment and quietly told Gaby and Greg where I was at. I felt a bit disappointed for a moment as I wanted to be told how dilated I was, but I knew that I must have been under 6 cm (apparently, I was only 4cm!) but I again remembered some words of wisdom Gaby had said to me -

'Never relate to the dilation number in a negative way, as every centimetre in dilation is fantastic and should be celebrated as a big achievement'.

With that thought I just geared myself up mentally for a bit more labour; I knew I could do this.

Meanwhile Gaby had run the tub and I got in, grateful for the immediate comfort and relief the hot water provided. Alas, it was not long lived. About 30 seconds after getting into the tub, Gaby recalls me sitting bolt upright and saying, "I'm doing a wee; a big one!" Gaby suggested it might be my membranes breaking and sure enough, when it kept going on and on and on, she checked the water for any discoloration (absent) and suggested to me that things might speed up now! Did they ever! The cushioning of the membranes had allowed me to labour feeling challenged but quite able to handle the discomfort. Not now!! The contractions came one on top of the other and were much stronger than before - I just remember saying on more than one occasion, "I just need to let you know that I can't do this for a long time, I am REALLY NOT enjoying this!!" I think it was when Greg got in trouble for putting the cold flannel on the back of my neck, not my forehead that Gaby indicated to him that I was getting close to being fully dilated and acting like a woman in true transition.

Sure enough, the midwife was right when she had told Gaby and Greg that although I was only 4cm dilated, fully effaced and ready to go. My first feeling to push came only 45 minutes after being in the tub and it scared me because I had been thinking I had a long time to go - so my initial reaction was there must be something wrong. After being reassured, I was helped out of the bath and back across the corridor and into our labour room. It was here that I got up onto the bed on my hands and knees. I went into automatic mode, piling pillows up under me, kneeling on all fours as I had done with my first birth - it must just be my thing!

All I really remember of the next amazing time was Gaby's gentle instructions, the feeling of Tahlia's head crowning and then withdrawing back up inside of me every time a contraction finished. I remembered thinking and saying, "please don't go away!" So, I pushed with even more determination when instructed to. "Nature is being kind" was the comment from the obstetrician as my contractions let me rest for five minutes in between. "I'm going to meet my little girl soon" I thought to myself as I paused to rest, ensuring I was present to the miracle of what was happening. As much as my position wasn't the easiest for the staff to see what they were doing, I never felt pressured to move which was just perfect as I found this position so comfortable.

373

I didn't see Tahlia being born but I heard Greg's excitement as she came out of my body. She was almost immediately placed in front of me on the bed, and due the quickness and energy I had given to birth her I had no strength in my arms to pick her up. All I could do initially was stroke her and say "Hello beautiful girl, you're perfect, you're perfect!" And she was (no bias of course!). The membranes had done a wonderful job of cushioning and protecting her for most of the pregnancy and labour and looked completely blemish-free and perfect.

I then lay watching in wonder as my baby, only minutes, suckled on my breast. My obstetrician reminded me that there was one more important thing to do and that was to birth my placenta! Last time this had been a huge ordeal, nearly resulting with me having the placenta surgically removed - and I so did not want to experience that again. In contrast to my previous experience, and as with everything about this birth, it all worked out perfectly well. My placenta arrived as it should, complete, in about 5 - 10 minutes after the birth of Tahlia.

Finally my labouring was done and I could sort of let go and rela - well that was the plan. Due to the speed of the delivery though my body went into a bit of shock – suddenly shaking while my teeth chattered for a good half an hour. To try to overcome this I had warm blankets placed on me, and I drank warm tea with lots of sugar to try to lift my blood glucose up. I received reassurance from Gaby who eased my concerns about what was happening, and within an hour the shaking had passed. I was feeling on top of the world - just in time for the arrival of Abi, my first born, and the Mums.

Finally, Tahlia was taken for a few measurements and a weigh in. Not long after she returned, and we had a very special family time before Abi went home to bed.

Meanwhile Gaby our doula showered and got dressed up for her night out. This was a pre-organised engagement that fortunately she was still able to attend given the speed of my labour/birth - I was so glad we did not interrupt her evening plans! Apparently, she was on a natural high all night, so no drinking catch-up was needed!

When people ask me about the birth, I respond by giving them this answer – it was honestly as good as I could have dreamed and wished for. I was so proud of myself and so grateful for the opportunity to have experienced a drug free, natural birth, thanks mostly to the amazing support of our doula Gaby, my husband Greg and the wonderful midwife I had on the day. Having a support person meant Greg was left to join me on the journey in his own way, knowing I was in safe hands. Even Mum said that she thought it was the most relaxed, calm space she could have imagined; perfect for giving birth in.

I believe women are being deterred from the joys of an intervention free birth as the fear of pain and complications leaves them doubting their own ability. While medical assistance is vital when required, a birthing mother needs little more than trust in those around her, encouraging words, and belief in herself. A doula provided all of this for me, and I will always be eternally grateful for such a special gift - Thank you Gaby!

Natasha French

7.

EMPOWERED VBAC-HBAC-NBAC VAGINAL/HOME/ NATURAL BIRTH AFTER A PREVIOUS CAESAREAN

Belle Verdiglione's Birth Story

I didn't intend on having a homebirth. I thought that women who gave birth at home were amazing and incredibly brave - I put them on a pedestal - something I admired but that "I" could never do. To tell Isabella's birth story I have to start at the beginning, 22 months ago when I had my son Orlando - my first birth.

When I found out I was pregnant I began reading all that I could about natural birth. I chose a birth centre because we wanted to have a waterbirth and I didn't want the temptation of drugs as pain relief. I knew the hospital was in close proximity 'just in case' and it seemed like a warm, beautiful and safe place to give birth.

It was a Friday when I went for a routine ultrasound at the hospital. The sonographer sounded nonchalant when she said, "Oh, a breech baby". What the...?!

My heart sank as my hopes of birthing at the birth centre were crushed in those four words. I was 40 weeks +10 days with a decent sized baby. This was not good. I was inconsolable as I spent the rest of the day trying to work through my options. I begged the doctors to perform an External Cephalic Version (ECV) to turn bub. They explained it was painful and dangerous, and that we had to wait until an operating theatre became available in case bub went into distress and I had to have an emergency Caesarean. We decided it was worth the risk. Two doctors performed the ECV, and my husband said he could not see either of their hands when they were doing it. It was extremely intense and uncomfortable being manipulated in that way, but I practised hypno-birthing during the procedure and the doctors could not believe how well I coped throughout it.

Unfortunately it was unsuccessful. I then requested to talk with the doctor who performs vaginal breech deliveries at the hospital. She spent an hour with us explaining the facts and how I did not fit the "criteria" for a vaginal breech delivery. In a nutshell, I was too small, bub was too big, and it was too risky.

I was deflated and exhausted when the resident asked me "so what do you want to do?" Hmmm... like I have so many options! She continued chatting about women who find it "easier" to have caesareans, that it's a safe option these days and asking why women would "want" to have a drug-free vaginal birth anyway! I was promptly scheduled for an "elective" caesarean the following day.

I shook my head. I didn't spend the last nine months researching natural birth to be booked in for a caesarean! This was not part of my birth plan! It hadn't even occurred to me that I would need a caesarean and I did not know anything about the procedure at all.

I explained to the doctors that I would present to the hospital after the weekend. I needed to get my head around what was happening and try to process it. I then proceeded to spend the next few days trying everything possible to turn bub around; chiropractic care, hypnosis, acupuncture, ice packs on my belly, music and light and I spent hours on all fours. Bub was 4.3kgs and he did not turn. I had a caesarean on the Monday and birthed a chubby little boy to the melodic sounds of Jose Gonzalez. He was healthy and divine. Orlando Jarrah Salvatore was placed directly on me and we were over the moon with our new arrival.

After surgery I was wheeled into the recovery room. I was dazed and a bit overwhelmed about what had just happened. Looking back, I know I must've been in shock. I was told my husband could not be with me, nor my girlfriend who was my support person and my newborn baby was swiftly taken away from me. I was not strong enough to fight this battle and we did not think to challenge this "protocol". My husband did not leave Orlando's side while he was being weighed and measured. However, I was groggy and left all alone in a hospital bed with no husband, no friend and no baby! What just happened?! It was my husband who told the midwives to take Orlando back to me so he could begin to breastfeed. He attached beautifully and we enjoyed lots of skin to skin contact over the next few days.

I was so happy with my boy, but I secretly mourned the loss of a vaginal birth experience. I didn't even know about a trial of labour! I vowed that next time would be different and I would never be separated from my little one again.

I quickly fell pregnant again. What a wonderful surprise. I immediately hired a doula who would assist me with my Vaginal Birth After Caesarean (VBAC) in hospital as I was now considered "high risk" for the birth centre. The midwife at the VBAC clinic was supportive of my decision and listened with empathy to my previous story. She understood the importance of a vaginal birth to me, and I felt like I was in a safe place. My doctor's appointment at 24 weeks was a different story.

The doctor had never met me before and her first comment whilst flicking through my chart was "4.3kgs, bet you're glad you didn't push him out". I could not believe how dismissive she was about my previous birth. I was in complete shock when I responded "actually, I'm really disappointed I didn't get to push him out". I waited for her to acknowledge my heartache. Nothing. I know now I should have walked out the door right then but a part of me was clinging to the hope that I would have my VBAC at the clinic. Over the next half an hour this doctor proceeded to instil the fear of God in me about having a VBAC. Although she said I had a 70-80% success rate of having a VBAC, I now had to adhere to all the hospital protocols for VBAC including; no eating or drinking during active labour, insertion of an IV drip, three hourly vaginal exams and constant foetal monitoring.

My VBAC hopes were slowly squished with each 'protocol' being rattled off but they were crushed when I heard constant foetal monitoring. I knew the ramifications of foetal monitoring meant not being able to use water for pain relief. Defeated, I thought to myself "so basically the protocols are setting me up to have another caesarean". When she finished, I challenged her about constant foetal monitoring, suggesting that I could have intermittent monitoring. She explained that this was not an option until I showed her hospital information that clearly stated I could ask for intermittent monitoring. She rudely snapped that I would need to speak with a consultant about the dangers and sign a consent form.

My mind was racing as I struggled to take in all of this information that I had not considered when dreaming about my wonderful VBAC. This doctor could potentially be on duty when I was having my baby. This is not a doctor who I would want to see again for a prenatal appointment let alone someone who I wanted at my birth! I knew I couldn't birth my baby at this hospital. It was no longer a safe place.

I left the hospital feeling disempowered and very emotional. I drove straight to the Independent Midwifery Centre. I introduced myself and then could not contain the tears any longer. I was a blubbering mess. I was met with open arms and the midwife sat me down and listened to me as I divulged all my fears and frustrations. I smiled through my tears, and she explained that it wasn't a typical day unless a pregnant woman stood at her doorway and cried. I felt nurtured and safe. I spent the next three hours talking about my feelings, things were coming up that I didn't even know existed, about my disappointment over my previous birth, about my fears of a homebirth and my fears of birthing in a hospital. I felt like I was in 'no man's land'. However, after a while of talking and getting it all out I regained my sense of power. I was emotionally drained but felt lighter with the knowledge that there was another option - a homebirth.

I was just about to leave when another midwife came in. One of the midwives pulled on my arm and said that I had to meet her and introduced me to her. During our conversation this midwife gave me a fresh perspective on Orlando's birth, and I instantly felt a part of me heal. I knew then that I had found her. I also knew that I had a long way to go if I was going to make this idea a reality and I would need to confront my fears about birthing at home. Would my husband support a homebirth? Would my family and friends be supportive? Was I brave enough to have a homebirth after having a previous Caesarean (HBAC)?

Over the next few months I researched HBAC's. I read books and embraced HBAC stories, and I decided my scar was not going to define my next birth. There was a lot of deliberation in our household about whether to have a HBAC or whether to brave the hospital system as my husband was just as new to this idea as I was. When we finally decided that we would hire our independent midwife for a HBAC, I was in my third trimester. It became apparent that people we talked to are fear-based and not well informed when it comes to homebirths and so we kept our decision to have a HBAC private.

At 40 weeks +8 days I woke up with lower back pain and cramping. I felt the rush of anticipation with the thought that "today's the day". I didn't want to get too excited as I had read contractions can come and go but pretty soon it was obvious that the surges were regular and getting more intense. Over the next few hours, I checked my emails, wrote a shopping list, tidied the house and played with my toddler. When I couldn't move or talk through my surges, I knew I had to wake my husband so he could help with Orlando, and I needed a heat pack on my back. Today was the day.

By mid-afternoon the surges were seven minutes apart and my husband called out while I was labouring in the shower "I forgot the champagne, I'm going to get a bottle and I'll be really quick". If I wasn't having such intense surges I probably would've laughed! He was only gone for one surge. When the surges jumped to two minutes he rang my midwife and I climbed into the birth pool. What a relief. It was instant. When my midwife arrived at sundown I felt like I had run a marathon. I remember saying "if you tell me I'm only 4cms I'm going to kill myself". I know I know, how dramatic. She didn't examine me until two hours later, at which time I was 4cms but like any good support person, she did not tell me that.

The room was cosy and warm and softly lit by a Himalayan salt lamp. I laboured in the water to the sweet tunes of Cat Stevens and Harry Manx. After each surge I fell back into the comfort of my husband's arms. In between surges I completely relaxed and felt so much energy rushing through my body. I couldn't speak or open my eyes. I felt beautiful and loved and nurtured. There were moments when I became emotional, and I resisted the labour. Instead of the offer of drugs I heard words of encouragement. I was told that I was a strong woman, that I could do this and when I moaned that I couldn't do this I was told "yes you can and you are doing it".

I knew that my baby was coming and I would meet him or her soon. When I was fully dilated, I had a moment of clarity. I opened my eyes and with a newfound spark announced that

I needed to move and get out of this pool right now. As I waddled over to our bed, I felt our bub move down with me. I was coming to the end of a long journey and I was exhausted. It took all my inner strength to help bub enter the world and I knew no one else could do this work for me. It was up to me. It was the most intense and humbling experience of my life. One that was truly amazing. No words can express what it was actually like for me to give birth; it was as if I was the only woman in the entire universe and at the same time, I was a part of all women. I breathed and roared and pushed with my body. At 1:30am Isabella Olive Lula was born. Alive, chubby, healthy and beautiful. I was healed.

I didn't intend on having a homebirth, but I'd do it all again in a heartbeat.

The Vaginal Birth of Richie Nathan Robert Potter

My first born was born in January 2015, via caesarean section. Private hospital, private obstetrician, and cascade of interventions including an early epidural and after only 3cms of dilation I was given a caesarean section. Complications written in the purple book "failure to progress".

In November 2015, we found out we were expecting again. We returned to the same obstetrician. I hired a doula and said she would support me in a Vaginal Birth After Caesarean

("VBAC"). I toyed with the idea, but secretly I was terrified. At 20 weeks, I went to have a pregnancy massage and the masseuse was a doula and had been for 20 years. After the massage I purchased a book called "A Labour of Love" written by Gaby (the masseuse). I was mesmerised. I finished it in 2 days, and I remember closing the booking and thinking to myself "I want what they're having!" I immediately bought her second book, and I began to attend her weekly antenatal fitness classes. She became my 'secondary doula' although I really wanted her as my doula! I drew on Gaby's expertise each week at Aqua and I attended her centre as often as I could. My husband and I attended Gaby's Childbirth Education, which felt a little silly being 'second time parents' but we loved every single minute of it. I now only buy expectant mothers a copy of Gaby's book. It's all they need. I know now for sure that I was meant to meet Gaby that day. Gaby changed the entire trajectory of my birth and for that I will be forever grateful.

I attended monthly birth rite meetings listening intently to women sharing their awesome VBAC stories with independent midwives and I thought "wow, what are these and where can I get one!" With the BEST birth team behind me at 30 weeks I decided to seek a second opinion. We contacted 'My Midwives in Perth' and were put onto Linda. We loved Linda but decided due to the outlay in costs to stay with our obstetrician.

I am woman, hear me roar

At 35 weeks I presented my birth plan to my obstetrician. I had been researching, reading and making decisions for the last 15 weeks. He proceeded to 'mark' my birth plan. I took it away and amended it. I returned at 37 weeks and said "I want to negotiate" - he said "I don't negotiate". I had asked for a spontaneous rupture of my membranes (water breaking) to which he said he would break them on arrival (if they hadn't already gone). As I felt it was one of the many things that caused my original caesarean section, I asked why it was done and he said to speed up labour. I requested it only happen in the event of it stalling. He told me that my birth plan cared more about vaginal delivery than the safety and wellbeing of my baby and he refused to care for me any longer and said that I could no longer be his patient.

Thank you, Linda, thank you for agreeing to take me on at 37 weeks even though you thought "oh gosh, how bad is this birth plan?!"

My estimated due date was the 3rd June 2016. I went into early labour on the 22nd May. I texted Linda to tell her that I was in early labour. She called immediately to explain that this could go on for a while. My daughter came at 39+6 so I assured her it wouldn't. How wrong I was!

On the 10th June 2016 (41 weeks!) at 8pm I called my doula. I was sure it was the real thing. Linda arrived around 10:30pm and did a vaginal exam and as per my birth plan. Linda did not tell me my dilation (I was 3cm and not yet fully effaced, it was STILL early labour!). The contractions spaced out and Linda put me to bed and went home. At 1am after 3 more contractions, I felt a pop! I am crying remembering how beautiful it was to feel my waters breaking naturally, on my terms, not his.

I arrived at Armadale at 1:30am. Linda again examined me and did not tell me (I was 6cm and fully effaced, yeah baby we are really doing this!). At 3:30am. I felt the urge to push. I thought Nope. Not yet. I haven't been through transition yet! I haven't shouted at everyone, told them I can't do it and I'm leaving…. Linda said to me at some point "you are doing SO WELL, you have gotten SO much further along than you did last time, you should be so proud". Oh, Linda, how you gave me strength I didn't know I had.

I asked for the gas. Linda calmly explained that most women have the gas taken off them at the pushing point. "What do you want the gas for now anyhow?" she asked. "I don't know!!!!!" I cried. I just felt exhausted.

At 5am after trying every upright position imaginable as per my birth plan, Linda came into the bathroom and calmly explained bubby was getting tired too. We had one last position to try and if this didn't work the Doctor was going to have to give bubby some help.

I ended up flat on my back with my legs up in the stirrups (not in my birth plan!). I pushed and I pushed. It felt like forever. I heard my husband excitedly saying "I can see the head!" The excitement and pride in his voice said it all.

It is said women in labour leave their bodies...they travel to the stars to collect the souls of their babies and return to this world together...

At 6:40am on the 11th June 2016, my VBAC baby Richie Nathan Robert came to earthside. I held him first. He heard my voice first. He looked into my eyes first. At that moment all my broken pieces were stuck back together.

'Like a superwoman who had won the lottery' is a pretty accurate description of how I was feeling.

My wish is that women find a 'Linda' and they don't fall prey to a private obstetrician with their own agenda and private hospitals. In healthy pregnancies YOU are the expert, NOT THEM! Thank you Linda, I don't think any amount of words could ever sum up how much you gave me, you gave me more than just midwifery care.

You showed me I was stronger than I ever thought possible, you showed me birth is raw, beautiful and amazing, when you just trust in it.

There is only one quote which I feel sums up our journey perfectly Linda:

"I believe everything happens for a reason. People change so you can learn to let go, things go wrong so you can appreciate them when they are right ... and sometimes good things fall apart so better things can fall together" ~Marilyn Monroe~

The HBAC Waterbirth of Archer- by Katie Chinnery

My son was born into a birthing pool in the middle of the afternoon at the end of March. It was mostly silent; I could hear the sounds of the school kids walking past and the sound of my dogs barking at them as usual. Life was going on around us outside and here I was, about to give birth vaginally for the first time. My first birth was an emergency caesarean; I hadn't experienced a normal vaginal birth before. I never wanted to feel a baby taken out of my stomach ever again and now, here I was having the total opposite experience for my second birth. No hospitals, no doctors, no interventions, no hospital rules, no limitations; just myself, my partner, my doula and the mid-wives.

Here is the story of my labour and birth...

10.30am - After an unusually decent night's sleep (you know how it is when you are in those final days!) I grabbed some breakfast and sat down on the couch and jumped online.

I had a funny feeling - like a cramp - and I went to the toilet. I sent my partner Scott a text message telling him to stay close to the phone, I think something might happen today. After a few minutes I needed to go to the toilet again and I had a bloody show. I rang Scott and told him to come home as I was having a contraction. Ouch ouch OUCH! I rang my Midwife, Emma, to let her know that something was happening. The pain was so bad I dropped the phone mid-conversation. I had this incredible urge to push. Emma tells me she is still on the other end of town but is on her way. I was scared she wouldn't make it in time!

I then rang my doula, Jodee, to tell her what's happening. I describe my contractions to her and she tells me she will get to me within thirty minutes.

11am-11:45am - While I waited for my husband I laboured away in my bedroom. I didn't feel like there was much time between each contraction. Every one that surged through me was hard, intense, and gave me the incredible urge to push. I was worried that I was pushing too early, so I squatted with my head on the floor and bottom in the air as suggested by Jodee over the phone. I called Scott again and almost yelled down the line "you have to come home right now!"

11:50am - Scott got home and quickly came into our room to check on me.

12pm - Jodee arrived and told Scott to start the pool. She put soothing oils in the oil burner as soon as she arrived. She calmed me down and started helping me cope better with the pain. I felt more focused. I tried to breathe through each contraction as they intensified. After 30 minutes Jodee suggested I try the shower, so we moved to the bathroom and I spent some time in there with the hot water on my back, leaning into Scott during each contraction.

12:38pm – Emma, the Midwife, arrived and started setting up. Someone suggested that I move back into the bedroom as we needed to use the hot water to fill up the rest of the pool. While the shower was helping, the urge to get into the birth pool was greater so we went back to the bedroom and I knelt over the bed for the next hour. Every 10 minutes or so Emma checked the foetal heart rate with the Doppler - perfectly normal.

1:40pm - After labouring away in my bedroom (and after a mishap where the hose filling the pool flew out and sprayed water all over our TV), the pool was announced full! I made my way down there and climbed in; it felt wonderful. I decided it was most comfortable to keep kneeling and lean over the side of the pool, holding onto Scott or Jodee's hands. Each contraction seemed to be getting more intense and longer. I was getting longer breaks between them where I was able to breathe slowly and recoup. I found the flickering lights of the electrical equipment around the TV were something to focus on. I asked out loud if this was really labour? (I get a few laughs!) The labour seemed to be settling down into a groove. I wondered what was going on. Everyone was telling me that I was doing well.

I requested no internals, so I had no idea what my body was doing. I had been trying not to push but I asked if I could push now. I get told to go with it. Looking back through my labour notes, I find that I was having a contraction once every two to three minutes lasting 60 seconds long. It sure felt intense!

2:30pm - I started to feel a little bit of stinging at the end of each contraction. WOW! I thought calmly to myself...My baby is going to be arriving soon! So, this is where I get back to the start of the story. I remember thinking my hair was all over the place. I was glad it wasn't too hot as my air conditioner didn't work that well when it was hot and humid. I even wanted my dogs to stop barking. I never once thought about that scar on my uterus!

2:56pm - I kept getting longer feelings of stinging. Then I felt a pop and a stretching sensation, and his head was out. Wow! I remember thinking "that means the rest of him will follow!" I felt his head begin to rotate. It was the most awful feeling. Not painful, but it felt like someone was behind me pulling him around, and I asked if someone was pushing down on him. No, the midwives told me, that was him turning all by himself.

3:03pm - I felt one last push and whoosh he slid out. Emma was behind me and told me to get my hands down whereby she pushed him under my legs. I reached down and pulled him up and out of the water. Oh my gosh! I stared down into his eyes, he stared up into my face and we gazed at each other. He is covered lightly in vernix, the rest floats around in the pool. He looked a little grey straight away but slowly started changing colour. I think, yep, I just birthed my baby, as you do. I thought straight away that yes, it hurt, but it felt...easy and normal. I then finally sat down after 4.5 hours and held him to my chest. I started to process what I had just done. I chatted away with Emma, Jodee and Scott while we waited for the umbilical cord to stop pulsating and the placenta to come away. I offered the breast.

4:00pm - I experienced mild cramps but no contractions. The backup midwife had a quick check and told me that I had to push the next time I had a contraction, like I did during labour. When it finally happened I pushed, and then- whoosh- the placenta came out intact. By now the cord had stopped pulsating so we clamped the cord and I asked Scott to cut it, which he did. The water was getting cold, so I handed over Archer to Scott for his first cuddles while I headed to the shower. Best shower ever. I remember standing in there thinking "I have just birthed a baby and I am walking around having a shower!" I felt pretty invincible right then. I went back to the lounge and got checked for any tearing. We found a 2nd degree labial tear as Archer came out with his hand over his face. I didn't care though; I had an amazing and empowering birth experience.

4:30pm onwards - I cradled my baby on my chest and started to call my family. I had already decided that I wasn't going to let anyone know until after the birth, so it was wonderful to be able to call them up and say "hey mum, dad, I had my baby not long ago!" I moved back up to the bedroom and got comfortable in bed. We then weighed and measured Archer.

By 4:30 both Emma and Jodie have left. Scott's parents brought our daughter back home to meet Archer. She sat on the bed next to us, reached over to tickle his head and laughed. He fits seamlessly into our lives.

Shane and Anton's amazing and beautiful VBAC

My first impression of Shane was one of that of an Amazon goddess, so tall and beautiful with long flowing hair, who had such conviction and inner strength.

Upon our first meeting, it became apparent to me that she felt like a victim of the hospital system during the birth of her gorgeous little boy Kit. It was clearly a case of the dreaded 'cascade of intervention' which when started you can never get off the inevitable road of more and more procedures being offered and thrust upon one.

The beauty of being a doula for me is that women like Shane have the opportunity to debrief themselves and open up and express themselves verbally so they can clear themselves of their previous birth experiences and how it was for them. For many women like Shane, having someone who will listen without judgement and really be heard is what they need. Especially important for women who have had a Caesarean and are wanting to experience a natural, vaginal birth the next time around.

So here I was, sitting in Shane and Anton's house listening to the familiar story of the previous birth experience that ended in a Caesarean but knowing that Shane's tone was dictating very clearly to me that this was not what was going to happen again. The one thing really struck me about Shane was right from the outset I could see she was so determined to not be led down the same pathway of birth again, and that she would do anything to assure a more favourable and positive birth experience. Almost immediately I could see her strength and determination to do things differently this time around. This is what sets some women apart from others who perhaps want to experience a VBAC – vaginal birth after caesarean. There is definitely an inner drive and mental focus and hunger for knowledge and information so that they can do it differently the next time around.

It was the case now of seeing Alison, Lisa and Shane on a rotational basis, (Alison and Lisa's stories follow on from Shanes) - all strong determined women who met at a Birthrites meeting and decided to have me as their doula and childbirth educator throughout their pregnancies leading up to the birth of their babies. How lucky I was to be given this opportunity in supporting these great women, all whom I really admired and loved for their passion and drive and above all else friendship and trust in me.

Over the next eight weeks leading up to the birth Shane and I had many discussions over cups of coffee to define what she would really like to take place during this birth. At each and every gathering I tried to get Shane to be as clear and specific as possible with the knowledge that she would have to have constant foetal monitoring (the hospitals policy!) which meant being continually connected to a machine whilst in labour. A form of intervention which a lot of VBAC women dread as their mobility is severely compromised, however Shane knew that by having me present and constantly massaging her back, encouraging her and supporting her 100% this was not going to be an issue at all. This is why so many women who are having a VBAC do employ the services of a doula as it can assist them tremendously to stay focused and in labour regardless of being 'hooked up' to a machine being limited in mobility.

The other issue I found very disturbing during the weeks leading up to Shane's labour day was the way in which she had

397

to fight for her right to have a VBAC experience, even though her chosen hospital had a team of Midwives specifically dedicated to assist women to have VBACs. It really amazed me and frustrated the hell out of both myself and Shane. After every appointment, I felt like I had to pick Shane up mentally and emotionally from the blow she had just received in her confidence and commitment to have the birth she wanted so badly for her baby. The blows came with each time in the form of Obstetricians suggesting that she was ridiculous to attempt to 'trial her scar'! And "why on earth don't you just have another Caesarean section? It will be a lot safer you know!" And the real clincher! "What on earth would you want to go through all of that pain for and end up with another Caesarean anyway?" ARRRGHHH!!! I was so unimpressed and so disappointed that this is how Shane was treated. Talk about dis-empowering a woman before her labour/birth experience. I know women all over Australia on a daily basis deal with this type of dumping from their care providers irrespective of whether they are having a first baby or VBAC experience, and it just makes me so mad.

Thankfully Shane was strong enough to pick herself up and shrug it off, re-focusing on what she really wanted to create. It really was a credit to her that she could do this as it is not easy by any means to remain so strong and positive when you are being told to doubt yourself, your ability and your body. I was truly in awe of her.

On the 21st of September 2006, Shane went into spontaneous labour late in the evening. I received a phone call at about
10pm and headed straight over to the house, arriving at about
11pm. It was here that I found Shane labouring in a very dark
room with just a little lamp on, rocking her body like a woman
possessed and needing to move. I could see that her contractions were coming on thick and fast however she was so focused
and strong and very much in the familiar labour state of being
present but not present. Shane was indeed in good strong labour and focusing within herself. I noticed also she had found
her rhythm through rocking and leaning forward on contractions and breathing deeply into her body.

I am not exactly sure how much time passed by before
Shane began to move about the house going to and from the
bedroom to the toilet to the bedroom, however I got a sense
that things were really starting to move ahead, and it was nearly
time to travel to the hospital. So with this thought going on in
my head I suggested that we get going and Shane felt that was
also a great idea.

After Anton and I packed the car we assisted Shane to climb
into the back of the car where she went onto all fours and continued to rock and move her body on contractions as we headed
for the hospital. Shane was truly amazing as she was just so
strong and determined and just kept quiet as we drove along
remaining at peace with herself and calm. We had had many
conversations about turning the need to go to hospital into a

positive experience and one which meant she was getting one step closer to receiving her baby into her arms and skin to skin for the very first time. This assisted Shane to feel positive and happy about moving to the hospital.

Upon arrival at 1 am in the morning we were required to stand in the cold of the corridor for about 20 minutes while the staff found Shane's file. This did not perturb Shane at all as and we turned this into a positive as it gave her a chance to stand up and walk the corridors stopping to lean on the walls with each and every contraction. I was actually very thankful for this as I felt it was assisting Shane's baby to come right down into the pelvis and onto her cervix.

Finally we headed to the labour room where we were greeted by a Midwife on the Aqua team dedicated to supporting women having a VBAC. To our dismay we found her very un-accommodating and not supportive at all in the fact that Shane didn't want to get on the bed but stand and lean forward over the bed. Both Shane and I knew however that this is what her body wanted and what she needed to do to get this baby born vaginally. It was also suggested that she have a vaginal examination to see how far along she was. We had previously discussed that any dilation is a good thing and that no matter what the number was it was all positive.

Before we had left the house that night Shane had asked me "how dilated do you think I am" and it was then I asked her to close her eyes and tell me what she thought her body had opened up to. At that time, she gauged that she was about three centimetres open. Women always amaze me how they are always so right about their dilation. So back in the hospital here we were with Shane about to have an internal examination in which we asked just for the number to be spoken with no other dialogue. To our joy and excitement Shane was five centimetres in which we were all delighted.

I know this propelled Shane onwards to just keep going and she did so beautifully, however she found the cords a real pain from the foetal monitoring machine, so I went to look for the telemetry. A telemetry is a portable unit that a woman in labour wears around her neck that monitors the baby's heartbeat and contraction strength just like the fixed machine does, however it enables a woman to be able to walk around within a certain distance from the machine that is picking up the measurements. It gives a labouring woman some space in which to move about and go to the toilet etc. There are also waterproof telemetrys that can be used under water so women can get into the bath or take a shower.

Unfortunately for Shane I could not find the telemetry so she had to soldier on. One thing that Shane did have was Kit's (her first born child) soft baby blue blanket in which she held and buried her face into during the contractions. This really was a comfort blanket as it continually reminded Shane that she was getting closer and closer to meeting her baby and somehow having that blanket and smell helped her on her journey.

It was in next to no time at all that I remember Shane getting onto the floor where she then started to rock back and forwards while she was on her hands and knees making some pretty powerful noises. I remember thinking to myself this sounds like transition! Sure, enough in next to no time Shane was beginning to push. Push she did, with and without noise in the most powerful and beautiful way. I felt so happy and relieved for her as her dream of having a baby vaginally was becoming a reality. I always get so emotional when VBAC women are giving birth because against all the odds (so it seems) and adversity they receive along the way they achieve their desired wish of giving birth, which is so very healing and profound.

I really lost track of how long it took to push Scout (Shane's beautiful baby) out of Shane's body at 3.13 am with the assistance of a little episiotomy. However, I do remember her coming into the world with a big gush all soft and slippery and so alert. It was here that Scout was placed skin to skin on Shane's body and we all cried tears of joy and happiness. It was a wonderful moment and one I will always treasure. Anton, Shane's husband was truly amazing as well as he completely trusted in Shane that she wanted to experience a natural birth this time around and wholeheartedly supported her and just let her get on with it supporting her physically, mentally and emotionally. We all worked together as a wonderful team. Shane's birth was a wonderful VBAC as was Alison's and Lisa's and I feel so blessed to have been a part of these women's journeys – thank you, thank-you.

My Birth Stories...... Alison White

Well, there we were, our dream had come true - we had sold the house and were taking the trip of a lifetime 4-wheel driving around Australia! We were in Townsville after completing the full-on 4-wheel drive trip to the tip of Cape York, Queensland. Sitting around the BBQ out the front of our camper I said to my husband Scott "well, we made a deal remember. We agreed that after we did that part of the trip we were going to start to try and have a baby". "It might take 2 years" were my famous last words - I fell pregnant that night, and so the next part of our journey was only just beginning......

I was excited to be pregnant so quickly and we decided we would continue to travel around Australia. However, I just got sicker and sicker. It was a combination of living in a camper trailer in sometimes up to 50-degree heat and lots of long hours sitting in the car between destinations. I really shouldn't complain because regardless of it being the most uncomfortable time, I was just so excited to be pregnant that I didn't let anything negative enter my mind.

We completed the trip to Perth, Western Australia just as we planned, and I was 17 weeks pregnant. We had seen doctors in nearly every state as we travelled, each confirming I was fine,

403

so I didn't think I had any worries. At the 18 weeks ultrasound it was confirmed we were having a boy. We were very excited and happy that all was well.

After a little research I booked into a local hospital; one close to the house that we had found and were going to call 'home' for our family of three. At a routine appointment at 30 weeks my blood pressure was up, and they admitted me to the hospital where I was in and out for the next four weeks. Then one day they sent me for an ultrasound to confirm that our son was in a Frank Breech (like a diving pike) position. They outlined that I could have him turned at another hospital or have a C-section as they didn't think there was enough room for him to turn on his own being my first baby, so they sent me off with a piece of paper telling me the turning procedure and what the "miscarriage risks" were. It totally freaked me out.

That week I read up a little on C-sections and began thinking "whatever is meant to be will be". I was in and out of hospital with high blood pressure and fluid retention until one morning I woke at home with a light period pain feeling, and my body flushed itself out like I had eaten something it didn't agree with. I thought "this can't be it, I'm 5 weeks early!" But it definitely was...

After two hours of feeling these period cramping type sensations I rang the hospital. They said to come in so they could check me out as they were concerned about my high blood pressure. I went into the hospital not thinking too much about 'the birth' of my baby. I thought this was just a 'check-up', nothing more! Upon arrival they did a vaginal examination, and I was 3cms dilated (not that I really remember this detail until I got my medical records two years later; I think I was in denial).

They did another ultrasound and confirmed that my baby was still breech. I decided to go for a walk and found myself in the toilet when my waters broke. I remained very calm and together during all of this. However, I was then taken to a room where it was clearly explained to me that a C-section was advisable. I guess I felt OK about all of what was going on because I had had the previous week to think about the whole idea and get my head around it. I think that's why I coped ok with the news at the time.

Upon giving my consent my husband was taken away to change into the lovely theatre attire as I was prepped. I was shaved, informed and advised to sign all the appropriate paper-work; it was like clockwork and did not for one second feel like I was about to have a baby. I had no questions, or at least none that I could think of at the time. I put my total trust and life in the hands of the specialists!

So my drug-filled birth included my husband watching the entire operation as I just floated through the moment... My son was shown to me all wrapped up and I thought "he's aliv"'. I was told that he had the cord wrapped around his neck twice and that it was a very long cord. It was probably a good thing

I didn't go in and try and have him turned (follow your intuition I say!)

Kaj Cooper White was 6 pounds 1, a great size for nearly five weeks early. He lay in a crib for assistance with oxygen for five hours or so and was a true champion. I was in recovery when I looked down and saw a small sample container with something in it. The nurse asked me "what is this?" I was thinking at the time "are you serious? How would I know?" Apparently they had cut out some cysts whilst I was 'open' and neglected to tell anyone, including me! (This was another thing I found out through my medical records when I received them!)

My blood pressure had risen throughout the day (not that I was aware of this) and I was informed an ambulance had been called. I was to be sent to King Edward Memorial hospital in Perth, some 20 kilometres away. They weren't sure if my son could come with me! This news came as my husband had gone home for a shower, and I was hysterical. I refused to go, and outlined that if I couldn't take my son I was staying until they had a crib for him. As you can imagine, my blood pressure continued to climb and was through the roof by the time my husband finally returned. He got there just in time to see me being transferred to the ambulance bed. He said the look on my face was one of devastation and he thought something had happened to our son, like he had passed away. After a moment, I was able to tell him I was off to another hospital that could better equip me and my rising blood pressure!

So off we went (thank god my baby was in tow) with no feeling in my legs and no idea where KEMH was (we had only been in W.A for four months). I didn't even think to research the fact that they may send me to another hospital, as I thought they would be able to deal with anything - apparently not. My son's first ride in a vehicle was in an ambulance and all I recall thinking is "it isn't meant to be like this!!!"

I really had no idea what the time was or what I was meant to be doing with my baby and felt very confused and annoyed. When I arrived, we were settled into a room where Scott was asked to leave and go home as the nurse (or 'Matron from Hell' as I referred to her) thought he looked tired and exhausted and suggested he needed to get some rest. The very next comment to me was, "Have you fed your baby yet?" I couldn't even re-member if I had held my baby, let alone fed him. I sheepishly said "No". "Don't you know how to breastfeed?" she snapped in reply. I was devastated at her abrupt response. Breastfeeding was very important to me and it was the last thing I could an-swer for right now. I responded like a little schoolgirl in deten-tion "the breastfeeding classes were meant to start this Monday. My son is five weeks early and I haven't attended any classes yet".

With that, the 'Matron from Hell' grabbed my boob and threw my son onto my nipple and stormed out, saying some-thing like "well I will have to get someone else to help you be-cause I don't have time for this!" There I was lying in this alien environment in a hospital bed in a Perth suburb I didn't even know existed - no family, no friends. All I knew was that this was not how I wanted to remember the birthday of my son.

I spent the next two weeks in the hospital. My blood pressure finally went down after three days; however, my son was jaundiced, and I had a lot of trouble breastfeeding. My milk never really came in but the midwives kept saying "just wait, it will happen". So, I fed and expressed every three hours like clockwork. I was so determined to give my son a good start, especially after our initial day meeting each other.

Finally, after two weeks, we got to go home. It was magical to be in our own environment at last, for the first time in months. Kaj lost weight in the first four weeks as my milk still didn't come in. In the end I said "ENOUGH!" and put him on formula. I never looked back! He is now nearly three and is a very healthy, active little boy!

We were again blessed to fall pregnant quickly, this time in three months. Again, with the sickness. At least this time I had a toilet and air-conditioning and we were not living in a tent I would joke to my friends. So, I was feeling a whole lot better about this pregnancy. However, what was on my mind was how I was going to have this baby? I had a friend that had a second baby via a second C-section and was saying "it's the way to go, for sure". Given my previous experience, I was not convinced at all but I was not sure what I wanted. I just knew this time things were going to be different, and I was going to have a say in everything!

At about 12 weeks pregnant I was searching the net and came across a link to the Birthrites website which was the turning point to my entire second pregnancy. I was so excited to read so much information on VBACs (Vaginal Births after Caesarean) and the positive stories about homebirths and hospital births. There was also a forum where you could discuss your queries and fears. I felt inspired and empowered by these women making their own decisions, I was amazed to say the least.

At my next GP appointment, I was given information about C-sections and my comment was something like "I know what they are. I have had one remember!". The doctor said "well you will be having another one, won't you?" Yet again, that was another turning point in this journey. I remembered thinking at the time "who the hell was she making that decision for me?" I knew one thing for sure and that was I wanted to be the one in control this time; fully conscious and aware of my choices. I went straight home, got on the computer and started to research everything I could find on VBACs both here and overseas.

I set up a file and saved everything in it so I could teach myself and inform my husband. I went to the next GP appointment with the longest list of questions on VBACs. My female GP said "If your hospital is happy to look after you that will be fine, you don't need to come back and see me again". With that I informed her I wanted shared care and she advised me to move on. I was shocked that a GP had refused to see me because of my birth choices. I left in shock, but again that just made me more determined to find out more and to start surrounding myself with people that believed in the same thing as me. This is when I contacted Penny at Birthrites and found out the date for their next meeting.

I was nervous, not really knowing what was going to happen at the meeting, but I was so glad I went. I met some of the most amazing people and was able to share my journey with them. It is there that I met Sara David, a midwife from KEMH. She also runs VBAC preparation classes and had, had a VBAC herself. I joined and borrowed books and CDs straight away; the resources were fantastic!

It was at these preparation classes where I found out what a Doula was. I fell in love with the idea straight away since I knew with the birth of my son, I had no idea what was going on, and being the first time around, I think my husband and I just agreed with everything that was told to us. I really believed that we needed outside help if we were to get the birth we wanted. So that's when the search for a doula began...

I contacted the Midwifery service and they provided me with a few Doulas' names. I also searched on the net and emailed a few Doulas telling them why I wanted one. I had a list of questions I wanted to ask them, but no one contacted me back.

I was devastated. However, this one name kept coming up everywhere I turned, yet I just didn't get around to contacting her for four weeks. Gaby Targett was her name.

After leaving a few messages for each other, we finally spoke, and I was so excited to finally arrange a time to meet with her. Gaby came to our house to meet Scott, Kaj and I. As soon as she walked into my house I felt a calming presence, it was amazing. We went through some introductory information and she asked me about my first birth and why I wanted a doula for this birth. Again, I had my LIST of questions which became a bit of a joke in the long run - me and my lists – Hey, go with whatever works for you!

As soon as Gaby left, Scott and I looked at each other and said "thank god we met her. She is going to keep our heads together in labour". We met Gaby several times, each time discussing in more and more detail my feelings about things, my birth plan and what visualisations I could do to keep myself focussed. I made up my own positive affirmations poster and also used the one I got at Birthrites. Gaby also gave me her hypnosis/relaxation scripts and showed me what exercises I could do on the fitball to help my pelvis to really open and assist my baby to move down – head down this time! It was the best preparation I could have asked for.

I had been seeing a team of midwives at KEMH and all seemed to be supportive, no blood pressure problems this time and no fluid retention. I was cruising along feeling great. All of them answered my questions and supported my queries at each visit; my baby was in a great position. Our 20-week ultrasound confirmed we were having a healthy baby girl. We had a name picked out already (one that we were going to use the first time) so I called her that name every day from then on. From about 30 weeks I was measuring weeks ahead, so as time progressed, they were concerned about the size of the baby. I was not!

I attended Sara's VBAC preparation classes and they were fantastic. It was here I met two other couples, Lisa and Craig, and Shane and Anton who were also planning to give birth at KEMH. Shane had also booked Gaby as her Doula, so we had a lot to discuss. It was great to share the same thoughts, ideas, fears and excitement. Lisa showed excitement at the idea of a Doula and took that thought home to her husband.

It was also great to see our husbands chatting about their fears and expectations; so much came out of this class for all of us. Many, including me, had tears rolling down our faces at times throughout our sessions as the realities of our first birth experiences were recalled. This is when I realised we still didn't know when I actually held my little boy for the first time. So then and there I decided to apply for my medical records. When they arrived, it was 80 pages long! I cried and cried. I found out about those cysts (that no one could tell me anything about) and it had the exact time when "baby went for a cuddle with mother". According to the notes, he was six hours old to my amazement. Other information outlined that I had dilated three centimetres. It was important for me to know that my body had done that on its own and that I had felt natural labour before all the medical intervention came about.

When I was 34 weeks pregnant, I went for my routine check-up of my little girl. I had my usual palpation and when the midwife felt the position of the baby she calmly said "oh, she is breech". This was at the exact same stage during my first pregnancy that I was told my baby boy was breech! She sent me off with a piece of paper telling me they can turn the baby and to look into it. I was so upset. I was thinking "not again. Why do my babies always go breech? What is happening to my vaginal birth plan? No, this is not happening". I left devastated, and for the first time I thought maybe I was meant to have another C-section. This thought didn't last long though. After contacting Gaby, she set me straight and discussed with me several things I needed to do to get my thoughts back on track: positive affirmations, talking to my baby etc. I jumped on the net and looked up my options, including the pros and cons of having an ECV (known as External Cephalic Version) or manual turning of my baby from the outside.

After talking to Scott, I decided I was going to have the baby turned, and that if she didn't stay in that position after the

413

first attempt, it wasn't meant to be. I was also going to try natural ways of turning her, so again on the Net I went and researched ways. I used acupressure, visualisation, positioning my own body in a more upright way, lying on the left side only, using a fitball and massage. I went back a week later to advise the midwives that I wanted an ECV and they informed me that because the baby was footling breech (feet first already down and practically engaged!), it was too dangerous to perform and they wouldn't be attempting it!

I just sat there and cried and cried. Seeing my distress, the midwife decided to do an ultrasound just in case she had turned. As soon as she put the ultrasound device on my belly she smiled and said, "Alison, she is no longer Breech". Again, I was crying, but this time with JOY and elation - everything had to have helped; all the natural things had worked, and we were back on track for our vaginal birth.

At 37 weeks I had light labour pangs on and off for three days, then they stopped. I let Gaby know and she said to just keep her informed. Thank god for texting as I knew I could get her at any time. Also, at the back of my mind was the fact that I knew that Shane and Lisa were both due around this time as well. I was concerned that one of us may not get Gaby as our Doula if we all went into labour at the same time. It was for this reason I got Gaby to introduce me to her back up Doula, Toni, who rang me and put my mind at ease. After a great conversation, she assured me that she would be there if I needed her, so that was all fine and I stopped worrying.

I was informed by KEMH that I would have to see an Obstetrician 'once' at about 38 weeks to sign a VBAC consent form to have the baby at that hospital. So, I thought "well, how bad could it be?" Again, I went in with the list of questions on monitoring, active labour positions and of course a copy of my three paged colour coded birth plan (a copy was already stapled in the front of my file at the hospital). I would never use the Obstetrician's name but I will say that Scott and I called him 'Dr. Short pants' because I don't know what drycleaners he uses BUT he really needs some new pants.

He was nothing but sarcastic. After he measured my stomach, he joked about how this baby was so big that she was going to split me to high heaven if I attempted a vaginal birth. I was shocked that he thought it was ok to talk to me like that. This was the first appointment I had taken Scott to and he was left speechless. He then took my blood pressure and said it was far too high and I would be sent upstairs for monitoring and then he would assess me after that. I said that I wanted to sign the form first and he said "no need with your blood pressure like this. I may be seeing you in the theatre this afternoon".

I left shattered. As I walked out I rang Gaby and she said she was on her way if I needed her, then I turned around and for the first time since the VBAC classes I saw Lisa. I was telling her what happened and she assured me that everything was

415

going to be ok, and for whatever reason, I really believed her. We swapped phone numbers and have been in contact ever since.

I went for monitoring and within 20 minutes my blood pressure was back to normal. 'Dr Short pants' checked the results, sent me home and said "I'll see you in a week". The next week exactly the same thing happened. He was not supportive at all, although he said a VBAC attempt was ok but with a baby this size I must be mad. So he organised the visiting midwifery service to come to my house every 48 hours. I was fine with this as I would know if the baby was staying in a great position and wasn't in distress which meant my blood pressure would remain normal. So at 39.2 weeks, the midwife came to the house for the last time and all was well.

At 39.4 weeks I began to feel slightly stronger pangs. I had been feeling light pangs on and off for two weeks, but I knew this was it. At 5am I woke up to the same period pain sensations I had with my son. I had a shower and moved around the room for a few hours before my waters broke on the toilet (again – which is very convenient I think!) I was so excited. However, upon closer examination I saw I had green meconium on the toilet paper.

I screamed to my husband to bring the phone so I could ring Gaby to talk this over. After our conversation I decided immediately that I wanted to go to the hospital (which all along is exactly what I didn't want as I wanted to get into good established labour at home BUT.....) So we dropped our son off on the way and got to the hospital at the same time as Gaby.

I slowly walked to the monitoring area, stopping along the corridor during contractions to focus and breathe. The first thing the midwife said to me was "I have read your birth plan". I was totally impressed. I thought about all that time and effort and fighting for people to listen to me and my needs and choices and that was the first thing she said. This, I thought, was very positive. Once in the examination room, she went to strap me to a monitor, and I warned her that if she did that I would have to be able to move about so to make sure the cords were long enough so that I could get off the bed if I wanted to.

I remember lying on my side and moving around a little as the contractions were coming two minutes apart for the next three hours while they monitored the baby in that tiny cubicle. An Ob came in and said "I have read your birth plan, it's very detailed." Oh my gosh, people are finally listening. He went on to say "we will see how you progress and if you don't progress an induction may be needed". All I could hear was..... blah.... blah... blah... I really wasn't interested in his thoughts. I put my hand up and sai, "STOP, we will cross that bridge if and when we come to it" and then I turned away and continued breathing through my contractions as he left. Scott, Gaby and I smiled at each other and I said "there will be no induction".

Finally, I was taken to a beautiful big labour room. It was like a hotel suite where Gaby had organised the bed to be moved and mats to be put down and a fitball to be brought in. The lights were dimmed all of which was on my birth plan and like we had discussed long before going into labour. Scott put on some music and Gaby suggested to the midwife I have a shower, so that's what happened; no monitoring, just me and the shower for a little while - heaven! Gaby stood with me giving me dried fruit as I showered - it was awesome and I felt totally relaxed.

With the contractions still coming every few minutes I got out of the shower and tried to go on the fitball but it was too uncomfortable, so Gaby suggested leaning over a beanbag on the floor. While the midwife went and got that, I asked Scott to bring over my affirmation posters, one that I had made with a 3D ultrasound photo of my baby that was taken the week before along with my Birthrites one. I went through them as I laboured leaning on the end of the bed. The midwife put a telemetry monitor on me, which allowed me to move freely anywhere I wanted to go within our room and it could pick up my baby's foetal heart beat which ensured me the baby was fine.

Then the most amazing thing happened. It was the midwives shift change and in comes my guardian angel - Sara David, VBAC guru. This was the first shift she had worked for a month as she had been on leave and she got me! She knelt down and said to me quietly "Alison, it's Sara David. I was wondering if I could be here to help you birth your baby?" I remember quietly saying "yes" as if I was breathless, but I wasn't. I was just so focussed on the job at hand, I even surprised myself.

A Doctor came in after some time to do a VE. I was amazed they hadn't wanted to do one earlier as I had been there about five hours, but I did state on my birth plan "NO VE's unless absolutely necessary" and the reason was clearly to be explained to me. She began by saying "now, I have read your birth plan" and went on to explain why she wanted to do the VE to see if I had progressed. I also clearly stated I was not to be told how many centimetres I was dilated and that it only be whispered to Gaby, and she would know if I wanted to know. The reason for this was I didn't want to be put off or deterred from the way in which I was powering ahead. I could see excitement in Gaby's eyes, and she looked at me wide eyed and I knew then it was ok to know. I was 4cms. I leaned over the beanbag for about the next 2½ hours, labouring away. Scott and Gaby took turns massaging my lower back, it was magical (I know that sounds weird, but it really was, I totally believed in me and my baby).

My body started to push on its own; I was a bit shocked. Then, TRANSITION (not that I knew that at the time). I said to Gaby "I'm not sure how ------ long I can keep doing this." It was the first time I had stated anything like this and Gaby and Sara figured something must be going on. Apparently,

419

Gaby and Sara (who knew about each other but had never met before today) looked at each other and went "here we go...it's time".

Sara set up the bed and all the necessities, while Gaby suggested I go to the toilet and empty my bladder. So I did, stopping and starting in between contractions. They both helped me head towards the bed and then the weirdest thing happened. I could not get my legs to move and I had a flashback to when the nurse was helping me out of the shower the day after the C-section with my son. I had to snap myself out of it, so I literally slapped the side of my leg and said "stop this. You're not having another C-section. You are going to get up on the bed and give birth now – let's go".

Gaby and Sara helped me up onto the bed. I was on all fours, just as I wanted to be and Scott was there waiting for me. My body was already pushing; I just had to go with it. Sara checked how dilated I was and came and whispered to me "Alison, you are fully dilated and ready to go". I had to confirm with Gaby that it was all true and I was ready to push; it all seemed to be happening quite fast.

Gaby suggested to Scott that he take some photos. So two pushes a few minutes apart and I had a very strong feeling it was only going to take one more push as I could feel her making her way down. I visualised a good friend of mine Yvonne as a miniature person sitting on my pillow yelling out "come on, come on. You can do it", encouraging me with all her might.

Scott came up to me and gave me a kiss on the forehead, and with one more push my baby girl at 8' 3oz birthed herself into this world. Scott, Gaby and Sara all had their hands on her and passed her between my legs. I said "hello little girl. You're ok, Mummy is here". I moved over onto my back and placed her onto my chest; it was truly amazing. Everyone had tears, except me, which I again was shocked at. I just felt so calm, yet excited and so inspired by the whole birthing experience that my little girl birthed herself exactly the way she wanted and that we were all there to help her.

It took 10 minutes to birth the placenta and we all sat around and watched the cord stop pulsating. Then our little girl took her first breath of life on her own, Scott cut the cord and we all sat around chatting about the whole experience, knowing that a higher force brought us together that day.

I tore and needed stitches, but that was so insignificant. I actually joked an hour later "is anyone going to weigh my baby?"

I got to experience an 8-hour drug-free amazing birth where I was fully present and aware of everything that was going on. Better still, I got to hold my baby skin to skin immediately for the very first time which was fantastic. I had the birth that I had dreamt of and was home within 48 hours and breastfeeding with no problems at all.

As I write this, my baby is five months old, and I am still happily breastfeeding. I wouldn't have it any other way.

All I have to say to women reading this is...

"Believe in yourself, believe in your body and its ability to birth, you can have the birth you dream of if you - trust"

Lastly, I would like to say ...

Gaby, your support was just amazing. Thank you for believing in us, we could never have got through what we did in the pregnancy without you. You were a calming tower of strength during labour, three cheers for our Doula..........

Hip Hip Hooray!!

Sara, you're a true professional with a heart of gold, thank you.

Scott, thank you for trusting me, your support was amazing.

Lastly and most importantly to my baby girl

SEISIA KIAL WHITE - You are my inspiration and I love you to the moon and back!

My Powerful VBAC of Ronan

My VBAC journey began after the birth of my first child. When I fell pregnant with Lola, I assumed that because we conceived her so easily and the pregnancy was a breeze I would have a normal, natural birth. My future stepfather had just tragically taken his life so it was an absolute blessing to fall pregnant, I was sure it was 'meant to be'. It helped me and my family to move on from this tragedy and focus on a new life. It always seems to be the way, you always hear of new life after death.

After a minor amount of research, we chose to avoid the care of an Obstetrician and go with the care of a midwifery team at the Birthing Centre at King Edward Memorial Hospital. I attended the ante-natal classes, read various pregnancy books and magazines, and discovered a wonderful book by Janet Balaskas called 'New Active Birth'. This became my bible as it was recommended to me by a friend who had a homebirth. I loved the idea of hiring a midwife and having a homebirth but was not at all confident. It was my first pregnancy and I hadn't had any friends who had birthed before me so I didn't get to hear any of the harsh reality stories that you can only hear from your friends. Or the ones that make you really think about what you are prepared for.

At 40 weeks plus 10 days I had to meet with an Obstetrician who recommended I book in for an induction the following day. I declined to consent to this as this was not at all what

423

I wanted. In fact, I was in shock because I had not even entertained the idea of being induced let alone being forced to do so. I had heard so many horror stories about women being induced and I was so upset. I wanted to go into labour on my own without the artificial intervention of the drug Syntocinon.

I went on a mission to induce myself by trying all of the home tricks in the book; raspberry leaf tea, hot curry, homeopathic remedies, sex and castor oil. None of them worked. The castor oil was my last resort. I remember taking it on the morning of a weekend when Craig was home from work. We decided to have fish for dinner that night and I assumed we would be able to get to the fish market and back by the time the rush to the loo started! We had just reached the end of our street when I got the urge to 'go' and had to turn back. I couldn't leave the house, but no contractions started and all I managed to do was run to the toilet all day. I thought at least if I did go into labour I wouldn't poo when it was time to push, as I was totally cleaned out!

I felt so much pressure on me to get this baby out that I became extremely anxious. I began to lose faith in my body's ability to actually go through with it. I believe this anxiety held me back from going into labour sooner. By my 42nd week I had to face the harsh reality that if I did not go into labour that day, I would not be going to the birthing centre. Unfortunately I didn't, and that was when I wished I had done more research. I would be birthing in the hospital (which was unfamiliar to me) with the possibility of being induced and no birth plan. I felt like such a fool.

On my 17th day past my estimated date I finally started to feel some little twinges in the afternoon. I was so relieved. My contractions had started by the evening but were not consistent. They were all over the place. They ranged from two minutes apart to 10 minutes apart. I did not sleep at all. I tried to convince Craig to stay up with me, but he insisted upon getting some rest just in case we would be in for a long haul. I wished he would stay awake with me but I also understood why he wanted to rest. I just wanted some company!

I rang the hospital around 11pm and explained my inconsistent contractions. The midwife I spoke to said that it sounded like my cervix was trying very hard to dilate. She recommended I stay at home for the rest of the night and come in the morning. I was very restless and could not keep still or find a comfortable position. By around 6am I had a show and then showered and was ready to go to the hospital. My contractions were getting stronger and were now at the point where I could only focus on them alone. Around 7.30am we drove to the hospital. I checked-in in between contractions and we went up to the birthing suite. I was quite calm at this point but was unsure of what to expect when we arrived.

I was told to lie back on the bed so they could hook me up to the foetal monitor. Once connected, the midwife left the room. It was hard for me to sit up with each contraction, but

I said nothing, assuming I had no choice. I could hear her heart beating consistently until I had a contraction and it slowly dropped down to approximately 70 beats p/m. (I later found this out when I requested my caesarean surgery records). I immediately panicked and asked Craig to get someone quickly. He raced out of the room and returned with the midwife who immediately rolled me on my side and began to explain that I would have to go for an emergency caesarean due to foetal distress.

I was given the magic injection and the next thing I remember was waking up in recovery with someone calling my name. Hours or days could have passed. I had no perception of how long I was asleep. I asked if I had a boy or girl. She told me that I had a beautiful baby girl. I was so happy. I was crying with joy and pain. I desperately needed some pain relief and was cold and shivering, apparently a side effect from the anaesthetic.

The rest is a blur. I can't remember getting from recovery to the ward but found out that she was born at 8.31am, weighed 3.66kg and was sent to the special care nursery due to her swallowing some meconium. She had to have antibiotics. I was finally wheeled there by Craig and my mum. I didn't get to see or touch her until around 6.30pm that evening. I felt too sick from the anaesthetic to want to see her any earlier. I was holding a kidney dish, vomiting bile and still feeling quite 'out of it' but was so determined to see her, even if I had to crawl there myself.

She was laid down on her tummy with a dummy in her mouth and a Perspex box over her. It was a very surreal experience. I did not initially feel connected because I did not see her come out of me. I found it hard to believe that she was actually there and was real. All I wanted to do was pick her up and smell and kiss her but I was not allowed. I craved that skin-to-skin contact. I could only reach in and touch her lovely soft skin. She had the most beautiful, shaped lips; I thought they were like Craig's. I can't remember how long I spent there. She looked out of place in the special care nursery; all the other babies were so tiny and mostly premature. She looked huge compared to them.

She spent one and a half days in the special care nursery. Once I was able to hold her, I tried to breastfeed. She did not take to it so well initially. I was expressing the colostrum and having it sent to the nursery. The midwives were usually busy attending to the other babies, so I persevered on my own. I did not want to harass them, considering those tiny babies obviously needed much more attention than I did. It was only when she was finally able to stay in my room with me that I felt like I had become a mother and we both got the hang of breastfeeding.

I was prepared for the 'baby blues' considering my traumatic birth, but surprisingly during my five days in hospital I

427

was on a complete high. I wasn't too hard on myself for not giving birth vaginally because I understood her distress and the need to get her out in a hurry. The breastfeeding was going well. I managed to breastfeed her for nearly two years. I had heard other stories of caesarean babies not taking too well to breast feeding, so for that, I was grateful. I think it helped me get over a few of those guilt hurdles about not bringing her into this world the way it 'should' have been.

It did turn me off from falling pregnant again because I just assumed I would have to have another caesarean. It wasn't until I was at a friend's wedding and Lola was a couple of months old when someone asked if we were going to have any more children. I said it was too soon for us to decide and that I couldn't handle having another caesarean. Coincidently, she had birthed her second child vaginally after a caesarean and she was adamant that it was possible. She made it very clear to me that to go through it again I would have to be well researched and strong. She planted the seed in my head about VBAC, although at the time I was not aware of the term.

As we started planning another baby again, I made a phone call to The Community Midwifery Centre in Fremantle and enquired about birthing vaginally after a Caesarean. It was only then that I became familiar with the term VBAC. The midwife I spoke to was extremely helpful. She made it quite clear that a VBAC was possible and gave me the contact number of the midwife, Sara David, who would be able to give me more information. My confidence rose after that conversation, and I kept Sara's number safely tucked away until it was needed.

Four years later and after another easy conception, I was pregnant again. I knew the exact date of my previous period and the exact date of conception. I was concerned that my dates were possibly out with the birth of Lola because she was 18 days overdue, even though I tend to have longer cycles – about 35 days. I wanted to be sure of my dates this time. This pregnancy was a rollercoaster ride from start to finish though. It was not as easy, physically or mentally, as my first either. I struggled with trying to run half a business and be a mother. I was worried about how I would cope with two children but realised that we would get by, no matter what. I have an extremely helpful family.

I had a very strong feeling right from the start of this pregnancy that I was carrying twins. I am not sure why, perhaps it was because there was a good chance we could have twins. They were on Craig's side of the family. When I went for my 12-week ultrasound I found out that I was carrying fraternal twins, but sadly lost one around 10 weeks. I think I was in shock because even though I felt it, I still could not believe it. What a blessing to conceive twins naturally. Yet, we felt so robbed and had a few very sad weeks.

I learned that amazingly my body would absorb the other placenta. I kept on focusing on the fact that I had one healthy baby and that was all that mattered. This helped me a lot. I

429

did not want to get down about it because it obviously wasn't meant to be. I reminded myself that I should count myself lucky. There are plenty of couples who have such difficulty falling pregnant. Every now and then I still get that feeling of being 'robbed', but as each day goes by and I look at my two happy, healthy children that feeling passes quickly and I am grateful for what was meant to be.

Around the fourth month of pregnancy, I developed a condition called Symphysis Pubis Dysfunction. This is caused by hormonal changes in your body and makes your ligaments soften in the pelvis, causing severe pain. This made it difficult for me to walk; I could hardly put any pressure on one leg. I found it difficult to get from sitting to standing and it was even very painful to roll over in bed. I hobbled around for a couple of weeks before deciding that it was not getting any better on its own. I consulted a Physiotherapist and after a few sessions, the problem was fixed. I was so relieved because the thought of putting on extra weight and it not going away was quite daunting.

At around my fifth month of pregnancy I started wheezing. I was coughing a lot and was having what seemed like symptoms of Asthma. I saw my GP and did a spirometry test and discovered it was in fact true. I needed medication to treat it which was such a relief. I didn't realise how hard it was for me to breathe at times. It must have been gestational because fortunately, during my last few months of pregnancy it disappeared and has since not returned.

Because of my previous caesarean I was unable to go to the birthing centre again. I was still not confident with the idea of a home birth, so we opted for the care of the team Midwifery at King Edward Memorial Hospital. On my first clinic appointment I discovered just how supportive my team of midwives were of VBAC. It was a wonderful feeling to not be judged, and my confidence grew from that moment. I was determined now. I was on a mission and if all was progressing well with my baby, I WAS going to have a VBAC. If for some reason I did have to have another caesarean I was going to be mentally prepared this time and be aware of my choices.

I eventually contacted the midwife, Sara David, and she informed me of a wonderful association called Birthrites. I became a member and was given a lot of VBAC and caesarean information. I was also informed of their wonderfully supportive monthly meetings which were attended by other women attempting a VBAC and women who were having empowered caesareans etc. I attended my first meeting and got to tell Lola's birth story along with what I hoped to achieve with this birth. It was wonderful to tell my story and not be judged. A lot of people outside of my small circle of support would ask me what type of birth I would be having. When I mentioned a VBAC, the general comment was "I didn't think you would be allowed". So I chose who I told and who I would keep it from.

This helped me stay positive. I only wanted to surround myself with positive birth stories and support. I would simply brush off anything negative.

I discovered through Sara David that she conducted VBAC preparation classes for couples and she strongly recommended we book one. It was held over two Saturdays and I attended the first one on my own as Craig had to work. At this stage I don't think he realised just how important this birth was to me. I would tell him my feelings at various stages of the pregnancy and he would listen but I would not get a lot of feedback from him. I knew he was thinking about his own trauma he experienced with Lola's birth and he made it quite clear that he did not want to go through that again.

It was at this class that I met Alison and Scott, and Shane and Anton. I noticed our bellies all looked around about the same size and we later discovered that we were all due around the same time. Shane and I actually had the same due date, the 1st October and I think Alison was due about 1 week after that. We all shared our own versions of unwanted caesareans and once again I got to tell of Lola's birth. The great thing about this was that we were asked to point out the positives of our caesareans, not the negatives. Craig was able to attend the last session the following week and we met another couple who did not make it the previous week, Mandy and her husband. I recently discovered she had a wonderful homebirth.

It was only after this class I think Craig realised what I set out to achieve. He was thankful he decided to go along because he got to overcome his main fear which was worrying about the baby's heart rate dropping. He got to ask questions and was reassured that I would have to be constantly monitored. This, on the other hand, bothered me as I did not want to be stuck to a monitor throughout my labour. I wanted an active labour, to not be restricted, to move around freely and have the option to use water if needed.

I also discovered that Alison and Shane had hired Gaby as a doula. I had not really thought about the idea but after meeting with a negative obstetrician during one of my clinic appointments and after hearing stories of successful VBAC due to a doula or private midwife, I considered it. I expressed my view to Craig about this and knew that I just had to do it. I needed all the support I could get while in labour and he happily agreed. I contacted Gaby and expressed my concern about our similar due dates, and she confidently reassured me that we would work it out because she had a back-up doula. I assumed she would say no because of this reason and was amazed that she agreed. She told me of her 'A Labour of Love' book and suggested I read it before meeting with her. She put it in the post that day and as soon as I received it, I could not put it down. I read it in two nights. This became my new bible. Gaby's voice was very calm and reassuring. I looked forward to meeting her face to face because I had a really great feeling about it and once again, I felt even more empowered.

When I met Gaby, I visited her at home and told her my story. She seemed to agree that my anxiety before Lola's birth held me back and stopped me from letting go. I had to get over that hurdle if I wanted to go into labour again. At least I had experienced some labour so I knew what to expect at the beginning. She asked me to visualise and write down what sort of birth I would like to experience this time around. I was to keep reading it every day. She expressed the importance of visualisation and gave me a copy of affirmations and a relaxation script that she asked me to listen to everyday. I kept a copy in my car and listened to it every time I was in there on my own. I especially found the relaxation scripts great for listening to before a clinic appointment. It helped me stay strong during those appointments where I would have to talk to an obstetrician during my third trimester. She gave me a hug goodbye, which I did not expect, but was warmed by. I knew she would be there for me and sensed she had a special insight or some excitement about these three possible VBAC's she would assist with in the near future.

The pregnancy was progressing well and we found out that we were having a baby boy. I could not have been any happier. I secretly wished for a boy. There are a lot of women in my family, so it was a blessing. I would have been equally as happy if it was a girl though. He was posterior so I had to spend a lot of time on my hands and knees. It was relieving because I also had some sciatic pain.

Gaby helped me prepare a birth plan. I was not going to the hospital without one this time! It was about four pages long and I felt silly for doing so but it was the only way I could express the type of birth I wanted to achieve. I also prepared a separate one for a caesarean birth but put it aside once complete.

Around my 38th week, I had to see an obstetrician to sign a VBAC consent form. I was well researched and aware of the risks but was not looking forward to it. I had heard the Registrar of Obstetrics was very supportive of VBAC's and she would be the one to see when signing the form. At my appointment I was not sure who I would get but when she entered the waiting room and called out my name, I was relieved. She informed me of the pros and cons of having a VBAC and the hospital policy and I showed her my birth plan. I still felt silly for having such a long one but she did not bat an eyelid at it. She just said that there would have to be a couple of things that might have to be negotiated. I asked about how tolerant they were of being overdue and she said that 10 days was when they would look at induction. I still did not want to be induced and had discussed with Gaby all of the ways we could try to induce naturally. I was certain that I would not go so far overdue this time.

Gaby told me that Shane had her VBAC, just before her due date and how well it all went. I was so happy to hear the story. It gave me even more hope and now it was up to Alison and me to achieve the same. I also felt less pressure knowing

435

that there were only two of us with births that might clash! I bumped into Alison and Scott at the hospital and discovered she was having some clashes with the obstetricians too.

I had been having some strong Braxton Hicks for a few weeks but nothing that would kick in. On my 10th day over-due, I had to meet with another obstetrician who was not so supportive of a VBAC. I was surprised because he did tell me of his wife having a VBAC with their second child. Everything he was saying became a blur. This was my first meltdown. Tears were streaming down my face as he was explaining all of the details about induction. I could not believe that he kept on going because it was obvious I was not really taking it all in. He just wanted me to sign the induction consent form and was not at all concerned about stopping to let me calm down. I basi-cally was forced to book an induction date. I did not sign the form and I had no intention of turning up for it. I told him I wanted to take it home and read it through more carefully.

On my way back to the car after this particular appoint-ment, I had once again started to doubt myself. I had stayed so strong throughout my pregnancy, but I was now sobbing un-controllably. I phoned Craig but it was pointless talking to him because I was a blubbering mess. I felt sorry for him because he was at work and could not make out why I was so distressed. Once we were both home and I was calmer, I expressed my fear to him of not being able to give birth. He told me to stop being silly and negative, and reminded me of all of the research I had done and that we had Gaby for extra support. I poured myself a large glass of wine that night and slept like a baby. The next day I woke up positive and decided that I had to take each day as it came.

On the day of my induction, I rang and said that I would not be turning up and was transferred to a midwife. She told me that I would have to go in for daily monitoring and I happily agreed. This was the start of me taking each day at a time, and as long as my baby boy was OK, I was happy to wait until he was ready to arrive into this world.

During my daily visits to the Foetal Monitoring Unit I was informed by Gaby that Alison had her VBAC as well. Both her and Shane birthed baby girls. I asked Gaby in great detail how it all went and it was all positive again like Shane's birth. I was excited now because I knew if these two strong-minded women could do it, I could as well.

The daily monitoring was taking its toll and was starting to wear me down. I met Gaby for a coffee and we discussed my overdue date. We decided that I was probably one of those women who had a 42-week pregnancy considering my last one and as long as the baby was OK, what was the rush? That afternoon I had a show. I was feeling a lot of pressure from my friends though. I shut myself in my room for the last couple of weeks prior to the birth, watched daytime TV and slept. Craig and mum took Lola to school and I did not talk to anyone but my family and Gaby. I was sick of people asking me when this bloody baby would come! I was having contractions every now and then but nothing that would kick in. However, one evening I started contracting and they were consistent. I believed it was finally happening but when I awoke in the morning it had all subsided. I tried not to be disappointed, but it was starting to become a real mental game.

Gaby told me that she had given Alison my number and told her of my story and the pressure I had on me. I received a wonderfully inspiring text message from her and I cried and cried. What an inspiration she was. She told me how Sara David happened to have her shift at the hospital the day of her birth, saw Alison was booked in the birthing suite and asked if she could switch shifts to attend her birth. Amazing! She told me how I could do it and it was the most amazing experience of her life and told me to keep on staying positive. She became my rock that last week prior to this birth.

Each morning I had to visit the Foetal Monitoring Unit. I went prepared with my book and a big bottle of water. The traces were always good and I did not have to do much to get him to move. The hardest part was facing a different obstetrician after each visit and the fact that I had to go through the same story every time. I was confident with the trace results; he was moving constantly, and I had a few extra ultrasounds to check my fluid. He wasn't fully engaged but I was led to believe that he probably would not fully engage until I was in established labour. The obstetricians always reminded me of this and tried to scare me because he was going to be a big baby. I made it clear that I did not care what size he was, I would try no matter what. Because Lola was 18 days overdue, I was willing to wait that long again and the obstetricians hesitantly agreed. Anytime beyond that though and I would have to be induced. They would not be happy to monitor me daily anymore; they just wanted to get my baby out.

I was still trying the entire home-inducing techniques in the book. Nothing really set me off so I had to agree to being induced on my 19th day overdue. It was a Friday, and we went fully prepared to hospital in the afternoon around 4.30pm. They were going to insert the Foley's Catheter that evening to try and get things started, and if nothing happened, I would have my waters broken. It was amazing. My due date was the 1st October and my birthday was on the 21st. Realistically, I was going to share the same birthday as my baby. It was very exciting. I never thought I would have to wait 20 days to meet him!

All of my anxiety disappeared because by this stage I was OK with the idea of being induced. I was ready to have my baby and I had played a mental game for far too long. I realised that I would have to change a few things on my birth plan but was OK with that too.

The birthing room was larger than I had envisioned, and we had a lovely midwife who knew some mutual friends of Craig's from the Goldfields. I had a portable telemetry

439

machine which allowed me to stay mobile. Once the Foley's Catheter was inserted, I asked if I could move around. We were told that we could go for a walk into Subiaco but only for half an hour or so. Once outside, I rang my mum to keep her updated and she was excited for us. She too knew that she would be meeting him soon. I also called Gaby and she would come in the next morning once things started happening. We walked and it was a beautiful balmy evening. I wished we could stay outside because it seemed to me to like my first taste of a summer night for the year. We held hands and chatted; we were both very relaxed. I was very uncomfortable though. He was pressing on my bladder and every so often I would get a really sharp pain. I guess I waddled, not walked!

Once we got back to the room, I had a cool shower. It felt wonderful and I did not want to get out. I got back onto the bed and we watched some TV. Since the baby pressed on my bladder so much, I was off to the toilet constantly. When I got up to go again the catheter fell out. We called for the midwife and she said not to worry, it was a good thing because that meant I was already 3cm dilated. There was no need to insert it again; they would just wait until the morning to break my waters. I was contracting all of the time and I could see it on the trace printout. I thought the constant monitoring would be a burden, but I found it reassuring. I could hear his heartbeat, and as long as it was consistent, I found great comfort in that. Craig decided to go home around 10pm to get some rest. I was grateful the catheter was out because it wasn't very comfortable so I could now try to get a decent night's rest. I went to sleep with the sound of my baby's heartbeat.

I was woken around 6am and found it hard to get any more rest. Before I knew it, Craig arrived. I quietly reminded him that he forgot to say happy birthday to me but quickly forgave his forgetfulness. I understood that it was quite insignificant compared to what we were about to go through. The obstetrician also arrived, and she seemed to WHOOSH in and flick the lights on which were quite startling. I had met her during one of my monitoring visits and liked her. I was thankful she wasn't a male. She told me it could be quite uncomfortable breaking the waters, but it was no problem at all. I had a couple of stretch and sweeps during my monitored visits and she did another one. I was still contracting so they gave me until lunch time to go into labour. I was quite calm and felt no pressure. By this stage I was OK with the idea of being given the syntocinon. I knew I wouldn't need much as I felt I was so close.

Our midwife for the morning shift was wonderful. I felt comfortable with her and she was very supportive of VBAC's. I knew she would be on our side. My contractions were getting stronger, and I had started to breathe with them. I was standing near the door when I saw a familiar face. It was Sara David. I could not believe it. I wondered what was going on. How could she happen to be there for Alison, and here she was standing in front of me? She saw my name on the list and could not believe it herself. She was aware of my due date and found it hard to believe how overdue I was as well. She apologised to me because she would have swapped shifts if she knew I was booked in. I totally understood it was out of her control, but she did pull a few strings for us though. She said she would talk to the obstetrician and see if she could get me off the monitor and get us out for a walk. She came back smiling and told us to do so and when we got back, I should get in the shower and try some nipple stimulation. She was nearly ready to finish her shift, so she gave me a huge hug and expressed her faith in me.

We just walked around the block but this time it was slow going. It was a warm day, and I felt those sharp stabs in my bladder. I was still blown away at the fact I had just seen Sara. It was fate and I felt empowered once again. When we got back, I showered and tried some nipple stimulation. I almost rubbed them off! Kristyn, our midwife, popped her head in to see if I was OK. I was concerned about wasting water! She told me to not worry about it and to stay in for a bit longer. Gaby had arrived and tried to stimulate some pressure points on my lower legs to see if that would help. She seemed concerned that I had not let go. I was not sure and started to doubt myself again. I got over that fairly quickly as we all discussed the possibility of having the syntocinon. I was OK with it and Gaby was sure all I needed was a tiny amount to get me going and that it would not be a bad thing.

I was not able to bring my labour on in the given time frame so at lunchtime I gave in and had the syntocinon. It took about an hour for the contractions to kick in strong and regular. I had a good feeling; his heartbeat was stable, and it was reassuring. I tried sitting on a fitball and rocked with each contraction but in the end, I found it most comfortable on my knees leaning over the bed. So much for my active labour, I did not want to move from that position!

Because of the syntocinon I was not having long breaks between my contractions; they were mostly a couple of minutes apart and very intense. I was coping well and breathing through each one. Being induced was not as bad as I had heard. I was making groaning sounds that I had never heard come out of my mouth before; it seemed very primal, so I just went with it. At no stage did I think of asking for pain relief. I just breathed through each contraction, in for four and out for six, just like I was taught. I was amazed at the power of them. It was very intense.

Gaby and Craig took turns in massaging my lower back which I found very relieving. I did wish I could get into a bath, but the monitor did not allow for it. It was all a bit of a blur from there because I went completely into myself and was not really aware of what was going on around. I was just focusing on getting through each contraction. I do think the amount of syntocinon administered was turned up at some stage though. Gaby kept on giving me sips of water and wiped my face with a wet flannel. It was hard work and I felt really hot.

The obstetrician came in a couple of times and I could tell she was anxious. She seemed to want to intervene and not let me go. As far as I was concerned things were progressing well. Because of his position and the way I was leaning over the bed, it was difficult for the monitor to pick up his heartbeat. She suggested that we use a monitoring clip that is attached to the top of bubs scalp. I did not want to do this at first but reluctantly agreed the second time she suggested it. I had to get on the bed and lay on my back. She had a difficult time attaching it and it was harder to get through a contraction this way.

As I said it's still a bit of a blur, but I heard some discussion about how dilated I was. I remember Gaby leaning over and saying quietly into my ear that I was fully dilated, and I should get up onto that bed and push. I could not believe it and asked if she was sure. She was smiling and seemed excited. She told me that she could see his head and it was full of dark hair. I could not believe it because I had gotten through the hardest part and I was nearly there. With each contraction I pushed as hard as I could. I kept on pooing with each push, and I remember laughing with Gaby about it. She told me not to worry and that she was taking care of it!

The obstetrician was in again at some stage and she was concerned I would not be able to push him out on my own. She said that I would need some help with suction, and she wanted to take me to surgery and give me a spinal block just in case I had to have a caesarean. All because his heartbeat dipped a bit when I was pushing, I thought surely this is normal and I tried to stay calm. This was not what I wanted to hear at all. I felt I had no choice because I did not want to put my baby at risk. I had not even considered pain relief and now I had to face the fact that I may have to have an epidural, perhaps un-necessarily.

I was wheeled to a room where they were to put the epi-dural in and was trying very hard not to panic. I didn't want to leave Craig and Gaby but was reassured they would see me in surgery. I had to sit upright on the edge of the bed with my feet up on a stool, knees bent. This was the most uncomforta-ble position to be in when I had to push and I was getting frus-trated because the anaesthetist was telling me to keep still. I wasn't sure if I was supposed to stop myself from pushing or not. They told me to keep pushing but it made me angry. How was I supposed to keep still and push? I am amazed how skilled these people must be, to be able to insert a needle in the spine quickly.

I was starting to feel like my control of the situation was being taken away and I think Kristyn, my midwife, sensed how I was feeling. She was so supportive. When we were having a hard time getting the monitor in a good place, I think she sat on the floor and held it there by hand for a couple of hours. Her shift was supposed to finish at 7pm but she stayed on to be with me, holding my hand most of the time. She was very re-assuring. Eve, the other midwife who was taking over her shift, was there as well and I had previously met her during one of my clinic visits. I was glad she was there too.

Once in surgery Craig and Gaby joined me. It was great to have them by my side as well as those two wonderful midwives. I dreaded having another caesarean, but the midwives reassured me that I was still going to push him out, I just needed some extra help. I could not feel when I was contracting at all so I was told when to push. Everybody was cheering me on. It was bizarre not to feel anything after the intensity of what I had just been through. I could not tell how hard I was pushing so it took me a few contractions to get there.

When he was finally pulled out at 7.30pm, I got to hold him straight away on my chest. It was something that I craved to experience the most. It felt incredible. He was warm and bloody, but I noticed there was not much vernix on him. He also looked rather blue. He was taken to a crib after my short cuddle to get some oxygen. I was trying to watch what was going on and I saw Craig standing over him, watching as well. He wanted to know when I could get to hold him. They just wanted to make sure that his pink colour returned, and his tongue was pink. He was screaming; what a good set of lungs he had. I could not wait to hold him.

The obstetrician was concerned that I had lost more blood than normal because I had torn internally quite a bit. I also discovered that she gave me an episiotomy. I dreaded this as I knew it would be a painful recovery. She spent a lot of time stitching me up. I believe the recovery from the episiotomy was just as bad as recovering from a caesarean. My episiotomy scar is about an inch long and it took me a few weeks to build up the courage to look at it once I returned home.

He was finally brought over to me and placed on my chest. I was congratulated. He was wrapped in a blanket and I was relieved because his colour had come back. He looked amazing. He had very dark features and heaps of dark hair. I looked inside the blanket and saw that he had a hairy back, shoulders and bottom! He looked like a little man. I was instantly in love. I didn't experience this with Lola's birth because of my emergency caesarean. She is the light of my life now but it did take me longer to bond with her. A positive birth definitely makes a difference when bonding with your baby.

I tried to put him to my breast, but it was awkward because of all the tubes in my arms and I was flat on my back. I had to keep one arm stretched out. He was trying to suckle, and I had a good feeling that the breast feeding would go well. He managed to latch on and I got to keep him with me from then on. It was a great feeling. Once in recovery I had started to shiver uncontrollably. It was a side effect from the anaesthetic, and it was very unpleasant. The epidural line was still in my back and blood had started to leak into it. This meant that I had to have it removed and I was grateful for that. I hated it being there. Craig had gone to make the phone calls to family and friends. They were all eagerly waiting to hear from us.

I was starving but was advised not to eat because I might have had to go back to surgery if the bleeding did not subside. I wasn't even allowed to have a drink of water. I was wheeled back to our birthing room and it looked different. The feeling had slowly started creeping back to my legs. I kept on trying to wiggle my toes. Craig, Gaby and I discussed what we had all just been through and I felt a great sense of achievement. Even though I had more intervention than intended, I still managed to birth my baby vaginally; something I had to experience and can truly say was the most amazing experience of my life. The obstetrician returned and informed me that the bleeding had subsided. I could finally have something to eat and drink. Nothing touched my sides; I had built up such an appetite and thirst.

Gaby, exhausted herself, left us around 10.30pm and Craig and I were left in our room to enjoy our baby. He was finally weighed and measured and was a big 4.11kg and 51cm long. We still had not named him. He initially had a hard time attaching to my breast, but once on, he stayed suckling for hours. I hardly took my eyes off him. Craig had to go home to get some rest himself and I was taken up to the ward around 3 or 4am. I felt slightly delirious. I think it was a combination of the anaesthetic and my natural high. I slept so well that night in between waking to feed him. I knew that there would be no chance of the baby blues, not after this birth.

The next morning, when I got out of bed, it felt as if I had been hit by a truck. I was very swollen around the episiotomy site and I had a huge amount of gauze stuffed inside me to stop the bleeding. I was advised to stay horizontal until it was removed. I had a wonderful visit from Kristyn, the midwife. I gave her a huge hug and thanked her for all of her support. She thanked me and said that she went home and could not stop talking about our birth. She said it was one of the most inspiring births she had experienced. She loved the idea of pain relief free births and was very pro VBAC. She also said how wonderful it was to have Gaby's support. She said sometimes during labour, she felt like she could not do enough to help the birthing mother because of paperwork etc. She said she appreciated the help of a doula because she felt less pressure and knew the birthing mother had good support.

I only spent a couple of days in the hospital and was looking forward to going home. We finally named him the day we left. He was to be known as Ronan James. Lola loved the name Jack so when we got home we changed it to Ronan Jack to keep her happy and make her feel involved.

If we decide to have another child, I will definitely consider a homebirth with the support of Gaby again and a private midwife. I now have the confidence in my body's ability to give birth. I could not have done it without Gaby's support before, during and after Ronan's birth and for that I am forever grateful. Her own birth stories were inspiring. She will always have a special place in my heart. From Ronan's birth I gained the friendship of Alison as well. We have a connection now that will never leave us and I'm sure we will both be self-appointed advocates for women attempting a VBAC!

Every woman's body is different. We were not all meant to birth in the same way, not according to an obstetrician's schedule anyway. We need to understand the value of woman-to-woman support and that birthing is women's business; we have been doing it for millions of years. Nobody will understand the type of support a birthing mother needs more than that of a doula or midwife. These women need to be more recognised and celebrated because if it wasn't for them, empowering births would not be achieved, and natural childbirth would be a thing of the past.

Nathalie's VBAC story

My first baby girl was delivered by caesarean in 2014. Although it was a beautiful, gentle caesarean (as it wasn't an emergency and they put the baby on me skin to skin straight after the procedure), it was still not the vaginal birth that I had been dreaming of for so long.

I'm still unsure about whether the caesarean was really necessary and regret not having asked enough questions of my obstetrician at the time. Essentially, at 36 weeks the obstetrician said baby was measuring a bit small and because of that, he didn't want me to go past my estimated due date at 40 weeks as he said that could put the baby at risk. It also didn't help that my estimated due date was just around Christmas (with lots of hospital staff on leave), so not very "convenient" for my obstetrician. Therefore, in my 39th week the obstetrician attempted to "induce" me with a few stretches and sweeps and some gel, but my cervix wasn't ready and my baby hadn't dropped, so there was no way it was going to work. So he told us he recommended a caesarean and trusting him, we just agreed without question. But we had a beautiful, healthy baby girl and she is the love of our lives.

And there began my VBAC journey.

In many ways, having the caesarean was a blessing as it resulted in me going down a path I never thought I would have (i.e. not using a private obstetrician) and having the most incredibly amazing and empowering vaginal birth. An even better labour and birth experience than I had ever hoped for. Following the caesarean, I did a lot of research about how to give myself the best chance at having a successful VBAC. My husband and I met with Gaby Targett and had a post-birth debrief where she helped me to feel confident that my body was able to birth vaginally and helped me to trust my body and understand that I hadn't really been given the chance to labour. I attended VBAC information sessions and read many VBAC birth stories and knew I could do it for my second labour/birth.

451

When we fell pregnant we decided to go with a private midwife rather than an obstetrician. Something I would never have done before (purely because I didn't know it was an option and because I thought that just everyone used an obstetrician).

I decided I wanted to birth my second baby in a hospital but wanted to labour at home for as long as possible. Because my midwife had admitting rights at a public hospital, this was possible.

All went well with my second pregnancy, as it had with my first. The midwife came to our house for our appointments, and we attended a few appointments at the hospital with an obstetrician (hospital policy). In my first hospital appointment (with my midwife in attendance), the obstetrician spent the whole time running through the risks of a VBAC compared to an elective caesarean and told us how likely she thought I would be to have a successful VBAC. She also mentioned that I was quite short and looked like I might have a small pelvis (!) and therefore this might affect my ability to have a successful VBAC. But we were prepared for the appointment to go this way and we just smiled, told her we were aware of the risks and I didn't allow it to create any doubt or negativity in my mind about my ability to birth vaginally. To my relief, our following hospital appointments were much more positive.

It was always my plan to book in for a natural induction massage with Gaby towards the end of my pregnancy. It just so happened that she was leaving for a trip two weeks before my estimated due date. I still wanted to have the massage, so I booked in with her for two weeks prior knowing that my body was still a while away from going into labour but knowing that it would still be of benefit. The massage was amazing and really helped me to relax, focus my attention on my body and to actually picture in my mind how I envisaged my labour and birth to go. I really do feel that the massage helped to start things going (physically, emotionally and mentally).

Labour and birth

On the night of my estimated due date, I started having contractions/tightenings throughout the night. They were uncomfortable enough to keep me from sleeping well but were very irregular, ranging from 15 minutes apart to 5 or so minutes apart. They continued throughout the night and started tapering off by morning. These nightly contractions continued for the next 3 nights. My midwife attempted to do a stretch and sweep on my estimated date but couldn't as although my cervix was starting to soften, it had not yet started to dilate. My midwife was not at all concerned and put absolutely no pressure on me about the fact that my estimated date had passed, saying that this was all part of pre-labour and that my body was doing exactly what it needed to do to prepare for labour and birth. This gave me the confidence that I needed to trust my body and the thought of having another caesarean never crossed my mind. I felt safe and in control.

453

A few days before the baby was born, I had the "show" and I also started to feel a bit nauseous. I had read that these were often a sign that labour wasn't too far off, so this helped my confidence to grow.

Three nights after my estimated date, my midwife did another check and I was only just 1 centimetre dilated and she was able to perform a stretch and sweep. My body was doing the work it needed to prepare for my labour and birth (albeit slowly). Four nights later my nightly contractions grew in intensity and were getting closer together (despite still being very irregular). I couldn't sleep at all as I was needing to concentrate with each contraction. I was unsure if this was the start of labour but decided to call my midwife in the early hours of the morning. She told me that it sounded like things were possibly starting to ramp up and asked if I needed her to come over to our house. But I felt calm and was happy to get back into bed and continue letting my body do what it needed to do until morning.

At 7am in the morning, the contractions were really starting to take my breath away and I decided I wanted to get into the bath which was such a good idea. It helped me to relax, and I continued to breathe through the contractions until about 9:30am when I asked my husband to call the midwife and ask if she could come over. The contractions were growing in intensity and were getting closer together but were still quite irregular. At this stage, my mum had come over to our house to keep my 2-year-old toddler occupied. The midwife arrived and performed a check and to my (and her) surprise, I was already 4cm dilated. I was so proud and relieved that my body was in active labour and that I had managed so well up until that stage.

The midwife asked if I wanted to go to the hospital or to stay home and I was happy to stay home for a bit longer (hoping for things to continue to progress as well as they had so far). I got back into the bath and continued to labour on my own for another couple of hours. I felt confident and had allowed myself to go into a completely different 'zone' where I wasn't thinking of anything other than what my body was doing and my baby. I then reached a point where things were really starting to build in intensity, and I was feeling a lot of downward pressure. I knew that if I didn't get out of the bath at that stage that I wouldn't want to make the journey to the hospital and my husband and I just felt more comfortable birthing in the hospital. So, we decided to leave for the hospital and decided to wait to see how dilated I was until we got to the hospital.

Thankfully, the trip to the hospital was short and we managed to get a parking spot right in front of the entrance. The midwife met us there and we walked to the labour ward (with me having to stop and lean against a wall a few times to breathe through my contractions). We got to our birth suite and the midwife made it feel so comfortable, warm and as homely as possible, keeping the lights dim. It was exactly how I had pictured it to be.

The midwife performed another check, and I was 7cm dilated! We couldn't believe how quickly things had progressed and knew we would be meeting our baby soon. The downward pressure was growing in intensity, but the thought of an epidural never crossed my mind (and in fact, it might have been too late at that stage for one anyway). I started off standing beside the bed and leaning over it, but then decided I would be more comfortable lying down on the bed (which I never thought I would have done). So, for the next hour or so, I laboured on my side on the bed. It was just our midwife, my husband and I in the room, with the occasional midwife and obstetrician from the hospital quietly popping in to check things were ok and then leaving. My waters then broke and from that point, things progressed very quickly, and I started to feel the urge to push. Within about 15 minutes, our beautiful baby girl was born in the July of 2017.

My VBAC was the most empowering, beautiful, extraordinary thing I have ever experienced. I knew I could do it and I did. And the thought of potentially needing another caesarean never crossed my mind as I had complete trust in my body's ability to birth and just let go of any fear that I may have had and let my body do what it needed to do. I felt so safe and that was mostly due to having such an incredible midwife who made our hospital experience feel as close as possible to a homebirth. Our bodies are amazing and I am so grateful to have experienced such an incredible VBAC.

Keeva Marybelle Morgan – born on 1.01.2016 at 1.17am, 3.42kg

An Amazing VBBAC – Vaginal Breech Birth After Caesarean

Well, my birth story really begins with the pregnancy and birth of my first child in Feb 2014. Skye was born via 'elective' c section after being confirmed breech at around 2 8weeks. I tried everything to get her to turn...inversions, moxibustion, homoeopathic remedies etc...but she wouldn't budge! She also was suspected of Intrauterine growth restriction (IUGR), so from 28 weeks I was in hospital 2-3 times per week for CTG monitoring and ultrasounds, which turned my low risk stress free pregnancy into quite the opposite. No issues were found on the ultrasounds but this didn't take away the stress of the unknown. As I reached full term and she was still breech. I was given no other option but C section, even though I really didn't want one.

I was told an ECV was not an option due to the suspected IUGR. My dream of a drug free waterbirth went straight out the window and I felt helpless and cheated. So, on 20.02.2014 I arrived at the hospital for my C section and Skye entered the world a few hours later. All my wishes for a more natural C section were refused (immediate skin to skin, music etc). However, I had a beautiful and healthy baby girl weighing 2.68kg (small but not IUGR!) I found the first few days of recovery quite overwhelming. It was a struggle to even pick up my baby and the drugs I was on did not agree with me. However once

457

we were home I recovered pretty well physically. Mentally though, the birth made me feel sad and it was something I did my best not to talk about.

In April 2015 I discovered I was pregnant again! I was so excited this time, planning for my VBAC and looking forward to the experience of having a natural birth. However on my first VBAC appointment I was told I wasn't allowed to be in the birthing pool and that I would need continuous monitoring...once again not what I had in mind. At this point I decided to look at some other options such as an independent midwife. I got in touch with a private midwife through The Birth House and decided that I would change my care from the hospital to them. I felt so excited as their approach was much more natural and supportive. However, at this point (around 30weeks) it was once again confirmed that my baby was sitting in the breech position. I tried to stay positive as I know there was a much higher chance of this baby turning than not.

Once again I tried all the techniques to help the baby flip, including weekly chiropractic sessions, but further ultrasounds at 32 and 36 weeks showed the baby was still head up. Unfortunately, this meant that once again my birth plan was slipping away. I felt angry and cheated for a second time. The midwife was unable to assist in the birth of my baby and would have to refer me back to the hospital. Luckily, I had kept in contact with the Vaginal Birth After Caesarean Head Obstetric consultant at the hospital, who had actually been very understanding of my labour plan and determination to avoid a repeat C section. So I attended appointments at the hospital with my private midwife (in case the baby turned head down).

After reaching 37 weeks and with the baby still breech, the Obstetrician agreed to try an ECV- manual turning of the baby (reluctantly!). He knew that unless there was an emergency, I was going to have a natural birth. So, at 38 weeks I went in for the ECV, but unfortunately it was unsuccessful. Although I shed a small tear or two, I soon felt like a weight had been lifted...I now knew the situation and was able to start planning rather than floating in limbo!

I had already been reading all the pro natural birthing books that I could. Now I researched everything on breech births that I could get my hands on. I began to feel quite excited again at the thought of having a natural breech birth, though I understood the risks involved. I decided to keep my midwife as a support person for when I went into labour, as I knew I would need more than my partner there if I was going to go against hospital policy and birth this baby vaginally. It was a comfort to know that she was going to be there to support both my partner and I through it all.

I wrote up a birth plan for my natural breech birth and also for a natural C-section, should an emergency arise and I had to go down that road again. I felt relaxed and excited about my birth again and of course to meet my baby. My Obstetrician advised me of the hospital policies but also clearly stated that at the end of the day it was my choice and they could not force me to do anything. He happily made notes in my file and took my birth plans. Now we just had to sit back and wait...

My estimated date was 30.12.15 and in the small hours of 31.12.15 I was woken up with some tightening. I had to breathe through them but I went straight back to sleep after a while. I got up around 8am and had another couple of tightening before I headed off for an acupuncture appointment at 9am. (the acupuncture was to help get labour started!) As the day continued, so did the tightening in my uterus although I continued to tell my partner and parents that it was probably just false labour and not to worry! Having not been in labour before, I didn't really know what to expect. We continued to make plans for our New Year's Eve family dinner.

At around 6pm I realised that the tightenings were increasing in intensity and also frequency (around every 8 mins) so I decided to get in touch with my midwife and also send my toddler off to her grandparents as she was starting to get stressed seeing me stopping to breathe through the now surges. My midwife said it sounded like it was happening, and that I should get back in touch once the surges had increased. I couldn't believe that I was actually in labour! At 8pm she came over after I called. By this time, I was in the shower to help with the intensity, which it did.

In between surges I was still very relaxed and able to chat normally, so she decided to leave us until they had increased more. I continued to try various positions, used stress balls, massage and also laid down to get some rest. By 10pm my partner called the midwife again, surges were now around every 4 minutes and were pretty intense. I was also vomiting in between them. We decided to do a vaginal examination just to ensure I was dilating (I didn't want to go to hospital too early and risk interventions and pressure from staff). Luckily the VE showed I was 6-7cms and my waters were bulging! It was time to get in the car and dash to the hospital. Thank goodness, the roads were quiet!

We arrived at the hospital around 11pm and I was introduced to my birth team. They had my folder and knew my plan, however the pressure was put on me to follow hospital policy and have a caesarean. I repeated that I would be having a natural birth unless there was an emergency at which point the 'on-call' Obstetrician that night standing in front of me said something along the lines of "well you may well end up with a dead baby on your hands then". I was shocked by this comment, and in my head I started to feel nervous. I turned to my partner to see his reaction.

He looked to the OB and said in a calm voice "we want to have a natural birth." In an instant, I got my confidence back and knew that we were not going to crumble to the pressure. Luckily, he disappeared shortly after and I was left with the hospital midwife and registrar who had a much better attitude. I decided to have a cannula so that I could have some fluids as I

461

had been sick so many times (I think they got it in on the 3rd attempt!) I was also hooked up to the CTG machine which was originally against my wishes but to be honest I really wasn't aware of it once it was on. After we were all set up, my independent midwife who was still with me encouraged me to go to the toilet to keep me active. Afterwards I got up on the bed and onto my knees, facing the head end with it lifted up so I could lean over it. I had my partner on one side and my independent midwife Pia on the other, both of them keeping me focused on my breathing and encouraging me. I was vocalising so much I'm sure the whole hospital could hear me...but I didn't care!

I was aware of the pressure increasing in my bottom and visualised the baby moving down. The surges were now really intense with almost no break and I started to think that I may not be able to continue much longer (I assumed this was transition!) The registrar asked if she could do a VE to see how I was doing...I told her there was no way I could lie on my back but luckily, she was able to do it without me moving and I stayed on my hands and knees. I was almost there...just a tiny bit of cervix at the rim she stated! I just had to keep doing what I was doing. Soon though, the urge to push was uncontrollable...I was trying not to push but my body just took over. Then I heard the best words in the world "if you feel the urge to push then go ahead". YES! I knew then that we were almost there. The baby's bum could be seen. On the next surge, I pushed as much as I could and the baby emerged...bum then body, with its legs up towards its face. One leg dropped out and then I gave a little push to help the other leg drop out.

The registrar then asked Pia and my partner Michael to support me under both arms and help lift my body back away from the head of the bed to help the head out. On my next surge, I pushed with everything I had to get the head out...and the next thing I hear is you've done it! I opened my eyes and there in front of me on the bed was my beautiful, perfect little baby. I was overjoyed and in shock I couldn't do anything but just stare! The happiness in the room was amazing. However, the baby was a bit flat so my partner quickly cut the cord and she was taken to a table across the room to be given air. She responded quickly and her newborn cry filled the room. I was so so happy. She was brought straight back over to me for skin to skin (only now did we actually realise that she was a girl!) This moment was everything I had wished for.

I decided to have the injection to birth my placenta as there had been some bleeding and the registrar strongly advised me to. I was able to breastfeed my baby the whole time. I also needed a couple of stitches but nothing major. Soon after it was just me, my partner and our new baby girl enjoying the moment and watching the sunrise on New Year's morning. It was beautiful. We decided to leave the hospital as soon as we could. I had given birth at 1.17am and by 7am we were in the car heading home with our new addition and pinching ourselves that we actually DID IT!!!

463

Although I didn't get the relaxed waterbirth I had always wanted...I think I got so much more! It wasn't easy and didn't come without a lot of hurdles but when I think back to it now it fills me with so much joy and I just know it was the right thing for me to do. I did not conform to what people thought I should be doing. I was informed and educated on natural breech births and I was supported by an amazing partner and independent midwife who believed in me. I went into it with my eyes wide open, but more so with the unwavering belief that I could do anything I put my mind to. "She believed she could, so she did". <3

Laura Beveridge

The Birth of Soren Ray Ravaei 30/11/17

At 41 weeks pregnant and as the days wore on, I was getting edgy and losing my confidence. I had felt empowered and ready but the last couple of weeks of pregnancy are hard and even harder when you go over the 40-week mark. The pressure came not from myself but from those around me. The well-meaning texts, messages and phone calls from excited family and friends, although lovely, made me want to hide away completely.

On Tuesday morning 28/11 I had some powerful acupuncture and felt Soren respond to this immediately. He was kicking hard and punching me as if to ask "what's going on Mum?!" Although this definitely got a response from the baby, he still just wasn't quite ready. In the evening I had a beautiful induction massage with Gabrielle Targett (Author of A Labour of Love). I was wrapped in deliciously warm towels of clary sage and massaged from head to toe as Gabrielle talked me through a guided visualisation and some positive affirmations. I visualised Soren in his optimum position, descending down the birth canal and being birthed naturally. I visualised my support team and the energy in the birth space. I told Soren that we could do this together, to work as a team, and that it was safe for him to meet us now. I told him how important it was for me to experience natural birth and that I trusted him completely.

On Wednesday morning 29/11 I woke up in an emotional wreck. A hot mess of hormones. I took my son to school and then went for an ocean swim. The sky was dark and grey, but the air was humid.

I cried, sobbing as I lay on my back in the cold water and held my massive belly... unsure as to why I was feeling so crappy and so over being pregnant. I spent the rest of the day crying on the couch and watching Offspring on Netflix.

My mum picked my son Jett up from school thank goodness and gave me a big hug as she left. I told her to keep her phone close in case I needed her to have Jett that night. By the time my husband came home, and I had done the homework and dinner routine, I was in a bad mood. I kicked both the boys out of the house - they went to play soccer, and I felt relieved that I had some space to just be. I had a long hot shower, diffused some oils and settled back on the couch. This labour had to start soon!

I noticed the windows needed to be cleaned (nesting will do that to you!) and so went to get some lemon juice and news-paper... I stood on a stool to clean the highest window when POP! Water started running down my legs... had I strained my-self and wee'd? Or was this it? I jumped down and more water came out, and then some more. I wasn't sure if it was my water breaking because with my first son, they had burst and gushed like a tidal wave over the bedroom floor.

This was gentler. At 8pm I texted my midwife "I'm pretty sure my waters just broke... I'll be in touch" and called my doula.

Then the adrenaline kicked in. I excitedly called my husband, three of my best friends and my mum. I had a shower, washed my hair, shaved my legs and put a bit of makeup on (ridiculous I know but I had a birth photographer coming)

I wasn't having contractions yet but I put on my beautiful labour beads from my blessing way, and set up a comfortable birth space by the altar I had created full of affirmations, crystals and beads that had been gifted to me and inspiring pictures, words and images. I wasn't birthing at home but planned to labour at home as long as possible before heading to the hospital.

My husband arrived home from soccer and both him and my son went to bed. I told them to rest and relax as the baby was sure to arrive if not tonight then tomorrow.

By 10pm my surges had started rolling in, steady but gentle. I started using the breathing techniques I had learnt at yoga and Hypnobirthing. I wanted to get into a rhythm and zone from the get-go. I did some yoga and laid down on the mat with a bolster and rested, half awake and half asleep, not quite able to completely switch off. By about 12.30am I was really having to focus on my breathing and couldn't ignore the surges, as they required all of my attention. I was repeating in my mind "breathe through it and then let it go. Breathe through it and then let it go". This really helped me to focus on each surge as an individual hurdle rather than labour as a huge, long marathon.

I started timing the surges and realised they were coming in strong and consistently. I called my doula, birth photographer and my midwife who listened to me have one surge over the phone and decided that we should all meet at King Edward hospital instead of at home. I was well and truly in active labour. I woke my husband and called my Mum over to watch my son.

By the time Mum arrived it was about 2.30am and I was in labour land. Unable to talk and desperate to get to hospital to set up space. Throughout my pregnancy my greatest anxiety had been about the transition from home to hospital. My

467

husband drove calmly and quickly through the eerie stillness of night as I was vocalising loudly in the back seat. Breathing in for 4 and "om-ing" out for 6 on every out breath. The surges were getting intense.

My beautiful doula Kelly met us at the car and escorted us inside where we met Cat, our photographer. We checked in and were ushered to a birth suite once Mel, our midwife, had arrived. As I focused on each surge, my birth squad worked quickly and quietly around me, setting up and holding space as we all settled into a steady rhythm, taking each surge one by one.

To me, the energy was calm and controlled. Everyone held space so beautifully. I was aware of my husband, quietly observing in the corner but also there for quiet and strong reassurance every so often. My doula, whispering words of support and providing physical support by way of massage and hip squeezes, the photographer snapping away -I barely noticed her as she moved so seamlessly around the room, she knew how to be present in a birth space without intruding. And my midwife, a pillar of strength. Sitting, observing and offering words of support. She held space and kept the hospital staff away.

We moved between the bathroom, sitting on the toilet, hip swaying and eventually ended up on all fours on the bed. We carried on for a couple of hours in a cycle of surge, breathe, peak, let it go, relax, rest. I remember being so proud of myself that I was doing it! I was labouring! Naturally! No drugs! And so, in control. A vast difference from my first birth experience.

Until I was having two surges in a row and my vocalisation became intense and primal, uncontrollable roars from deep within. I could feel Soren moving down the birth canal and the pressure felt so intense I remember asking everyone "is this normal?!" And "this is fucked!" And they all just smiled and told me yep, it's normal and I'm birthing my baby beautifully.

After a while I was urged by the hospital to have some monitoring as Mel was having trouble picking up a heartbeat with the Doppler and with the straps. Not surprising considering I was moving around and finding it hard to keep still. I eventually consented to electronic foetal monitoring as I knew the risks of having a vaginal birth after a c-section and could understand that it was important to monitor Soren.

Meanwhile, the pressure was becoming more and more intense! And I was making noises that I had no control over. I was birthing my baby!

The next 20 minutes or so were a blur as the hospital weren't happy with Soren's heart rate and started to prepare for Caesarean. This was disheartening because it was sudden and disempowering after I had felt that both Soren and I were doing so well. I knew he was about to be born so I was pissed off that the hospital staff had forced their way into my birth space to burst my bubble.

Upon reflection, this just highlights for me the importance of having continuity of care and trust in your care providers. Without this, women have little hope of no intervention. I have no doubt my pregnancy and birth experience would have been vastly different if not for the amazing support of my midwife who was with us throughout our entire pregnancy.

The doctor requested a VE first to which I consented even though I found it incredibly hard to move onto my back for it. I eventually did between surges and the Dr was surprised to feel Soren's head! He was nearly here!

That gave me all the inspiration I needed! I had laboured so well, with such loving support! I was NOT going to have a repeat caesarean. With my birth squad surrounding me, and the words of my midwife "you're doing it!!"

I gave birth to my beautiful boy in four minutes. The sting of his head emerging felt incredible! A baby was coming out of my vagina!! In three almighty pushes. With not a tear.

Soren was placed on my chest in a flurry of camera snaps and tears and elation and emotion.

I did it! I got my VBAC!

Soren Ray Ravaei arrived at 6.04am Thursday 30/1/17. The same birth date as his cousin Noa (who also had the same midwife).

The first hour of his arrival earth side was beautiful and peaceful as we delayed his cord clamping, had a feed and had skin to skin with Mummy and Daddy while I waited to birth the placenta (those surges though were just as intense as labour contractions)

We were in a bubble of love. My Mum and big boy, Jett, came to meet Soren and we had beautiful photos as a family.

Mel worked hard to clean the space and I had a shower while my husband held Soren and we got ready to leave. Soren was eventually checked over and weighed and measured. 9 pounds 11 oz of pure health and perfection.

I felt so incredible on a natural Oxytocin high and so happy that I had fulfilled my dream that I had worked so hard for over the previous nine months.... or closer to eight years since my first traumatic birth experience.

By 10.00am we were back at home, all cuddled up in bed and snuggling as a family. I was so elated that I was able to birth my baby and leave straight away to begin my fourth trimester at home. Again, this was with the support of my incredible midwife. We were so happy and couldn't have dreamed of a better birth experience.

In my opinion, a VBAC is something that you have to work for. It takes education, empowerment, the right care providers to be with, supporting you and preparation.

I am forever grateful to my awesome birth squad who knew how important it was to me to have this experience, to my husband who trusted the process and to Soren... my beautiful VBAC baby, who knew exactly what to do. This birth truly healed me and has only made my passion for women and their birthing rights stronger.

Dani's Positive and Empowered VBAC

I got my VBAC!!! I wanted to share my story hoping it will help anyone else that needs to hear a positive VBAC story. My first was born 2 years ago via a C-section due to 'CPD' at the time I didn't know any better and they made me labour on my back and failed to wait to let me give birth naturally. During the surgery I tore downwards as they were doing the incision, so they told me I was 'not allowed' to have a natural birth next time. The experience was very traumatic and still scares me to this day but got me motivated to get informed and made me realise that this is my body and I get to decide what type of birth I would like to have next time around.

Fast track to today and at 40+1 weeks I gave birth to my beautiful daughter Abigail on 13th of April 2017, naturally in a 3-hour labour from start to finish with no drugs. She weighed 3.58kgs and had a decent sized head on her, yet I managed to push her out even though I was told my pelvis would be too small to do so and that I would risk my baby's life due to increased risk of rupture! I stayed in an upright position which I think made the difference.

For me the most important part of my journey began when I met the most amazing doula Anaya Watts. Without her, I can guarantee the outcome would have been different. She was so important during the pregnancy when all the doctors were trying every scare tactic -she kept me strong and believing in myself and ability to birth and to keep me going during the labour to achieve everything I wanted.

So, for everyone out there please remember the female body is amazing and we just need to believe in ourselves and support each other.

8.

EMPOWERED
LABOUR INDUCTIONS

Michaela's Birth Story of Nyx, 4th June 2006

I was 11 years old when I attended the birth of my first sister, and 13 when I witnessed my second sister being born. I have wonderful memories of my mother's pregnancy, preparation and births. It was a peaceful, calm and beautiful family experience. I don't know what inspired my parents to do this back in the 80's but I'm glad they did. I remember my mother's strength and determination being a strong birthing woman, empowered and having her own natural births.

My second birth inspiration is my aunt who had three successful home births. She is a journalist and advocate for women and their right to birth naturally. Having such strong female mentors and role models to look up to, it never occurred to me that when I finally had children, birthing naturally would be negotiable or questionable. Growing up I found myself just as strong and determined with the same expectations my mother and aunt had. I was against the medical profession which I call 'the establishment' and its tendency to interfere where it's unnecessary. Like many others, I'd heard loads of terrible stories and about many bad experiences. I was fiercely determined not to fall under the establishment's spell and be persuaded to have the birth someone else wanted or dictated as to what they thought was best or more convenient. I wanted my birth, happening to my body, to be done my way and to be surrounded by people only who unreservedly understood and respected that. End of.

It was a Tuesday and my sister, and I had been racing around organising painting, re-upholstering and carpeting for my house which was gutted and being renovated. I had an appointment scheduled for my 36 week check up at the Family Birth Centre that afternoon, so I left my sister at the house to supervise. A few weeks earlier I'd had a little high blood pressure, but a check 48 hours later was fine and showed that everything was normal. On this day though I went to my appointment feeling a bit frazzled and puffy but feeling ok, nonetheless.

When my 15-minute appointment turned into 45 minutes and the midwife was delaying and talking to keep me there to re-check my blood pressure, I knew something was up. She explained that things weren't looking good and that she thought I might have pre-eclampsia. She told me I needed to go to the hospital for foetal monitoring and more checking immediately. But I'd left my sister at my house with no facilities, so I told them I had to go. They reluctantly let me but we agreed that should there be anything wrong in the test results, they would call and I'd go straight to the hospital.

Two hours later they called and told me to be at the hospital within an hour. I was sitting on the edge of my bed crying, devastated. It was a lonely moment knowing that something was wrong and that all of my preparation and hopes for a Family Birth Centre birth without 'the establishment' and without 'interference' and without 'being told' how my birth would happen, were gone. But I and the family around me tried to stay calm and positive – it might just be fine, and a little monitoring might reveal that. But we loaded the car and went prepared anyway.

A few hours of foetal monitoring revealed that I had pre-eclampsia and it was progressing quickly. I was feeling ok I suppose, a little worked up and uptight maybe, but I thought that was because we were so busy with the house. The first Midwife warned us that I might not be going home before my baby was born. The second Dr told us our baby would definitely be coming early. The third Consultant told us our baby needed to be born NOW. My husband and I were in shock. I was only 36 weeks, we thought we had weeks left, we were worried about the baby being born early, we wouldn't be moved into the house in time, and I was terrified of hospitals, Doctors and the establishment. I wanted to get up and run.

My aunt, who'd had three lovely homebirths, had previously said to me "there's always time". I remembered it, said it over and over to myself and wasn't going to be pressured. My Doula, Gaby, was on the phone to us with support and guidance also making sure we weren't being swept away. I asked the Consultant if I was in urgency or an emergency? When she said that it was urgent but not dire yet, and since by now I knew I was staying in the hospital and would need to be induced anyway, I asked if I could sleep the night and if we could start the induction the next morning. I just needed to get my head around it; everything was moving too fast and despite my preparation, determination and strength, I was scared.

By the time I got to bed it was after 1am and I didn't get much sleep. After all that, my induction wasn't started until about 4pm the next day anyway. And when it started, I found out that even though I hadn't felt a thing, I was already 4cms dilated. So my baby was coming anyway !!! Up to this point, I hadn't felt anything more than what I thought was baby movement. For weeks I had been feeling the baby pushing hard down on my cervix and it would often stop me in my tracks. I just thought it was more of that too.

The Foley's catheter fell out after about 45 minutes and I knew that once the drip started things would be happening hard and fast. I asked the midwives if they would let me progress into my own labour rhythm naturally – since I was already dilating and clearly my body was preparing itself for birth. After two conversations with those in charge, they agreed and for the next three hours they left me alone to progress on my own. By about 8pm and with the concern growing over the pre-eclampsia, they started the drip, and my contractions were only about 2-3 minutes apart.

I had wanted a natural birth in the Family Birth Centre with my husband and Doula. I didn't want drugs and I didn't want intervention. But now all I could do was focus on my yoga breathing and get through every wave as it came. My husband and I were so prepared for all this. We'd been to my doula's birth workshop, we had yoga mats for the floor, sponge mats for the bath/shower, fit ball, bags of salt, towels, blankets, music, food, drinks and my list went on. We had the massage routine practised, affirmations written, and we used none of it. When it was all happening, I couldn't stand any noise and I didn't want to be touched. I was on my knees leaning over the fitball, focussed on breathing with nothing else on my mind.

I had set a goal for myself to call my Doula when I felt it was getting tough and was reaching the point where I thought I might ask for drugs. This was hugely beneficial. It gave me something to think about without distracting me from my job. With every wave, I reminded myself that if I got through that one, I could get through the next one; I did a good job, just keeping going.

By midnight I was feeling pretty ragged. Every contraction was really tough now and they were coming so close together. I wanted to vomit; my body wanted to heave but I just couldn't. I remember moaning, 'why can't I vomit, why can't I vomit' and the midwife saying 'it's just the pain'. Every few minutes I could hear the drip pushing more Syntocinon into me. I was resenting it but I was in control of my breathing, so I was calm and comforted. My husband was so great and amazing.

My husband called my Doula Gaby just after midnight and she came straight away. I was ready for her to get me over the line now. I wanted some help and was softly moaning 'help me' as a kind of mantra. What the hell, I didn't connect with it, it was just something to say to get me through the contractions without thinking. Everything in the room changed when Gaby arrived. She was calm and took over. I looked to her. She was to me a huge comfort and relief, stroking, whispering encouragement, supporting. I felt by now that I wanted to sit on the toilet because I remembered that it was a good position for the baby to descend. We sat there for ages, it was dark, quiet, relaxed. Gaby had given me a cave to find peace in, and I did.

A while later Gaby suggested I sit on the fitball and I tried but I couldn't. I could feel the baby very close now. I went back to the mat and stayed on all fours as I had been. By now my legs were weak and my knees were sore, but it was the only place I could stay in and be alright. I was desperate now; the intensity was overwhelming, and I asked for the gas. It seemed to take a while to get it sorted and I only got to have one go when I felt the incredible force to push. At first, I didn't know what it was. The pain of labour changed in an instant and the push was immensely satisfying.

I looked forward to the next one, it was like the biggest most incredible rush and then the biggest relief. I remembered Gaby's workshop where she said to use every opportunity to push that baby out. Don't hold back, relax and ride the wave. I did and again imagined my body pushing down and pulling tightly around my baby as it descended more and more. I kept asking Gaby if she could see anything yet. I thought surely with each push my baby must be half out by now, but no. When my baby's head did start to appear, Gaby took my hand and put it on my baby's head so I could feel it. I felt total amazement, I had touched my unborn baby and I so badly wanted to hold it.

I pushed and pushed with everything I had in me. I was exhausted but I knew I was going to meet my baby any moment. Everything was quiet, too quiet except for me. All I could hear was myself, groaning and exerting. I told everyone "it's too fucking quiet in here!" Then Gaby started explaining to me everything that was happening. I could feel the peek-a-boo happening where my baby's head would slide back a little in between pushes and I was getting frustrated. I was working so hard for so little reward.

After a few massively intense pushes where I felt I wasn't making progress I was told the baby couldn't come out any further, Gaby told me my perineum was stretched to its absolute maximum and I could feel every bit of it. That was when it was suggested I would need an episiotomy by both the midwife and Gaby, and I knew if my doula was suggesting it – it was for real. I trusted their judgement and call. During all of my preparations I was strongly against this and had wanted to tear naturally. But in the moment, and once my Doula had again agreed that it's what I needed, I was almost shouting "do it, hurry up!" With the next urge to push I gave it everything and slowly, with the help of the midwife, my baby slid out of me.

It was a few moments before I got to hold her and unfortunately my husband didn't get to cut the cord. Our daughter was having a little trouble breathing, was swept into a crib and surrounded by about eight people. It was a terrifying few moments and I felt my whole life pause – this could not be happening. It took a few minutes for her to come around and breathe for herself and then she was handed to me. I remember reclining back on my husband and into his arms with our baby daughter on my chest. She was beautiful.

While it hadn't been what I'd originally planned, I'd had the natural birth I wanted with a minimum of intervention. My experience was hugely positive and I look back on it happily. I'm glad I stood up for myself when it mattered even though it was intimidating and frightening to do so and I'm so lucky I had chosen the right people – my husband and my doula Gaby - to be around me to make sure that happened.

An Amazing Journey

Ruby Fossey (Yeates) was born on Saturday 1st at 4:30pm. I know Matt rang you Gaby after I got a hind water leak and got admitted to KEMH on Wednesday night. Thank you for the advice and information you gave him, it was good to get info from someone other than a doctor. At the time (and up until Friday afternoon) I was adamant I didn't want to be induced or at least to leave it as long as possible. The doctors weren't that supportive, stating examples of babies dying etc.

Anyway, I tested positive for Group Strep B and they said I really should be induced once I reached 36 weeks, and they were happy with the baby's size etc. So on Saturday morning I was taken to the labour ward to be induced. The doctors had told me I would have to be monitored the whole time, no showers, waters broken and then immediate synto through the drip. However, my midwives were far more understanding and really listened to what I wanted. They delayed the start of the drip to see if I would start labour on my own as they wanted to see if I could start labouring naturally from my waters being broken. They also agreed that when the drip did go in to extend the time before each increase in dose to give me time to adapt to the contraction intensity.

They found a portable foetal heart rate monitor for me so I could move around, and after an hour or two of monitoring they were happy to just monitor every 20 minutes out of each hour. So then I asked to use the shower - they said of course. Just as I was about to get in I thought I'd chance asking about the bath. A doctor was in the room at this point and turned to me and shook her head. However the midwife didn't see this, told me it would be fine and went off to fill it! The bath was AMAZING. I spent an hour there and I felt the most relaxed I have ever felt - almost out of body! Towards the end I started to feel I couldn't do it anymore and wondered if it was too good to be true and I was in transition (4 hours from the start of the drip) or if I was just needing pain relief.

Thankfully, at the same time I felt the need to push. At that moment the midwife said I should get out of the bath - which I wanted to do, and head back to the room. Once in the room, I spent about 25 minutes pushing while standing/squatting against the bed and out came Ruby. She was absolutely fine at 6.2lbs. We had skin on skin contact and then she went on the breast right away. I was also fine, no tearing or other injuries which was also amazing. I used your breathing Gaby, all the way through, eyes closed while Matt massaged, and mopped my brow. I made some horrible deep groans when pushing that I think shocked both me and Matt, but it was what my body wanted to do!

Anyway, because she was four weeks early they made us stay until she started to put on weight, but all the midwives are great, and it is giving me a good relaxing start to looking after her so I don't really mind.

I just wanted to thank you for everything that you contributed towards me having an amazing birth!

Dr Chrissie Yeates, Teacher of Mathematics

Sabrina's Birth of James

Even before I fell pregnant, I never considered anything but giving birth vaginally. To me it was the normal process for a woman to go through, and also because I had an incredible fear of the epidural so having a caesarean was not an option. That is until I fell pregnant. One of my friends started talking about the so-called 'negatives' of vaginal birth and that the things 'down there' would never be the same. After this discussion, I was so fearful of enduring a vaginal birth that I started contemplating having an elective caesarean like my friend. I spoke to my obstetrician about my concerns that I had for both vaginal and caesarean births. He provided an unbiased opinion on both and really just left it to me to decide. I pondered for a few weeks and was very much headed for the elective caesarean option as the fear of the epidural was something I couldn't quite get over.

Then I met Gaby at the aqua-natal classes. I mentioned I didn't want to go down the path of birthing vaginally as I didn't want to have incontinence issues in the future. Gaby laughed and told me to read her first book. So I did just that. Reading Gaby's book, and attending the aqua classes, hearing the various journeys that the other women were going on with their birth made me feel so empowered. I knew that I could also have a wonderful experience of birthing vaginally if I chose to. The fears I had regarding post birth issues were so minor that I stopped thinking about them. Consequently, here is my story about my amazing pregnancy and birth journey.

Through-out my pregnancy I made sure that I was fit and healthy. Looking after me was a priority as I was caring for this tiny person inside me who meant everything to my husband and I. I couldn't wait for each Wednesday to come as I knew I would gain more insight into labouring from Gaby and the other women at the aqua-class. I visited Gaby through-out my pregnancy for massages and also had a hypnosis session. I have always been good at visualising so I felt I had a good idea of how I wanted to give birth. Yet, doing this work with Gaby gave me even more confidence in myself and body.

As I neared my estimated due date, the 15th December, I began getting excited as I knew it was around the corner that I would finally meet our little boy or girl. On my estimated due date I had an internal examination by the obstetrician and to my surprise he said I was already 2-3cm dilated and 75%

effaced. He said he would be surprised if I didn't go into spontaneous labour by the end of the week, and that he would book me in for an induction on 19th December if I hadn't gone by then.

Initially I was very positive and kept telling myself that my body would just do things naturally. Every movement had me on edge as I was waiting to go into labour. As the next couple of days passed, I started to worry as induction was not in my plan at all. This was an intervention I did not want as I wanted to avoid any sort of drugs, and worse still, I didn't want to end up with a caesarean if things didn't work out.

The day before my induction date was horrible. My body had not shown me any signs of going into labour and I couldn't understand why, when earlier in the week my obstetrician had given me hope that I should go into labour spontaneously. After much debating in my mind and speaking with my husband, we decided to cancel the induction. My husband knew how much I wanted to do this on my own and he was so supportive, particularly during this time. My obstetrician advised me that he would re-book my induction for 23rd December as he could not let me go beyond this date. I felt relieved in my decision and knew that it would happen on its own.

That night and the following night, from 4pm until midnight, I had contractions five minutes apart and felt that my labour journey was imminent. It wasn't until Monday afternoon had come and gone that I felt a sense of loss. The induction was only hours away and even though I knew that I would meet our little one soon, I couldn't help but feel disappointment in myself that my body wasn't doing what I wanted it to. I continued to think that I would go into labour that night but as my husband and I woke to the alarm at 6am on 23rd December, I knew I was headed for the induction. We had our usual breakfast and at this point I was relatively calm and knew I couldn't have done much more to go into spontaneous labour. This was after two weeks of massages, acupuncture, plenty of sex, eating pineapples, drinking raspberry leaf tea, primrose oil, eating hot foods and walking kilometres every day!

We arrived at the hospital at 7am. We sat in the birthing suite and I was trying to focus on what was to come. The midwife, Julia, came in to introduce herself. At this point I explained that I wanted to have as natural vaginal birth as possible, which meant no intervention unless the baby or I were at risk unless I asked for something such as pain relief. She was very understanding and explained that she would be here to support me during my labour in any way possible. Just before 8.30am, my obstetrician arrived and did another internal examination where he advised me I was 5 cm dilated. I was then given the Syntocinon and within minutes my contractions began. Instantly, I felt the contractions were stronger than that of what I had experienced earlier.

I decided to sit on the fitball and felt relatively comfortable in this position as I breathed through each contraction and used the hypnosis to visualise the opening of my cervix. After about 45 minutes I decided to stand up to go to the bathroom. As I sat on the toilet, I had an intense contraction and knew the contractions were beginning to shorten to about two minutes apart (the clock in the room was right in my view! I don't recommend you have a clock as it makes time pass very slowly!). As I returned from the bathroom I decided to try standing and leaning over the bed. I only managed one contraction in this position before I asked to lie down on my side as the intensity was increasing rapidly.

At 9.30am I made my first sound with the urge of wanting to push. The midwife asked if I was feeling pressure and I explained that I was. She let me go for a couple more contractions and my vocals increased with each one. At this point she did an internal examination and advised me I was 7cm. She told me to keep going and that within the next half an hour I would likely be ready to push. Half an hour felt like forever and the midwife was advising me to stop the urge to push until I was fully dilated. At 9.40am the contractions were so intense. At this point the midwife offered me some gas which I accepted as I needed something to calm me down. I didn't want to have the intervention of any drugs, but I knew I was in need of something as I was transitioning and very close to pushing. I knew that my turning point was when my husband had put some hand sanitiser on and the smell was so repulsive that I yelled at him to go wash it off!

At 9.45am, I couldn't resist the urge to push, so the midwife conducted another internal. I was fully dilated and ready! The midwife positioned me upright on the bed and told me to pull back on my legs with each push. This wasn't the position I had planned on birthing as I wanted to go on all fours, but the midwife told me to try this position in the first instance. Along came the next contraction and I was told to push. It was such an incredible experience. It was almost instant relief that I was able to push through the contractions. After the first contraction the midwife made a call to my obstetrician. She told him that he needed to come up as the head was crowning and that the baby would be here in no time. I pushed through two more contractions before the arrival of my obstetrician.

I wasn't far off when I felt the burn. I knew this sensation as I had been using the Epi-No to help stretch my perineum to avoid any tearing. Then came the next push which the midwife talked me through to avoid any tearing and out was the head. With the next contraction I knew that the baby would be out, and indeed that is what happened! The obstetrician held my baby up and asked me if I could see the sex of the baby. I ecstatically said "it's a boy!". So after 1 hour and 40 minutes of labouring I welcomed my precious little boy at 10.10am.

Although I didn't experience what it was like to go into spontaneous labour, I did manage to have the perfect birth through induction. My body was obviously ready for the birth and needed that little push along. I couldn't be happier with how I laboured and even today when I think about my birth or talk to other people, I feel so proud and elated with my experience. I can't wait to do it all over again!

Katie's Positive Birth of Indica

On the Friday 28th of July, I was exactly a week past my estimated date of birth of my beautiful baby girl. I didn't mind at all though as I was enjoying this pregnancy and didn't feel or look ready at all, as I was very small and compact. I also knew this baby was going to be on the small side as I am not a big person myself.

On this Friday morning, I woke up from a very restless night of on and off contractions and period pains that got down to seven minutes apart, then just went away allowing me to go back to sleep for a few more hours before it all happened again. I also had my 'bloody show' come out in the morning, and I woke up hoping today was the day, but trying not to get too excited (as I knew it could be three more days yet!).

As the day progressed, I had the familiar period cramping here and there but nothing too dramatic. I had a 41-week appointment at the hospital, so we went in. Monitoring showed the baby's heartbeat was dropping as I had contractions and I

491

was quickly told that I would need to be admitted, waters broken and induced.

I had attended Gaby's 3-hour Intensive Childbirth Educational Workshop and we understood how this can lead to the 'cascade of more intervention' making it hard to get off that road once on it. We negotiated more time monitoring to see if the situation would improve. Having had an easy pregnancy and educating myself by completing a hypnobirthing workshop with Gaby, I was in quite a bit of shock being asked to be induced right there and then. It was hard knowing that I would not be allowed to move around, use the water and have a waterbirth. We did not even have our hospital bag with us!

Luckily for us, Fiona Stanley Hospital was busy that night, so I was not pushed and was left to be monitored for over six hours. However during this time my blood pressure became erratic and high, and it was decided that intervention was needed. Again, we asked for a step-by-step approach. Firstly, a saline drip was used to try to hydrate me and regulate my blood pressure and the baby's heart rate. Then my waters were broken at 11.30pm (24 hours after I had had my first twinges). We let Gaby know what was going on to give her the heads up. Our attending midwife understood our desire to take things easy and allowed me one hour of contractions before she would insert the synto drip.

The contractions began to escalate naturally, and I begged to be allowed to have a shower away from all the foetal monitoring and machines. I was giving permission and took myself and my IV drip and bag of Synto on a stand into the shower. Not long after, my body decided that it was time to purge, and I had a bowel movement on the toilet and a big vomit in the shower.

The Synto drip was given at 12.30am, but I had made the midwife promise to take it slowly. Meanwhile I was on the bed being monitored as the baby's heartbeat did strange things when I leaned forward so the only position I could happily stay in was on the bed in a reclined position. This was something I did not foresee at all. I had planned to be walking around, sitting on the fitball, standing in the shower, having a waterbirth... and here I was stuck in the most uncomfortable position with two monitors strapped to my belly and an IV line in my hand!

Gaby arrived at 12.40am. It was perfect timing. Gaby and I debriefed the day's events as I started to go into labour.

It was exactly half an hour later, and I could no longer talk to Gaby as I had to focus within. Gaby went from chatting to being really calm and assisting me to breathe, surrender and let go! It was really tough, and I am a strong woman, but this was a challenge. The hypnosis for birth scripts helped as I had to try and get my exhale sound correct and picturing my hypnobirthing trigger of my wedding ring expanding in the sunlight (like my cervix would be!)

The contractions really did go from 0 to 100 in that half an hour. I remember Gaby saying come on let's get you off the bed and sitting on the fitball. I knew Gaby knew what she was doing, and I trusted her judgement and wanted to be out of the semi reclined position. It was while I was sitting on the fitball I felt a shift into my pelvis from the baby and I had a big, bloody show again. Gaby looked very impressed as she felt it seemed to get the baby down even more which it did. I tried to stand for a while but had to get back on the bed as bub's heart rate went all over the place again.

Things really did get going after that as in next to no time I felt this huge urge to push, and I was so hot and the pressure feeling in my bottom was huge. I let out a deep primal noise that woke Dean up from a deep sleep and I stated out loud to everyone "I have to push now". With that the midwife did a quick VE and said I was fully effaced, and 9 centimetres dilated and said not to push as I still had a centimetre to go. I can tell you I ignored her and pushed like there was no tomorrow, there was no other option to hold back as every cell in my body was saying push, and I just had to go with it.

My intuition was spot on and not long after my baby's head was on view, and I could see everyone getting excited. Once I saw my midwife put on her plastic apron, I knew it was time and I could now see the end of the road. As Gaby had said, the pushing stage is like a reward. I was told to stop pushing with my voice, so I closed my eyes and focused. My support team was amazing, and I was coached to open perfectly as I engaged every piece of strength and pushed with maximum effort. I opened my eyes just in time to see my baby fly out into the midwife's hands in just one contraction and push.

She was placed on my chest and my husband was right there. The moment was surreal, and I was out of control, as I felt like I was out of my body. It took me about a minute to control my breathing and get my mind back. Our little girl was born at 2.43am, weighing 2.67kg. The placenta birth was very easy, and the placenta was very small and calcified (very cooked!). Indica was officially one week past her estimated date, but the skinny wrinkly body and small placenta indicated maybe two weeks overcooked. Due to the coaching though the pushing stage I had no tearing at all.

I feel so blessed and happy to have had this fast and straightforward induction experience. The knowledge that my husband and I had gained prior to birth allowed us to use our voice and have some control over our situation and resulted in this beautiful and quick ending to my pregnancy and labour journey.

9.

VAGINAL BREECH STORIES

Edie's Breech Birth Story

O ne night, at around 35 weeks, I woke up in the middle of the night with a jolt – I was used to the baby kicking at night but this felt different – there had been a huge movement. I went back to sleep and didn't think much more of it as the baby kept moving normally, but a few days later when we went for a routine appointment at the Family Birth Centre, King Edward Memorial Hospital, they felt my belly and told me that the baby had flipped and was now breech. Both Tim, my husband, and I were breech babies so it had always been in the back of my mind that this was a possibility. Tim turned during labour and was born head first but my birth was an epic natural breech vaginal delivery at KEMH back in the late 1970s.

As soon as we discovered we were pregnant, Tim and I started looking into birth options – we'd heard so many stories about how hard it is to find an obstetrician that we thought we'd better get onto it quickly. One weekend we booked to tour St John of God Murdoch (our nearest hospital) and the Family Birth Centre at KEMH. Before the weekend we didn't have a strong view about the type of birth we wanted – most of our friends had given birth at private hospitals, and one close friend had opted for homebirths, which sounded great but wasn't an option for which we felt ready. By the end of the weekend, we were very sure we wanted a natural birth at the Birth Centre. I was uncomfortable the minute we walked into SJOG due to the amount they talked about caesareans and other medical interventions - their focus definitely put Tim and I off.

The Birth Centre by comparison was almost like being at home, with soft lighting, comfortable rooms, and minimal intervention. We were converted! They also did water births which was by far my preferred option. We then started to look further into natural birth, including doing lots of reading and talking to people we knew who had experienced natural births. One option that sounded great to us was to engage a doula, so we had an expert on our side to advise and support us through the process. Gaby Targett was recommended as our 'doula who trained other doulas' and we were delighted when she was available to work with us. From our first meeting she presented giving birth as a positive and empowering experience, and this really framed our view of how we would bring our child into the world. We were lucky in that we had a really easy conception, and I felt great during the pregnancy: we could really focus on preparing for the birth. We also attended the birth classes at the Family Birth Centre which were great and gave us plenty of information about natural birth.

But now our baby was breech, and suddenly our plans were being seriously challenged. The Birth Centre is not allowed to do breech deliveries, and we heard from various people that most obstetricians would insist on a caesarean delivery for a breech baby. While I didn't have any fear about giving birth vaginally, I was petrified of a caesarean, so this news was alarming.

Working with Gaby we tried everything to turn the baby – moxi-combustion, visualisation, lots of getting into upside-down positions, handstands in the swimming pool, Pulsatilla naturopathic drops, even playing music via headphones near my pelvis! Unfortunately, while I could feel that the baby was turning into a transverse position, she would never fully flip to head down. I started to get the feeling that she had made up her mind to come into the world bum first and wasn't going to be dissuaded by any of our efforts!

By now I was feeling quite distressed by the combination of focussing on turning the baby so we could have a 'normal' birth and learning everything we could about breech birth so we could try and prepare for that if the turning failed. I had started maternity leave and had been expecting to spend my time relaxing and getting into the right mindset to surrender to the birth experience. Instead, I was preparing to negotiate the breech birth we wanted and reading everything I could try and make the case that it was a safe and a legitimate option.

The problem we faced was that after a study published in 2000 called the 'Term Breech Trial' led by a Dr Hannah (I couldn't believe the name), it was decided that it was safer to deliver breech babies by caesarean. A few years later this trial was peer reviewed and found to be flawed, but by then it was too late and most hospitals in Australia, and other western countries, had stopped doing breech vaginal deliveries - meaning most doctors no longer had the skills to support a breech vaginal birth. Some skills still exist in the midwifery community, but in WA, the Community Midwifery Program only delivers 'surprise' breech births. Tim and I felt like we were being punished because of some poor research and would be forced into an option with which we felt very uncomfortable.

Then, a glimmer of hope - we heard that Dr Anne Karczub, the Head of Obstetrics at KEMH, was prepared to support vaginal breech deliveries! Anne attempted an ECV at 37 weeks, which unfortunately yielded the same result as my other turning efforts – baby turned halfway, then back to breech.

After the ECV we asked Anne to support us for a natural breech delivery at KEMH. She agreed, with some caveats about the type of interventions that might be necessary based on her experience (the possibility of Syntocinon to speed up contractions in the final stage, and the likelihood of an episiotomy). It was a relief to know that a caesarean would only be carried out in an emergency – much like any other birth.

Of course, nothing could be straightforward – Anne was about to go on two weeks leave so I spent a lot of time telling the baby that she couldn't come out early – a possibility, given that when Anne examined me after the ECV she had said my cervix was already very 'ripe'.

A couple of days after my estimated due date, and once we knew Anne was back at work, we decided it was time to 'bring it on'. I went for a long walk (more a waddle) along the beach; we had sex and went to bed. I woke around 3am with some contractions but they petered out and I went back to sleep. The next day I got as much sleep as I could and went for another long walk around the neighbourhood, stopping to have a few contractions along the way. By about 6.30pm the contractions were getting regular, and I needed to lean over onto a fitball when they came on. As the contractions progressed, I could feel myself getting more and more focussed when they arrived and then moving into a state of relaxation between each one. At about 10.30pm I asked Tim to call Gaby because I felt that surely this must be the real thing by now- the contractions were getting pretty intense. I also had a bloody show around this time and was getting around with a cloth nappy in my undies in case my waters broke (good tip from Gaby!).

Gaby arrived and helped me to continue labouring in a couple of different positions, including in the shower, which was lovely, although it did remind me how much I had hoped I could birth in water. At around midnight I asked that we go to the hospital – I wanted to get the car trip over and done with, although it wasn't as uncomfortable as I had expected.

In the hospital, the midwife in the Foetal Monitoring Unit insisted I have a saline drip to rehydrate as they thought the baby was showing signs of stress, and it took ages to insert the cannula into my vein. I kept having contractions and wishing the medical staff would go away so I could focus. The registrar then wanted to do a VE to 'check that I was really in labour'! I wasn't keen but it was good news when they had a look and saw I was seven centimetres dilated. Suddenly, the medical staff were much more interested and got us straight into the labour suite.

The next five hours passed without me having any consciousness of time. All that was going on for me was focussing on a contraction, then relaxing and zoning out into a kind of dream state while I waited for the next one. Tim, Gaby and my mum Jody (who had arrived by then) took turns rubbing my back and giving me ice to suck. Esther, a student midwife we had met during the ECV), gave me advice and helped with some of the medical elements. We did what we could to use the labour suite to get into different positions and dimmed the lights as much as we were allowed, although we completely forgot about the music and essential oils I had carefully packed!

Another VE and I was told I was nine centimetres dilated with an anterior lip. I remembered something I had read by Ina May Gaskin (the 'mother' of spiritual midwifery) about a woman who had visualised herself opening up to birth her baby by repeating 'I'm gonna get huge!' in her head. So, I lay on my side imagining that my birth canal was a big smooth tube for the baby to slide down, and thankfully next time the doctor checked the anterior lip had gone.

I began to feel like I needed to push during my contractions and was making a noise like a motorcycle revving up! Fortunately, someone suggested I breathe and blow instead, otherwise I probably would have wrecked my vocal cords pretty quickly. One of the hospital midwives said to me "blow away the horrible pain" and I remember saying to her "it's not horrible!!" – she left me to it after that! Twice during the night different registrars came in and offered me an epidural – I asked one of them" have you read my birth plan?" which clearly stated I didn't want to be offered drugs. In retrospect, it surprised me that they offered drugs without first observing that I was doing fine and coping well with the pain.

The description Ina May Gaskin uses of 'clean' pain during childbirth makes a lot of sense to me – it is very intense during contractions but nothing like the pain of something like a bad toothache, that doesn't go away and makes you feel miserable

503

all the time. It also feels productive – it's happening for a purpose and each contraction takes you closer to the birth of your baby, so in a way I felt like I could welcome the contractions when they came along, rather than dread them as I would if they were pain that indicated being unwell.

Another consultant had been on during the night who had experience with vaginal breech birth so Anne had decided she didn't need to come in – but I was so glad when we realised the night shift had ended and Anne walked in – just as I was fully dilated and ready to really push. She had asked previously whether she could use the opportunity to train a junior doctor in how to deliver breech and we had agreed. I felt her confidence totally changed the attitude of the other medical staff in the room and everyone became more convinced that this breech delivery was actually going to happen.

She put her fingers on my perineum and told me to push into exactly where her fingers were putting pressure (I wonder if I could have done that with an epidural?) and soon I could feel the baby moving down. I could also see the looks on Tim and Gaby's faces as they started to see the bottom emerge! My contractions weren't coming quick enough, and I started to hear things about syntocinon. Luckily, Anne gave Gaby a chance to try acupressure and homeopathics first and they seemed to work, along with me giving little pushes without a contraction to try and remind my body what it was meant to be doing! Soon the baby was really pressing against my perineum and it felt like I was pushing into a brick wall. Anne said it was time for an episiotomy and I didn't object – as soon as it was done it felt like there was nothing stopping the baby from getting out, which was quite a relief. With some amazing manoeuvres (that I couldn't really see at the time but have seen now in photos) Anne showed the junior doctor how to deliver a breech baby and all of a sudden, our little Edie was out in the world.

I'll never forget looking at the joy and amazement on Tim's face when he saw our little girl being born. She was put on my chest but was a bit blue so they took her over to the resuscitaire. As soon as she got there, she let out a cry so they brought her back to me. I delivered the placenta while we tried to get her on the breast, then she nuzzled around on Tim's hairy chest while they stitched me up. The most amazing thing was the natural high that I was on for days after the birth.

The natural hormones were amazing and I'm so glad I didn't have any drugs to interfere with their effect. We chose to spend one night in the hospital so that everyone could get a good night's sleep before going home. My recovery was really quick, and I felt so confident and happy after the birth. One of the best things is that it felt like everyone involved with the birth, now has a better understanding and even a passion for supporting breech vaginal birth, so hopefully in the future the options for women with breech presentations in Perth may not be so limited. Doing the research and finding someone like

Anne, who is confident in delivering breech, seemed to be the key.

Jody's Story of Hannah's breech birth in 1977

It was the second half of the seventies and many of us in that decade were dedicated to trying to make the world a better and more peaceful place, to embracing natural means of creating health and happiness, to enjoying natural food, environmentally friendly products – and to opting for natural birth.

When I became pregnant on my 30th birthday I planned to have a homebirth. However, I also sought out an obstetrician whom I felt would be sympathetic to my views about birthing should I need to go to hospital. I was lucky to find all I could hope for in Dr Colin Douglas-Smith. A highly respected obstetrician and gynaecologist, he was also a dedicated Yoga practitioner and had full respect for what I was doing. I had been teaching Transcendental Meditation (TM) for nearly three years and had, in fact, taught his wife to meditate.

I visited 'Dougie-Smith', as we all called him, about once a month. He fielded all my questions about natural birth, episiotomies, perineal massage, a lack of intervention and of analgesics, with grace and a total absence of dogmatic or dismissive arrogance. And there was a fair bit of that around in the male dominated medical profession in those days. I continued to teach TM all through my pregnancy and in my little spare time I read every book I could lay my hands on about natural birth and home birth. These ranged from classics like Grantley Dick-Read's Childbirth without Fear to Frederick Leboyer's Birth without Violence, Ina May Gaskin's just published Spiritual Midwifery, and to anthologies of homebirth stories from North America, some including recipes for placenta stew.

I had a wonderful pregnancy with only occasional bouts of 'afternoon sickness' in the early months, quickly cured by practising TM. When we discovered that the baby had settled into a breech position in the third trimester, none of us was worried. Dr Douglas-Smith attempted to turn the baby externally, but once he had her halfway around, she declined to go further and flipped her head up again. My first thought was "good on you babe. You know what you want!" So we settled into knowing that this was most probably how she would be born (although at the time we didn't know she was a girl) and I resigned myself to a hospital birth. I never considered, or was led to consider, that it would be anything but a natural vaginal birth. I was very healthy and relaxed, and Dr Douglas-Smith was unfazed about delivering a breech baby. It was just seen as one of the ways babies can present to be born. And my partner, George, was prepared. We had been to ante-natal classes together and we were both confident we could do it. We were excited and positive.

My contractions began in the morning of the 28th of September – nearly a week after the 'due date', with a slight threat of induction spurring them on. I stripped off in the spring sunshine in our vegetable garden so the baby could get used to the light. The contractions became stronger as evening approached and around midnight, when we had been in bed for a couple of hours, they became strong and fast. An hour or so later, after a particularly strong bout of contractions, we headed to KEMH.

The usual protracted admission for those days ensued; paperwork, enema, no shave and then, at 2.30am, we were taken to the eclampsia room as we were perceived to be the most 'problematic delivery' of the night. It was coldly metallic and brightly lit, but luckily spacious. Unfortunately, I was made to lie down. Maybe I could have objected to this, but didn't, so my labour was accompanied by a lot of lower back pain and George was subjected to many hours of back rubbing. He was amazing, rubbing firmly through every contraction, and I couldn't have coped nearly so well without him. Between contractions I easily and quickly came back to a fully relaxed state. I felt 'positive pain' was a better descriptor for contractions than 'pain', as they had a constructive purpose – and the 'pain' disappeared completely as soon as the contractions stopped. At some stage I was connected to a foetal heart monitor, which turned out to be comforting to George, to hear the baby's strong, regular heartbeat but annoying to me, as it impeded easy movement.

At 6.30am I had a VE. My cervix was 7 centimetres, fully effaced and very soft, and the membranes bulged with contractions. The midwives predicted the baby would be birthed by 8.00 or 9.00am and rang Dr Douglas-Smith. George rang my mother. We wanted her to share the experience of a natural birth since she had been deprived of it, having, in her words, 'been knocked out' for both my brothers' and my births.

My labour continued – and the back rubbing. At 8.00am Colin came in and I requested barley sugar to suck for energy. The contractions were strong and regular, coming every two and a half to three and a half minutes, I think, and I was coping well. At 9.00am Colin felt the membranes bulging and then at 10.40am gave me a VE, as there was no evident progress. The cervix was 7-8cms, but contractions were slowing. The baby's bottom, not being uniformly round and hard like a head, hadn't managed to open the whole rim of the cervix.

Apart from the barley sugar, I hadn't been given anything to eat or drink, so my muscles were obviously getting tired and the barley sugar hadn't done the trick. At 11.15am I was set up with a drip in my arm and Dr Douglas-Smith felt that the only way to get the contractions moving again would be to administer synthetic oxytocin – Synctocinon - and dextrose. We began with just dextrose. Dr Douglas-Smith's communication throughout the day (he popped in every hour between lectures and rounds) had been wonderful – warm, natural, calm and inclusive. He knew that I wanted the deep level of experience that natural birth provides and that I didn't want this to be diminished by any intervention, if it could be avoided. Confident that he would only intervene if he judged it absolutely necessary, I accepted his decision to give me Syntocinon.

We found a sustainable level of Syntocinon so that I could cope with the contractions, which returned to a regular pattern, and we were doing fine. At about 2.00pm I was heading into transition and suddenly thought "I think I've forgotten the breathing". At that moment the door opened, and my dear friend Fiona Stanley walked in. She had had her first daughter a few months earlier and had been ringing the hospital since early in the morning. She knew how much I wanted to give birth naturally and when the hospital staff became reticent and wouldn't tell her what was happening, her husband Geoff suggested that she go and investigate while he minded their baby. She jumped on her bike, grabbed her white lab coat so that she would be given admittance and appeared at the door of the eclamptic room like a guardian angel. She acted as a birth coach, guiding me into a good breathing pattern during each contraction.

At some point during the day, a former next-door neighbour and close friend had also appeared. A medical student, she was doing her obstetrics and gynaecology prac at KEMH. We assigned her the task of official photographer and she was an assiduous recorder. My mother was an assistant back-rubber. Also at 2.00pm the midwives who had been on duty and were supposed to go off asked if they could stay until the birth, as they had never seen a natural breech delivery. The new shift came on and the old ones stayed. So it was fortunate indeed that we had a big room and that Dr D-S was used to an audience.

With George and Fiona's assistance, both supporting my shoulders as I was finally ready to push, the baby's bottom began to appear. We then knew she was a girl! Dr D-S followed the method Samoan women used to deliver their own breech babies and gently eased the legs out and up, and then I pushed out the head. She was a beautiful long-limbed baby with a lovely head and we were thrilled when her Apgar score was 9.9. I had thought Hannah might be her name when she was in utero, but her Dad, experienced in these matters, said "you have to see the baby first. They come out with their name on." He looked at her with love and awe when she emerged and immediately said, "hello Hannah". And Hannah she was and is.

So in summary, the things that really assisted us to have such an epic but special birth experience were; preparation – classes and reading, a total absence of fear, the ability to relax completely between contractions, a supportive and absolutely present partner, a wonderful obstetrician, and family and friends, especially Fiona. And, most importantly a strong baby who coped with such an extended labour, and who 33 years later repeated the experience in giving birth to her daughter, also breech, but with more knowledge, the assistance of Gaby as doula, and, therefore, with more speed.

Hannah's birth was the peak experience of my life. The process of the long labour was an important part of it and I remember feeling a little sorry for the woman in the next room who had only had a twenty-minute-long labour. There was something about the time – and the strange timelessness – of Hannah's long approach to the outside world that somehow prepared me for the new and uncharted role of motherhood.

Kathryn's Breech Birth Story

August 1, 2011

Well, it all started on Monday evening, August 1, when I started to get a sore lower back. It's a pain I hadn't experienced before and was rather uncomfortable. Daniel, being the lovely man he is, massaged me for a while. I then went to bed shortly after, not thinking anything else of it.

August 2, 2011

I woke up to the sound of the alarm. My plan today was to go to the gym down at the surf club, a few good hours of work, followed by pregnancy swimming classes, some more work, and then my favourite yoga class with Michelle.

I took off to the gym and got onto the bike for my thirty-minute stint, followed by some light arm weights. I spent most of the time on my bike chatting to friends at the gym and found it hard to ignore a niggling pain in the top right-hand side of my abdomen. This is the place where I had been experiencing a lot of pain in recent weeks – 'Billy' the name we had called our baby since conception would often stick his legs out into my right side as if having a stretch. It was quite painful, and quite frequent. I thought this pain was just some more of this 'kick and stretch' action.

I took off home, had breakfast and then went to the toilet where I noticed a slight bit of spotting. I was slightly concerned, but not too much as I had had the spotting at fifteen weeks, and it turned out to be nothing. I had also done a lot of reading which educated me in pre-labour spotting amongst the myriad of other prelabour symptoms – purely the body practising and getting ready for 'the real thing' in 3-4 weeks' time...or so I thought...

I called the family birth centre and let them know of my symptoms: spotting, slight menstrual cramps, and starting to pass bowel motions. They weren't too concerned, and said to me to sit down, relax, and monitor it for a few hours. I was to call them back in the afternoon for an update. So being the workaholic lady I am, I grabbed the laptop, and lay down on the couch, settling in for the day of what I thought was just a bit of relaxation while tapping away on the keyboard.

As the hours passed, my slight menstrual cramps continued, and as the midwife said to time them, and they were approximately ten minutes apart, like clockwork. My curiosity
got the better of me and I couldn't help but start using Google
to find various stories from women who had similar symptoms
to me. One story in particular was exactly the same as me, and
that lady was in fact in labour. "Surely I couldn't be in labour?"
I thought to myself. It just couldn't be?! My plan all along was
for our little Billy to arrive on 1st September, the first day of
Spring. This was one month too early for that!

3:30pm

At approximately 3.30 pm I called the birthing centre again
to let them know that I had been passing bowel motions regularly and had been having regular faint cramping all day. The
midwife conferred with a couple of her colleagues and came
back to the phone to say that to be safe it would be best to get
checked out just to be sure everything is okay – even though it
was more than likely just my body getting ready and practising
for the real thing – labour in a few weeks' time. As I had
changed my due date with the birthing centre to be August
27th , not August 21st , I was technically four days too early to
have a check at the birth centre, so due to protocol I had to go
to the main hospital next-door. I called Daniel to let him know
that there was a change of plan; our 4.00 pm appointment with
the naturopath was now 4 pm at King Edward Memorial

Hospital, in the labour ward. I called Gaby, my Doula and left a message giving her the update on what was happening.

4:15pm

Upon arriving at the hospital I felt more uncomfortable. As I sat in the waiting room surrounded by others who were sick, coughing and spluttering everywhere, I wondered to myself how I was going to last waiting to see the triage nurse! Finally, she saw me and I had a little chat with her. She thought that I was probably just having early labour signs but would sort me out with a midwife to get checked. Back out to the waiting room and luckily Daniel had arrived. To help with my discomfort, a midwife brought me a pillow to kneel on. Ahhh… that was a saving grace.

5:30pm

Shortly after the pillow, the midwife, noticing my discomfort, found a room for me to lie in until they had the time to see me. I was then set up on a CTG – a device that monitors the baby's heartbeat, my heartbeat and the 'contractions' I was having. All seemed fine. There were slight contractions happening, but they still didn't feel like much, and little Billy was hiccupping….which I recorded on my I-phone for safekeeping.

6:30pm

Just as a standard check-up, the midwife decided to give me a cervical examination. She fiddled around for a while,

515

humming away, and nodding to herself, muttering "I see, I see" a number of times. Finally, she pulled her gloves off and said "right…I see" again and then said to Daniel and I "right…now a couple of things. I have had a good feel of your cervix, and it all looks in order. You are actually 1cm dilated and fully effaced. Now perhaps this is better explained by drawing it for you…" So she took a pen and paper and proceeded to draw a picture of a cervix….and explained to me that my cervix had thinned out to the position it needed to be in to start dilating, and in actual fact she could fit her little finger into the cervix. This meant that whether I liked it or not, I was in labour.

Right. Labour. This wasn't part of the plan at all. I spoke to Gaby again, however we all agreed that this was very early labour, and it could go on for days like this, and if I was lucky, I may be able to move to the birth centre if I could stay relaxed and in this early labour stage for a while. That was my plan.

The midwife checked the positioning again of Billy, and like all the other midwives had said, Billy was head down, and the head partially in the pelvis…ready to engage it seemed.

7:00pm

So, Billy wanted to come early. And here I was at the hospital, not the birthing centre. It was then my mission to try and get moved to the birthing centre, and for them to recognise my first due date of August 21st (my scan date) not August 27th (my ovulation date). By this point, Sue Anne, my midwife from the birthing centre of whom I spent most of my time with for my fortnightly check-ups came up to see me. She was a welcome sight amongst the sterile hospital environment, and tiny little room I was sitting in. Sue Anne then served as my 'go-between', between us and the hospital staff. She was liaising with the Registrars on duty, and the midwife who had examined me. According to the midwives, the Registrar was adamant not to let me leave the hospital, either to go home or go next door to the birthing centre, where I was adamant, I wanted to be for the night. I hadn't met the doctor at this point, and it was quite distressing that they were trying to force me to stay in the hospital when that wasn't part of the plan at all!

7:30pm

My waters broke.

There I was, laying on the bed trying to relax, talking with Anne Wylie, our neighbour on the phone, and trying to decide what we should ask her to put in a bag and bring to the hospital for us. As I was talking away to her, I felt a massive gush of liquid forming around my vagina....uuuggghhh, it was my waters. They had broken and there was no turning back. I quickly hung up the phone, got off the bed, took my leggings and underwear off, and yelled at Daniel to grab the bin – that was the only thing in the room I could see that could take the gush of water. It was everywhere and didn't seem to be letting up.

At this point, deep down, I knew that it was inevitable that I wasn't going to ride this labour out for a few days, and I wasn't going to be going home tonight. I was going to have the baby either tonight, or tomorrow morning. I was a little upset, but it was all happening so fast I was mainly overwhelmed, trying to think clearly about what was happening to me. Daniel called Gaby with the update. Anne used her amazing initiative and packed a bag for me with what little information we provided and made her way to the hospital in between feeding her son Jack. While I was standing over the bin, Daniel ran outside to grab some help; the obliging midwives entered the room. The registrar then came in to have a chat. She said that I would have to give birth at the hospital. She then also said she would like to do a scan of the baby, just to double check the positioning, so wheeled an ultrasound machine into the tiny room.

Sue Anne had mentioned to me that this registrar, Lauren, was the registrar who didn't want me to birth the baby at the birth centre, so already I had my guard up when she had entered the room.

7:50pm

After a couple of minutes of looking at my uterus, Lauren said to me "the baby is actually in breech position"… My heart sank, really not believing what I was hearing. It couldn't be true, could it? Four midwives, including the midwife from only one hour earlier, had all said the head was down, and starting to engage. It had been this way since my thirty-three-week scan when I felt the baby move. What was going on? Thoughts were racing through my head; caesarean, drugs, epidural… all the words that had been really scary to me, words I didn't want to hear, flooding my mind like a wild torrent of water flooding the riverbanks.

Lauren spent a bit of time measuring the baby, remeasuring and looking at the whole positioning. The story was that Billy's bottom was sitting in my pelvis, so that's why it seemed like a head. His head was sitting up under my ribs, and his legs were jammed up against his body, his feet up near his head. This explained to me all those uncomfortable moments where he would let his legs fall over to the right side of my body – his little kicks would really make my stomach-ache at the most in-opportune times. How could they have gotten it so wrong?!

Lauren then took the scanner out again, said she would be back, and went to converse with another registrar – the shift supervisor for the evening. Sue Anne and another midwife, Taryn, came in and were talking me through what was happening. They said it didn't look good, and it may be that I might have to have a Caesarean. Lauren then returned and explained to me about the measurements of Billy – he had the head of a thirty-eight-week-old, the bum and legs of a thirty-eight-week-old but an abdomen of a thirty-three-week-old. This is what she was worried about. As the abdomen was so small she thought it would be a risky birth. While all this was going on, my contractions started to get a little stronger and more regular.

519

I knew I was getting into established labour now. This is what I had read about; this is what I had practised my breathing for. This was it.

The senior registrar, Tamara, then joined us in the room and they proceeded to explain to me about the risks of a breech birth, and how it was so dangerous etc. etc., and that basically I needed to have a think about what we were going to do. It was all happening so fast, it was all a daze, people were coming in and out of the room while I was trying to get through contractions and think clearly at the same time. The room then cleared which left myself, Daniel and Sue Anne to think about things. I wanted Sue Anne's advice. "What should we do?" I asked her. I had no idea what to do. She explained a couple of things to me. One of them was that the abdomen size wasn't accurate. Once the waters break and there is no amniotic fluid around the baby, it's harder to get an accurate measurement of the abdomen size. It's never accurate. This was interesting to hear. She also said we should call Gaby. We called Gaby with an update. Sue Anne and Gaby had a chat, and Gaby said well if they were saying that there really needed to be a Caesarean, then maybe it was what we should do. That was definitely not what I wanted to hear, but as Gaby had had so much more experience with this type of thing than me, I started to think….this can't be happening can it?

Gaby also said that Sue –Anne had said to fight to birth this baby vaginally as it was in a perfect position to be born and that Sue Anne had told her to come in as soon as possible to liaise with the staff and support a natural birth if it was to happen.

Even though they had said to us that it was our choice, I couldn't help but feel it wasn't. I felt like there was no way in hell they were going to let us have the baby breech, and later Sue Anne confirmed it. She told me that both Lauren and Tamara had said there was no way they were going to birth a breech on their shift, probably due to their inexperience!

I had done so much preparation for this birth, listening to hypnobirthing scripts, reading, yoga, massage, really slowing down (which is hard for me as I am such a busy person!). One of the most insightful things I did was to read the book by Ina May Gaskin, called Spiritual Midwifery. It is a book about a bunch of midwives who live on a farm in the middle of the USA, very hippy, but very natural in the way they support natural birthing and labour. Part of the book contained numerous birth stories, from the extremely full term, to premature, to breech – it seemed any type of birth that was on record, these midwives and their partners and supportive doctors had birthed them on this farm. As soon as the breech birth was mentioned to me I started to think about these birth stories. It was a source of confidence for me, and comfort. So many women had done this before me, and so many women had birthed breech babies, why couldn't I?

8:45pm

Anne arrived. I heard in the background that Anne was here, and all I wanted to do was see her. I needed to see a familiar face, someone who had only three weeks before been through this same thing. As soon as Anne came into the room I burst into tears. There I was, in labour, naked, in tears sobbing into Anne's chest. I kept muttering "it's not fair, it's so unfair".... while the doctors and the midwives, and Daniel, watched on. I must have been a sorry sight.

9:00pm

I am not sure on the timing as there were a number of things that were a little hazy to me...but Tamara had explained one thing to me. She had said that she needed to check with the consultant who was on shift as to what their thoughts were on a breech birth. I wasn't really sure what she meant by this but it wasn't until I was told that we were being moved to a birth suite that, in the corridor, Tamara said to me that the consultant had agreed to support me through a natural birth. I only partially comprehended it at that point.

The support staff offered me a wheelchair to make my way, between contractions, to the birth suite. The thought of sitting down or doing anything that was in any way slightly restrictive was too much to think about. I declined the offer, preferring to walk the short distance from the triage room to the birth suite. I was really hoping the birth suite was where I was going to stay, and they weren't going to rush me up to the theatre to perform major abdominal surgery on me... being a Caesarean!

While hobbling and waddling to the birth suite I met Taryn, the other midwife from the birth centre who was on duty that night. She had an immediate soothing voice and instantly calmed me down. She had to get back to the birth centre shortly as they had two births on that night (luckily I didn't end up needing the birth centre as there wouldn't have been any room for me!). I had wished she could stay, now that Sue Anne was needing to leave.

When we arrived in the birth suite I immediately relaxed a little more. The room was large, the lights were dim, and it looked more like a nice bedroom than a sterile hospital room. I was introduced to Rosemary, the midwife on duty, who Sue Anne later told me was one of the midwives trying to get me back to the birth centre as she knew that's where I really wanted to be.

Anne, our neighbour and good friend who had kindly brought in some essentials for me into the hospital (don't you just love women who know what to select that was perfect for a labour experience, without as much as two words mentioned between us) joined us in the birth suite – this was great as she was a comforting support, especially special as she had a three-week-old baby at home waiting for another feed. She ended up staying until 10.00 pm, just before Gaby arrived.

With the help of Daniel, Anne, Taryn and Rosemary, I started to settle into the birth suite, where I was going to spend an unknown number of hours having contractions. I wanted it to be as comfortable as possible, as I had no idea how long I would be experiencing labour.

I looked for a mattress, cushions and bean bags – anything that was going to make me more comfortable to labour away on the floor. I was finding the most comfortable position on my knees, and leaning forward over cushions, pillows, bolsters, whatever I could find. Although the birth suite was large and had dim lighting, it was still a hospital room, and had a hard floor that was freezing...not really conducive to spending much time on!! We pinned our 'birth plan' up on the wall, luckily, we had completed this only two days before...! We also had planned to have good food, and music to listen to while I was labouring, but alas all we had was my I-touch, with no speakers, so Daniel did the best he could, setting it up with music I wanted, right next to my ear so I could at least hear some of it. After a while it kind of faded into the distance where my focus and concentration of labour took over.

As I was surrounding myself with the small number of comforts available to us, Tamara started to explain the conditions upon being able to labour in the birth suite and continue with a natural breech birth. I had to have a cannula (an open port in my vein just in case I needed to be hooked up to a drip or something similar), and be hooked up to a CTG machine throughout the whole labour so they could monitor the baby's heartbeat. She also said that the labour needed to be progressing well, at a consistent rate – this meant I needed to become more regular with my contractions and my cervix needed to dilate consistently otherwise the doctors would treat that as a sign that something could go wrong. I may then have to go up to the theatre for surgery. This is one of the reasons they weren't really allowing me to eat food or drink much (however I did sneak a banana and drank water throughout).

I can confidently say now that by far the most frustrating thing throughout the whole labour was having to wear the straps around my body connected to the CTG machine. Not so much wearing them, but the midwives fussing with it all the time, when the positioning was slightly out. I remember thinking to myself often 'jeez why don't they be a little surer of themselves and position it properly in ten seconds, rather than fiddling around for what seemed like hours?" The time I had to spend in a still position while they tried to get it 'just right' was very painful, especially when contractions were coming on all the time and I needed to focus and get down into my comfort position leaning forward on the cushions on the floor.

9:20pm

I had asked to have a shower, and golly that was one of the best things I was able to do all night. Not only was I allowed to take off the damn CTG straps, I was able to stand there with the warm shower pelting down onto my back. My oh my it was relaxing, and I was able to lean over a chair during the contractions, chatting away to Anne.

It was at this point Jan Dickenson came in, the senior consultant on shift. She said she thought she should pop in and meet the lady in labour! She popped her head around the shower door and as soon as I saw her, I melted with relaxation. Her manner and demeanour was one of confidence, wisdom and experience. I said to her that I was so pleased she was here and thanked her so much for supporting my birth. She said that after seeing me she said I would be fine; I looked fit, healthy and alert – all things I knew I was, yet it was nice that she thought so too. It was the first point throughout the whole King Edward experience I felt confident that they were able to help me birth our baby.

I explained to Jan that there were two due dates - one was the 27th August and the other the 21st August. The first was the ovulation date and the latter was the Anthony Murphy twelve week scan date. The latter date meant I was at term, 37.4 weeks to be exact, and once Jan heard this she was even more confident. She also said to me that the baby was small, and his positioning was good, so I would be fine. I heartily agreed and said that's exactly what I was trying to explain to the other doctors! I was so relieved, and a wave of happiness and confidence came over me.

10:00pm

Anne had to leave, and I thanked her profusely for being there for us. She was such a rock of support.

10:20pm

I got dressed once more and was hooked up to the CTG straps once again, so the doctors could monitor the baby's heartbeat and my contractions. I took up my positioning on the floor again. Daniel was helping me with gentle reassurances and finding some relaxing music for me to listen to. It was hard as all we had was the little I-phone and no speakers. I was really struggling to hear it.

Tamara, the main doctor responsible for me, checked my dilation and I was three centimetres dilated. That indicated the labour was progressing well.

10:50pm

Gaby walked in. She was a welcome sight, especially as I had no idea how long I would be labouring for into the night. I felt that it wasn't going to be a massively long labour, but regardless it was good to see her. She immediately took control, checked I had enough water and food. Food was a bit of a sticking point as the midwives were trying to hold me off eating, just in case I needed to be rushed to theatre for an emergency caesarean. Rosemary, the main midwife, had gone on break and the other lady, I can't remember her name now, was lovely. She had a calming touch and voice to her and was really helping me with the contractions while Gaby talked with Daniel and got an update. Both the midwife and Gaby were talking with me, talking me through contractions, encouraging me to breathe. At one point Gaby started to massage my back which I found unbearable as the heat from her hands was so intense. I grabbed her hand and pushed it off, apologising but it was just too hot. I am not sure how I thought of it but I was worried that Daniel hadn't eaten anything substantial for hours, so I asked Gaby to stop by a fast food outlet on the way to the hospital and pick something up for Daniel. Burger, fries and coke. Just what the doctor ordered, so Daniel got stuck into the food. The poor darling must have been starving.

11:00pm

At this point, my baby's heart rate was stable, showing to be 140bpm, which was normal. I was contracting three times in ten minutes at this point and was really uncomfortable as I needed to pass motions. I ended up taking off the straps and going to the toilet and managed to pass small motions in the toilet. The motions continued from that point on until the birth, yet instead of the toilet I had the assistance of poor Daniel cleaning up my mess! I swear I must have emptied my bowels more than I had ever done in my life!

11:30pm

I continued to motor through the contractions, they were still three in ten minutes, yet I was having two contractions at once. They were lasting what seemed like two minutes each as I was definitely doing regular breathing cycles.

One of the most significant parts of my labour was one contraction in particular. On this contraction, Gaby asked me to visualise a flower opening, and although I had only listened to her hypnosis for birth script with the flower visualisation once or twice, I was able to really picture a flower opening, and just like that, I could actually feel my cervix open up - just like a flower. I would say the cervix at this point would have moved about three centimetres. I felt so in tune and in sync with my body, I knew exactly what it was doing. I knew I was close to being fully dilated. I could sense it, and almost breathe it in.

From here on I just kept in the zone, breathing in for four seconds through my nose, and out through my mouth for six seconds. Each contraction seemed to meld into one. Time just seemed to merge as well.

12:00am

It was at this point that Dr Adams came in – he was the anaesthetist and was trying to convince me to have an epidural. I found this quite amusing, as I had earlier when I was in the triage room, when asked about epidurals, of which I had a pathological fear...yet they still wanted to try and encourage me to have one. It's funny thinking back now, that the baby actually birthed only forty-nine minutes after Dr Adams came to visit me – surely he could have recognised I was in established labour by this point!

Anyhow, as I said above, I was clearly in established labour and it was hard for me to really listen to Dr Adams. He was patiently waiting for me to engage in eye contact. This was quite hard as I was contracting every other minute. One contraction would finish then another would begin again. It was relentless, and I was almost at breaking point as the feeling was extremely intense. It's hard to describe actually – it's such an involuntary feeling of not only the muscles tensing, but the pelvis moving open to allow the baby through the cervix and into the birth canal. With the help of Gaby and Daniel I was breathing my way through, in for four and out for six, like clockwork. I noticed sometimes I sped up the breathing but kept trying to remain focused on making sure the breathing was constant and methodical.

All while Dr Adams was trying to converse with me, Gaby stayed by my side, talking softly to me and quietly, keeping me focused and on track. She again asked me what stage of the marathon I was at...I had a real think about it, then answered '32kms'. To me this meant I was in the downward phase of the marathon, I had 10kms to go. Not enough to relax and coast to the finish, it was more the 'grin and bear it' phase, where I had to draw from that inner strength in my legs, rely on all the training sessions I had done to ensure I had enough endurance to continue powering to the finish. This was the 'hard yards' point of the race as Gaby called it, a time where the pain was intense, and I had to push through, just like I was right now in labour!

The marathon I was actually visualising was the Gold Coast marathon, the first marathon I had ever done back in 2003. It is a marathon I had actually visualised prior to the race, and during the race it was surreal – it was like I was acting out what I had visualised in bed all those nights before leading up to the race. At the 32km mark of the marathon, I remembered I had done all of that training, it was really hard, my legs were sore yet I knew I had the strength to continue. As long as I could push through that part of the marathon, I would be okay. If I could only get to 38kms then it was the downward slog home.

If you compare the 32km mark of a marathon to labour, it's actually right at the transition point. It's where you feel exhausted, hate the pain, unsure of how much longer it's going to last, coupled with how much longer you think you can last! I did have a fleeting thought at this point of labour – maybe I should consider an epidural...that thought only lasted about a minute.

The next contraction soon took over and I began to focus on the breathing again. My focus at this point really moved within. I became so driven, focused on my breathing and thinking about what I was actually doing – getting my body ready to push the baby out. It's really a wonderful thing, and I am really glad I had the chance or space in my mind to consciously think about this fact while I was in the throes of labour. It's like a combination of intense pain and a surreal reality at the same time.

12:25am

Now I was feeling like I wanted to push. The midwife Rosemary asked to do a vaginal examination and it was most uncomfortable, as I had to move from my safe position on my knees and the bean bag to be on my back. It was excruciating. The contractions at this point were coming very often. Tamara asked to review me once again to double check the dilation of my cervix.

Gaby asked again where I was in the marathon. I said the 38km mark and I knew I was close. So very close.

12:35am

So, only 10 minutes later, Tamara (Dr Hunter) came back in from her rest (she was on night shift and trying to get some precious sleep) and did another vaginal examination. Poor Rosemary must have gotten it wrong, as I was FULLY dilated, the full ten centimetres. Not sure how that can happen, but I was really glad that Tamara had requested a double check. I can say now that the urge to push is very real, and further proof that the woman is more in tune with her body than people give her credit for. If I had followed my instincts and pushed, the baby would have been born an hour earlier! Trust the woman I say. She knows her body better than any other.

Again, I had to roll over onto my back for Tamara to examine me. The contractions were coming in one continuous momentum at this point. They were non-stop. The pain of Tamara feeling my cervix was excruciating. My natural urge/reflex was to grab her hand and pull it out with force. It just hurt so much her touching and prodding what was such a sensitive area. My cervix had very quickly, in two hours, dilated from virtually nothing to ten centimetres. What is usually done by the baby's head, my baby's bottom effectively did by applying pressure on the cervix with the bottom and legs. I was already proud of my son who was still inside me, being such a strong little man.

Dr Dickenson was now contacted to come back into the hospital for the birth.

At this point all I knew was that I had to wait until she arrived before I was allowed to push. The pain of this was absolutely mind-blowing. Trying to force my body against its will to not push out a baby was so very hard. During each contraction, which as I said earlier, felt continuous, I lost my breath and almost hyperventilated. It was crazy...

I kept my breathing going with the help of Gaby and Daniel, both of them trying to direct my thinking towards different things. Gaby was great at keeping me visualising the marathon I was running which helped me to stay focused on where I was going and helped me to acknowledge just how far I had come in my body during this labour!

It was unfortunate that I didn't get the chance for my pre-doula meetings with Gaby, to really run through my birth plan, what I wanted to think about, visualise etc. I didn't get the chance to explain to her what would work really well for me. Thankfully she knew I had been a marathon runner and extreme sport athlete and knew I would be good mentally with what was thrown at me during the labour. We had to make do with what we had at the time and it worked beautifully.

At this point I moved to the bed and they allowed me to continue kneeling, resting on my hands. Daniel came up next to me at this point and I clung to his hand from that point onwards. Gaby was using a cold flannel to wipe over my back; a welcome relief to the extreme heat that I felt was steaming from my back. I felt red hot yet at the same time I didn't really notice.

Throughout the whole labour I was clasping a little stone with the word "trust" on it, that a friend had given me, who had experienced a lovely waterbirth in Brisbane last year. I kept hold of this stone for the rest of the labour, until our baby was born.

I am not sure if this fifteen-minute period waiting for Dr Dickenson was the longest or shortest period of the whole labour. It was a little surreal and seemed like one big contraction.

12:50am

Dr Dickenson arrived, yay! I was now allowed to push. And push I did!

With the first push that I did with the contraction I felt a definite movement. It was like Billy's bum was bracing itself and locking into the start of the birth canal. At this point the contractions slowed a bit from what they were previously.

In between pushing I could hear many voices; there was a definite calm that had descended across the room once Dr Dickenson walked in. Not only was her demeanour calm, but her experience was so vast that everyone there would have been happy knowing the delivery would go fine...

At this point the contractions had slowed down a bit and I started to wait for each contraction to indicate when I should push.

During the preparation for birth had I spent a lot of time reading about how to protect the perineum so it wouldn't tear. This included stretching it in the lead up to labour, as well as taking particular care in the birth process, resting the baby's head on the perineum so it would stretch slowly, easing out the rest of the body after that. The breech birth was a total reversal of this. All the preparation I had done went out the window. Instead of being asked to wait, pause, gently waiting for the perineum to stretch, I was asked to push, push, push.

Instead of my perfect planning, since the baby was breech, as my next contraction came on, what seemed like many voices behind me kept calling out, 'push, push, push'. "Push as hard as you can". So I did. I really tried and tried to push, it felt like all of my strength was focused on pushing. Every part of my body seemed to be working towards the same goal of pushing the baby down through the birth canal. I felt him sliding down through my birth canal. It was such an amazing feeling. It actually didn't really hurt like I thought it would. It felt like a really large poo, sliding through with each and every push.

After some great progress I had a short rest. It was a short relief for me. Everyone in the background was congratulating me on doing so well with my pushing. It was encouraging. Gaby was still patting a damp cloth across my back, while I was clutching Daniel's hand tightly. I kept my trust stone in my left hand and Daniel's hand in my right. It was like I had everything I needed and wanted at that point to get me through. It's funny though, I was so in the zone that there wasn't really any pain. There wasn't any excitement either. It was just a focus; a drive towards the goal – pushing my baby out of my vagina as soon as I could, and as safely as I could.

The second time I pushed I actually pushed through the contraction. I made a lot of progress. I could feel his little bum coming out of my vagina, then going back in again. I had read so many birth stories like this before, where the head would pop out, but pop back in again until the next contraction or two. I made a pact with myself that on the next contraction I would push the bum right out. And so I did. He came out and stayed hanging in that position. He was nearly born!

At this point Dr Dickensen asked me to move over onto my back, and lie back, to enable her to perform her manoeuvre once it was needed. She was going to hold the baby's head in position, so it didn't flex backwards and get stuck in the birth canal. From this point on the pressure was really on, to push the baby out as soon as I could. Gaby asked me if I wanted to touch the baby's bottom…I just couldn't think about that. I was too focused on getting the baby out. That was all that mattered.

1:00am

It took only two more contractions. The next one got him to the point where his body came out, and Dr Dickensen flicked his arms out. The last contraction I really gave it my all. With guidance from the support group around me, I pushed and pushed. I could feel the head, the hardest part of my baby, sliding out through my perineum. I felt a slight burning sensation but knew there was nothing I could do as I had to get him out as I was being instructed to do so. Everything they were asking me to do I was complying with as diligently as I could.

1:09am

The contraction stopped, I took a quick breath then let out another huge push, I pushed as hard as I could. It was so hard, yet so satisfying. He was out! Yay! I breathed a sigh of relief, as the doctors worked quickly to cut his cord and get him some oxygen to help him pink up.

I was in a little daze, just sitting/half lying there, resting. Daniel left my side and followed our baby over to the table where the doctors were working on him. Gaby stayed with me. I was in a spaced-out mode, and in the background, I could then hear him cry. It was such a surreal feeling. It was like I was outside of my body, observing all of this happening.

The third stage of labour is what they call it when women give birth to their placenta. My plan was to birth it 'naturally', or what they call having a physiological 3rd stage. However, as Billy had to go onto oxygen straight away, they had to cut the cord quickly. This meant our umbilical cord joining us wasn't able to pulse until it stopped the blood flow naturally. For this reason, I wasn't able to have the physiological third stage, so Tamara (the doctor) advised me to get a shot of syntocinon to assist with expelling the placenta. I was still hesitant as I wanted a totally natural birth, however as I had a tough quick breech birth it was easier to assist the placenta to come out by having a syringe of Synto to prevent any excessive blood loss. It all took about two minutes and the placenta came out.

Before I knew what was happening, Daniel brought our baby right back over to me, and we placed him onto my chest. Daniel had tears of joy in his eyes. My heart just melted seeing them both. I was extremely happy too, but the exhaustion was also there so I wasn't my normal bubbly self. I also did not really believe it as it was all so surreal. Wow. I had a son. Wow.

We spent a bit of time enjoying our little boy, looking at his eyes, nose, mouth, little hands and feet. Ahhh… he was so gorgeous. At this time Tamara asked if I was ready to get a couple of stitches as I had torn a bit – not much but enough to warrant a couple. I thought, 'why not?'…

Gaby then helped me to feed him for the first time. She basically took over my breast and nipple, and he was like a duck to water. He latched on really well for the first time. He was off! It was such a special time. Yet at the same time still surreal. So, so surreal, just like a dream come true.

It's just so hard to describe the feeling that one has throughout labour, and immediately after your baby is born. I truly recommend every woman who is able to carry a baby through pregnancy to go for it. The best thing I have ever done in my life, and now two months into it, life just gets better and better. We love our little Billy with all our hearts.

Soren's Breech Birth

On September 12th, 2004 I gave birth to my son Soren by vaginal breech birth. His birth has captured the imagination of many people, since it was a vaginal birth after a previous caesarean (VBAC) and a spontaneous vaginal breech birth. For me, I was simply doing what my body told me I had to do on the day.

I am ecstatic at the birth and the outcome, although nothing went according to plan! I give full credit to my support team (my husband Mick and private midwife Marilyn) and the hospital staff (midwife and obstetrician) who attended me on the day – I couldn't have done it without them.

So what happened?

The story of Soren's birth starts about four years earlier with the birth of my first child, a daughter Tessa on 1/9/2000. I was very ill with a liver problem (obstetric cholestasis) in the third trimester of my pregnancy, and she was presenting breech, so at 37 weeks she was born by caesarean section. We were thrilled to have our lovely daughter and my health improved immediately. However, my recovery from the caesarean section was long, slow and painful, and it took months to establish breastfeeding. Now Tessa is a delightful, happy, healthy 4-year-old.

When we decided to try for a second child, I knew I really wanted to avoid getting obstetric cholestasis again if I could, and I also wanted to birth vaginally rather than by caesarean section. After more than a year of preconception care under the guidance of a naturopath, we were brimming with health, and I became pregnant a second time.

I chose a private obstetrician who was prepared to support me for a VBAC. He advised that I had a 90% chance of the obstetric cholestasis recurring but was unable to suggest any preventative measures.

I had been advised that a knowledgeable support person such as a doula or midwife was important for a VBAC, so I also engaged a private midwife. She cared for and supported me throughout the pregnancy and was the best thing that ever happened to me. I also kept working with the naturopath to optimise my liver function through herbs, diet and reflexology. I was very fit and healthy throughout the pregnancy. No signs of obstetric cholestasis.

My broad plan for the birth was to labour at home and then birth in hospital. Towards the end of the pregnancy, I even started to consider the possibility of a homebirth.

I put a lot of effort into preparing myself for the birth. In fact, I gave up all notions of working this year in favour of birth preparation. As well as preparing my body – walking, swimming, yoga – I put most of my effort into preparing my mind!

I read widely and saw for the first time that birth was not all about pain and fear, and that someone like me – conservative, averse to pain, not overly maternal – could have a 'good birth'. It was a revelation, and at the same time very challenging – could I actually do it? I talked to women, meditated, went to birth preparation classes, sought counselling to deal with some 'old baggage', and went over and over the birth scenario with my midwife.

At 35 weeks the preparation stopped, and our thoughts went on a tangent – the baby was lying breech. The next four weeks were a time of great stress as we tried everything in the book to encourage the baby to turn – lying upside down on an angled plank, crawling on all-fours, handstands in the swimming pool, homeopathics, pressure on the little toes, moxa sticks, acupuncture, energy work and visualisation – all to no avail. At 39 weeks the obstetrician attempted to turn the baby by external cephalic version (ECV) but it was not successful. The baby did not want to turn. At this point I decided not to try anything further to turn the baby – it clearly did not want to be head-down!

Being pregnant with a breech baby is a rather lonely road. I was preoccupied with dealing with the breech situation, while the other pregnant women I met were happily getting on with their birth preparation. We had nothing in common at that time. I felt very alone, especially when I realised that the decision about what to do was entirely mine. After the ECV, even though unsuccessful, it was a great relief to move forward, to get on with the business of having a baby rather than focusing on the breech position. Of course, my birth options had narrowed down! A homebirth was out of the question.

The obstetrician was quite specific: the birth would be by caesarean section; a vaginal birth was not an option. He agreed to allow me to go into labour and then do the caesarean section, so at least the timing of the birth would be natural, if not the birth itself. I was pleased that at least my baby would be setting the birth agenda. We planned to give birth at Woodside Hospital.

My midwife's thinking was not limited to a caesarean section however. She advised me that a vaginal birth of a breech baby would be possible at King Edward Memorial Hospital (KEMH) if I wanted it and if we explored our rights and strongly insisted on it with hospital staff. I could not imagine being able to labour effectively if I was in an adversarial situation with hospital staff over my birthing choices, so I was not prepared to pursue the vaginal birth option any further. I agreed to the caesarean section, with the arrangement being that I'd labour at home for a few hours before coming to hospital.

Four days after my baby's estimated due date on a Saturday morning I woke up feeling different; something was imminent. I had a near-constant "hard stomach" with Braxton-Hicks's contractions. The day and evening passed uneventfully – Mick finished the house project he was working on and we put Tessa to bed. I was still feeling 'different' but had nothing to report when we went to bed at 11.30pm.

Labour started immediately. The contractions were about 15 minutes apart and I was able to breathe comfortably through them whilst lying in bed. Over the next four hours the contractions gradually got closer and more intense. I stayed in bed but was not able to sleep at all. At 4am on Sunday morning I was no longer comfortable in bed, and I went downstairs. I dressed and lit a candle. Outside it was a beautiful clear starry night. I pottered around putting the last few things in my hospital bag. I leant on my kitchen bench for each contraction and was then able to continue my chores. I had to go to the toilet between each contraction.

At 4.30am, the contractions were 5-6 minutes apart and intense, and I had a bloody show. I woke Mick and told him it was time to call our midwife Marilyn. Mick started to massage my back with each contraction. My contractions were intense and hard work, but I would not say painful.

Our midwife Marilyn arrived shortly after our call. I laboured on; I felt I was handling the contractions without distress, and I was relaxed and able to chat in between. In fact, part of me wondered if this was the real thing! At 6am, just before Mum and Dad arrived to mind Tessa, Marilyn did a vaginal examination and found that I was 6cm dilated. I was elated and amazed, as it had been relatively easy to that point.

Obviously, we would have to get to the hospital pretty soon for the caesarean section.

Marilyn phoned the obstetrician to fill him in. He reiterated that he would not support a vaginal birth. Marilyn reminded me of my options: we could go off to Woodside for the caesarean section as planned, or we could still change our minds and go to KEMH for a vaginal birth. A decision was required, and soon! It was down to me! Mick would support whatever I decided. For the first time I entertained the idea of a vaginal breech birth VBAC. I was progressing in labour and handling it well. I knew about the risks – I'd done my homework. I thought of coming home a few hours later with my baby or a few days later with a painful wound and my baby. Outside it was a beautiful spring morning.

For once in my life my brain was not weighing up pros and cons. Rather, I just knew what had to be done. It's hard to explain, but this baby had to be birthed vaginally. I felt this in my body very strongly. So I made the call. We would go to KEMH for a vaginal breech VBAC.

Marilyn was on the phone again, advising the obstetrician that his services were no longer required, and letting KEMH know that we were on our way. Then we literally flew to KEMH – Fremantle to Subiaco in 12 minutes – the fastest trip of our lives. Thank goodness it was 7am on a Sunday.

Sitting in the car was painful. It felt like I was sitting on the baby. On arrival at KEMH I was offered a wheelchair but couldn't bear the idea of sitting down. So, I walked to the labour ward; everybody jumped to when my waters broke on-route!

At the labour ward, we met our delightful hospital midwife who was more than willing to help me to birth my breech baby. She had organised a mobile foetal heart monitor so I could move and birth standing up. Baby was fine. I was now fully dilated with a slight lip, so I panted through a couple of contractions while we waited for the lip to go and for the consultant obstetrician to start her shift.

The consultant obstetrician was warm and kind and she very calmly advised me of the risks of proceeding with the vaginal breech VBAC, including that the baby could die. She offered me a caesarean section even at that late stage. (I noted that no-one outlined any risks of a caesarean section to me!) She then very kindly offered me encouragement in what I was doing and said that she thought things were proceeding well. She also told me she was experienced with breech births. What more could I want in the way of support? It was wonderful. I restarted my desire to birth vaginally. After that, I was down to business.

I was birthing standing up, hanging around Mick's neck to bear down. It was amusing to glance down and see the consultant and midwives crouching awkwardly on the floor, looking up at my nether regions! I took a while to get the hang of pushing. The baby's bottom was in view, but not out yet. After a while Marilyn could see that an episiotomy was looming, so she told me to give it my all. I held my breath and pushed with all my might. At last, the bottom was born. The rest of the body, the limbs and then the head followed quickly, with only minor assistance – the consultant's finger inserted in the baby's mouth to pull the jaw down and head forward. There was no time to get onto the bed to birth the head as the consultant had wished – I heard her ask for a cloth to catch the baby, and he was out!

After four hours of established labour and an hour of pushing, my breech boy was in my arms, on my breast, the two of us in a heap on the floor. I could not believe that the birth was over, that he was with us and that all was well. I was filled with wonder and gratitude. It was 9am. Our four-year-old Tessa came to join us and meet her brother at lunchtime. We went home at 3pm. And named him Soren.

Afterwards, I realised just how wonderful Marilyn, our private midwife, had been for us. She made all the phone calls to the original obstetrician and hospital and to KEMH, shielding us from the flak that I'm sure was flying. She advised the hospital staff of the wishes I'd expressed in my birth plan (and which, in all the hurly-burly, I'd forgotten to mention), including my desire to birth standing up and my wish to birth the placenta naturally, without an injection. She stated my wishes, and they were respected. I did not have to argue my case. And then her presence and care made it possible for us to go home the same day. She endured our freezing house while I laboured and did not express alarm at travelling at 120km/hour through suburban streets to the hospital!

The next day, when I reflected on my decision to go for a vaginal birth, I was shocked. Seriously shocked. When I looked at the situation from my rational (non-birthing) perspective, I could not believe I'd taken the risk of a vaginal birth. Just one day later, I was no longer driven by instincts, I was back inside my head.

I feel blessed to have a beautiful, healthy son and I'm so grateful for the journey and the experience that my pregnancy and Soren's birth have been.

Otis' Breech Birth Story, Baby No.3

To me, the last month of pregnancy seems to be the longest. The same questions keep coming up: did we know whether we were having a boy or a girl, when was I due, was I feeling well (did I look unwell? I love being pregnant!). We endured the myriad of opinions on whether we were having a boy or a girl, based on a number of theories, including 'carrying high or carrying low'. My sister and I were due within weeks of each other, and were quite different shapes, she was carrying high and I was carrying low. We both had boys. I wonder now whether the different shapes were more an indication of the way the baby was presenting in utero.

Apparently, it's not that unusual. My (second) son was born breech and I was born breech. It just seems to be a dying art. As in, fewer women are currently birthing naturally with their baby in the breech position. Many women are persuaded to have the baby turned manually before the end of term or have C-sections. As a consequence, fewer medical professionals ever actually witness a natural breech birth.

A routine check-up with the GP/Ob at 39 weeks resulted in an immediate visit to the hospital for an ultrasound: the doctor suspected a breech presentation. This was quickly confirmed by day's end. The doctor then organised an immediate C- section at the regional hospital. I asked the GP/obstetrician whether we could discuss alternatives to the C-section and was told that breech births were risky; the best outcome for the baby would be to have a C-section. There was no consultation with either myself or my husband as to whether we would agree to a C-section; it appeared to be normal protocol to conduct a C-section under these circumstances. But this was not at all what Warren, and I had envisioned. We had spent many hours considering a homebirth for our first pregnancy; a second home-birth was also our preference. We declined the C-section and went home for a little time to think and discuss our options.

Our first child was born in what would be considered a textbook natural birth, so I had, up until now, no concerns about this second pregnancy. Now we needed to consider two issues: whether to have this C-section or not, and if not, whether we would or could have this baby at home. I have always maintained that I was open to rethinking my strategy (birth plan) at any stage of the pregnancy. That is to say, I was prepared to listen to advice and do research, and to make a decision accordingly. I wanted to remain empowered in my pregnancy and birth by having informed choices. My husband and I consulted our independent midwife. We also conducted some internet research on breech birth and we had a night to "sleep on it".

In the meantime, I had not quite reached full term, and I wanted to try to get the baby to turn. I went to the local Chinese herbalist and tried moxa sticks, I went to the local swimming pool and spent time duck diving, I had foot reflexology and osteopathy and I rested and meditated with my head lower than my bottom. But still I felt no great somersault. Nor did I feel uncomfortable or that the baby was distressed.

As the estimated date arrived, we reconsidered our approach. The revised birth plan included trying one last time to turn the baby, this time by ECV (external cephalic version, a manual manipulation to turn the baby in utero). As long as the baby was showing no signs of distress, I wanted to continue with a homebirth. Option Two was to attempt a natural birth, but in hospital. As a last resort we would opt for a C-section if emergency conditions arose; I would not be emotionally blackmailed into it.

The ECV was unsuccessful. Once again, the obstetrician explained the risks of a breech birth, and stated that theatre was ready and waiting. I countered with the offer to wait for spontaneous labour, and then to come into the hospital to have the baby. This, too, was denied. Again, after more discussion between my husband, midwife and myself, I informed the obstetrician that I was going to go home and wait a few more days for spontaneous labour and a natural birth. I was upset by the doctor's attitude. When I calmed down I was proud that we had walked away with a strong decision that was right for us at that moment.

The next evening, while trying to round up the troops for dinner, my labour began. It began to rain hard, and my husband ran off to put tarps on the roof of our new house, still under construction. The midwife was still a half hour away. I bounced on the fitball for a few seconds then had a mouthful of food. If this was going to take all night, I wanted some sustenance. This worked for exactly four mouthfuls. My husband returned soaking wet. Our doula took Jasper off for a shower and tucked him into bed. When Jasper got out of the shower I hopped in for some relief. A few contractions later, the baby's bottom appeared. In the next two or three contractions some legs plopped out, followed by arms and shoulders and a chin. During the last contraction, the head came out.

With the full support of my husband and midwife, our son Otis was born, naturally, at home, in a breech presentation.

Holly's Surprise Breech Birth

My pregnancy so far has been a dream and I am thrilled to be nearing my due date to meet the little boy I have affection-ately named Arlo Lennox.

I am attending my 38week antenatal appointment at Fiona Stanley on Tuesday 4th of July, I'm 38+3 weeks pregnant and up until today, the midwives have told me my baby is head down which is all that I want as I have planned a water birth, minimal / no intervention and delayed cord clamping and par-tial lotus birth.

I was not prepared at all when the attending midwife Jess is unsure of his position only to later determine with the help of a senior midwife that he is in fact breech.

I'm given 3 options.

One having an ECV- manual turning of the baby, option two being, a C-section and three is, contacting King Edward hospital where it is more likely a Doctor would consider a vag-inal breech birth.

Two and a half hours later I'm heading home tired and emotional but armed with every spinning baby technique and plans to start making appointments for chiropractic and acupuncture sessions. I am due back at the hospital first thing the following morning for a scan to determine what exact breech position and speak to the consulting obstetrician about my options.

My scan confirms Arlo is Frank breech, four and a half hours later, I am attended to by a brand new fresh off the mark, straight from university young and eager male obstetrician. He confirmed what I already knew and advised that senior doctors were still discussing my case but was happy to reiterate to both myself and my doula that it was ultimately my body, my decision and although the doctors are there to advise me, that none of them can force me to do anything I did not want to do! Sadly, the senior obstetrician, an older South African male was quite intimidating and had quite a different opinion.

He held nothing back, arguing the baby could get stuck, end up with brain damage, broken bones you name it - he said it. He also informed me, he had delivered breech babies, but due to this being my first baby, and my pelvis having not been 'tested' that should I present in active labour, he would decline to see me or assist in delivering my baby! My experience with this doctor was overwhelming, he made me feel fearful of wanting a vaginal birth but luckily for me I had my beautiful doula Tara with me and she was able to ask the questions that I wasn't able to and support me in a time where this particular doctor was relying on my lack of knowledge and weakness.

He really put the pressure on me, wanting me back at the hospital the following day for an ECV. After hearing, what it involved it just wasn't sitting right with me at all and I needed time to think it through so I agreed to come back to the hospital on the following Monday which would have me at 39+2 days gestation for a scan, allowing me time to explore every other option and technique to spin Arlo naturally before intervention taking over.

I tried everything, acupuncture, moxibustion, sound healing, heat and cooling, light and sound, inversions, breech tilts and reiki. I threw everything at it to try to turn my baby, but he did not budge!

By this stage I still had complete faith in my body and Arlo, knowing that when the time was right, he and I would know what to do. My instincts were telling me that my little man was not in distress and was very happy where he was.

Sadly, I felt like the hospital tried to trick me into a number of things telling me that for the ECV on Monday, I'd need to fast.. I hadn't agreed to an ECV just a scan, but soon realised the only reason I'd been advised to fast was due to them pre-empting doing a caesarean section soon afterwards. When I arrived for my scan, the receptionist advised me I was booked in for an ECV - and asked if I had I fasted and I said no, I'm here for a scan. I then filled in mountains of paperwork followed by paperwork for Medicare which stated I was being booked in for an induction. This infuriated me, and I pointed this out to the receptionist again who sheepishly stated it was just a mistake.

You can understand why at this stage I was ready to call it quits with the process and walk out!

After finally being taken into a room for my scan, and luckily having my best friends Tara and Eve with me for support I am introduced to Eman who is the consulting Obstetrician. Instantly I warm to her, she's from Egypt and has a beautiful maternal vibe about her.

The scan reveals that my little man hasn't moved at all, he is in exactly the same position. I feel a little defeated at this stage, knowing I had gone into the hospital on this day truly against having manual manipulation to turn this baby.

Once again, after the warm and caring demeanour of Eman, she explains the ECV to me and I feel happy to consider it as an option because I still haven't come to terms with Arlo remaining breech. She allowed me time with my friends to process the information she'd given me and discuss it with them. No pressure at all.

After 5 minutes mulling it over with them I feel comfortable giving it a try.

The first attempt was unsuccessful with Arlo's bottom not moving at all, the procedure was uncomfortable, and my bladder was full, but I was determined to give it another go asking if there was anything I could do, perhaps I could get up and empty my bladder, and maybe moving around might help. The second attempt truly seemed like it was going to work, both women were using all of their weight behind them, slowly turning him from his bottom to his head to spin him around. I could feel him shifting and was so hopeful, but in the end, he just wouldn't spin head down.

By now, Eman sadly says to me I'm so sorry Holly, we've done what we can and he just won't move, we just can't risk trying again. I was devastated and it was a very emotional time, I felt like I had failed, and it was heartbreaking as tears started to well up. Once again, she left me alone to process the situation and returned five minutes later asking me what I'd like to do. I enquired about King Edward and how I had been advised it was an option, and she went straight to work getting me a referral.

While I waited, hooked up to the foetal monitors, Arlo showed no distress at all. Eman came back ten minutes or so later to tell me she was waiting to hear back and, in the meantime, also consulting with other doctors at the hospital about their availability to support a vaginal breech delivery.

When she finally returned she advised me straight away that King Edward had declined to receive me for a referral due to events that had happened earlier in the year, however after consulting with the head of the hospital at Fiona Stanley and emails discussing me with the other doctors that I would be able to present in active labour, and that anyone with breech experience would be on call and available to support me with my breech birth.

I was overwhelmed with emotion and so grateful at that moment. What an angel, after telling me she was off to Bali for five days the following day. I could only hope Arlo would wait for her to return to Australia and she could assist me and Arlo into this world.

This is a true testament to her as a woman, she could see and feel how important it was for me to have a chance at a natural birth before having to have a C section, a truly amazing woman going in to bat for me and my rights! Women empowering women.

I couldn't have hoped for a better outcome, I was going to be given the chance for a natural birth and couldn't be happier. Finally, I was able to put my mind at ease and no longer worry about a C section - my biggest fear!

I felt satisfied knowing I wasn't due back to the hospital for another week, then I would be 40 weeks in gestation, then I could relax. Two days later on a Wednesday which was the 12th I visited my chiropractor Taylor to try the Webster technique again, she did some myofascial release which instantly made me feel like she had created more space in my body for Arlo to move and after my session with her in the morning I felt like today was the day!

I had a constant nagging headache all day and hopped into bed for a nap in the afternoon hoping to sleep it off, by 4:20pm I felt a strange popping sensation in my tummy which I'd never felt before, followed by me trying to get up only to find out that my waters had ruptured!

My best friend and birth partner Eve rushed home to organise my labour things, while I took my time (although I was advised I needed to go into the hospital straight away) ringing my doula and my mum, showering and making sure I had everything in my bags.

We arrived at the hospital around two hours after my waters ruptured and I was sent straight in to have an examination to determine what stage of labour I was in, by now I was having manageable five-minute apart contractions.

The first attending midwife wasn't that friendly giving us a bit of a hard time about all of the bags and bolsters we had, taking up too much space and to be fair, yes, we were very prepared because we knew we weren't going home now, this was it.

My doula Tara arrived soon afterward even bringing me a burrito at my request ha-ha.

A beautiful Indian midwife popped her head in asking the other midwife to take me across to a labour suite. When the attending midwife mentioned my name, her face lit up in a big grin and she said "oh you are Holly! We've all been waiting for you and we are so excited to have you and will take amazing care of you" and this warmed my heart. I felt truly supported and knew I was in good hands.

We were moved into a birthing suite around 9pm, unfortunately a waterbirth was no longer an option for me but was able to have cordless foetal monitoring allowing for me to use the shower, the support people had set up my diffusers with clary sage, lavender and wild orange, and in the background, I had beautiful soft meditative music playing, I was calm and in the zone.

I really don't recall when I went from eating my burrito and laughing with my friends to being down on all fours breathing through contractions.

The midwives changed shifts and Jane arrived, she would stay with me for my labour and birth.

When Dr Raj Singh comes in around 10 - 10:30pm he did a scan to check to make sure Arlo was still in breech position.

We were all set for my VBB although it was a little unclear whether his cord was next to his neck or around but his heartbeat was strong and he was in no distress.

Dr Singh was incredibly informative, and I sensed he was very well respected by all of the staff as he went about drawing me some diagrams to explain the different birth scenarios.

Finally, we both came to the agreement that it was informed consent between adults and I had a full understanding and knew the risks involved, he went on to advise me that he would have some non-negotiables about delivering Arlo breech. I would need to deliver in theatre, should there be any complications and would also be in stirrups and have an episiotomy, while this did deviate away from my birth plan I was at peace knowing I'd have him naturally!

Hearing about his 22 years' experience in his profession delivering babies, in India, the UK and Australia performing around 1000 vaginal breech deliveries with only 2 bad outcomes I am satisfied we are in good hands.

Around midnight he returned to my room for a VE, where I am now five centimetres dilated, this is great news and I feel triumphant although starting to tire but continue in my meditative state with both Tara and Eve supporting me with cold face washers, back massages and hip squeezes.

When he arrived back to my room around 2:45am for another VE I'm now nine centimetres dilated and advised if I feel like pushing to try not to as Arlo's heartbeat is starting to drop and it's time to move to the theatre. I'm given a gown to put on and sign the necessary paperwork for any procedures that may need to take place, I vaguely remember how to sign my own name in such a hazy state.

Tara walks me through to the theatre where we stop just shy of the entry and I have a huge contraction while leaning on her shoulders. The pressure is unreal, and I know it's not long to go.

Before I know it I am up on the bed and my legs are in stirrups. Dr Singh is still joking with me about our conversation earlier on the strength that Maori women possess during childbirth and that I too had that strength and we needed to work together.

When he told me to push, I needed to push as hard as I could. I was exhausted and had no idea how I'd have the energy or strength but a huge contraction and a fierce roar and all I hear is Jane say, I can see your baby's bottom, he is here!

Another huge contraction and roar and another push, all that's left to come is his head and finally the last contraction and push and I hear his cry. The emotion I feel is indescribable, he is placed on my chest and it's a surreal experience.

All up it was about five minutes of being in the theatre, surrounded by doctors, nurses and midwives under that bright sterile light that Arlo made his way earth side, just as I trusted him too and he is perfect.

I laboured and delivered my little babe, drug free and in the end, it was my stubborn placenta that wouldn't detach that would mean I'd have to have an epidural to manually remove it. Some might have been disappointed getting all that way drug free only to have an epidural, but it didn't matter to me, I was so proud that I had stood my ground, firmly trusting in my body and in Arlo and knowing that my body was capable of safely birthing him. A woman's right of passage to be able to do what nature had intended.

Arlo was born on Thursday 13th of July 2017 at 3:27am weighing 3.6kg and 51cm long.

Our stay in the hospital was roughly 24hours in the end due to the antibiotics I needed for the removal of the placenta. During this time, I had many fascinated visitors who wanted to congratulate me on the first planned vaginal breech birth at Fiona Stanley Hospital. There was overwhelming support as I had really opened up the discussion for more women to have a choice about their birthing rights and decisions surrounding breech births.

It was quite humbling knowing Jane, my midwife had only attended one breech birth and she truly was moved and said it was amazing! Both Natasha who assisted and stitched me up, Dr Singh and Jane all came in to congratulate me on my courage and strength in birthing Arlo vaginally and to make sure that I was being looked after. What a team.

I want to say a huge thank you to all of the staff at Fiona Stanley, as I am so grateful for the way I was treated by everyone both during my labour, birth and post-natal time at the hospital. What an incredible experience and I can't wait to share my birth story with Arlo when he grows up!

Holly Stewart

Jerri's Amazing Breech Birth

It was the morning of my baby shower, lying in bed contemplating going for a walk when I heard a pop. My waters had broken.

This was so unexpected as our little man was four weeks early.

Being my first baby and having been told at the hospital birthing course that we don't need to come in until the contractions are 10 minutes apart, I decided to take my time. I had to finish packing, had a shower and within 45 minutes we were on our way. Jumped in the car and boom, contractions started 3 minutes apart. Needless to say my husband was freaking out, and regretting letting me choose a hospital that is 45 minutes away. I kept my cool, calling my mum to tell her the baby shower may be off but not to cancel yet as I wasn't sure, makes me laugh now! I was so in denial.

When we arrived at the hospital the midwife did an exam, she was very shocked when tiny toes grabbed her. We of course knew our little man was footling breech and we were actually booked in for an ECV attempt the following day. Obviously, he caught wind of this and had other plans.

The obstetrician came in and we headed to the theatre for a caesarean, except on the way down I felt a strong urge to push. I couldn't help it, crazy how your body just takes over.

We got down there, spinal block in and he took another look. Next thing I know he's asking me to push, our little man was already halfway out. Everything happened so quickly, 3 hours from my waters breaking and he was here. What just happened?!

My obstetrician was so amazing, kept his cool the whole time. He knew how badly I wanted a vaginal birth and still to this day I can't believe I got my wish. The experience for me although hectic was still super positive, and we now have a beautiful 2-year-old boy and an awesome story to tell.

Birth Story for Baby Luci Alyce

Back in early March, Gary and I decided it was time to stop being selfish and start a family. Luckily for us it wasn't so difficult and before we knew it I was pregnant. I felt I knew from day one that all was 'go' — my body just told me all was okay and the baby-making process was underway.

My profession is an aerobics instructor/personal trainer, so monitoring my heart rate was most important to me. I cut down on my cardio classes, especially the high-impact ones, and concentrated on the toning.

I went through my pregnancy very easily, but could not believe how much energy it used up. From being a person who was hyper and always on the go, I found it hard to slow down.

Now, looking back, Thursday was a big day. It started at 5 a.m. supervising in the gym, followed by a two-hour walk through Kings Park, including the Kokoda trail, back to the gym for lunchtime supervision followed by a circuit class in which the 'hula hoops' came out. Watching the participants wiggle those hips and try and keep the hoop up was so much fun — the laughing and banter was alive! Mid-afternoon I was on my way home — rather tired but with more to do that day. Waxing was the next priority, followed by the weekly shop and home to unload. Deciding that we were just too tired to cook, Gary and I took off for an early dinner at the local Indian. After a tasty meal it was home to bed, it had been a long day and sleep was needed.

Well, the sleeping soon ceased at about 10.30 p.m. All of a sudden I felt like I had lost control of my bladder, so I bolted out of bed not realising what was going on (this was all happening three weeks early!). Did the toilet thing and then went back to bed, but no sooner had I got comfortable and it happened again. You know how 'everyone' tells you that in first pregnancies the baby never comes early — well don't listen. I realised then what was going on, that labour was starting, but went to

565

the toilet again just to be sure. Now the other thing that 'everyone' tells you is that first pregnancies are prone to a long labour — again, not always true. I went back to bed and lay there looking at the clock trying to time my contractions, which were coming in four- to five-minute intervals. Within the hour they were only minutes apart, so I thought it was time to wake Gary.

It was amazing how quickly he moved. After weeks of me being hassled over packing my bag for the big day, guess who didn't have his packed? So the panic was on!

By midnight the contractions were coming hard and fast and with a quick call to the Family Birthing Centre (FBC) we needed to be on our way. Well that was easier said than done — trying to run between contractions when I could feel the baby bearing down was a challenge in itself. It took twenty minutes before I was kneeling in the front seat of our VW Polo (facing the back) and Gary zoomed off down the street. Six red lights and a section of roadworks later, our gorgeous little girl, Luci Alyce, was born in the car outside Karrakatta Cemetery. Of all the places to be born, it was outside the cemetery!

Yep, she was in a hurry, and in that much of a hurry she came out bum first. It was scary — birthing her myself was one thing, but when I realised I had her bum in my hand, that was something else. Then the feet came out. I started to worry about where that cord was going to be. I yelled at Gary to stop the car, which he did, and he came around to the passenger side. When he got there, I told him to hold 'this' — he did not realise just what 'this' was! It was our baby's legs and bottom. I tried to reposition myself and feel where the cord was going, as my biggest worry was it was going to be around the baby's neck. Then the penny dropped for Gary, who assessed the urgency of the situation and said that we needed to get to the FBC. Luckily, I finally felt the cord was free of Luci's neck and when Gary took off, in a bit of a panic, out she popped!

Arriving at the FBC I was now seated properly on the front seat with our gorgeous little girl in my lap still attached. As the door opened at the birth centre, Gary fell into the midwife's arms with all that had just happened, as it started to sink in. The midwife who greeted my husband at the door was Wendy, who came to the car to assist me into the birth centre. I said to her that Luci had come out bum first — "no" she said, "that can't be right", but then her eyes popped out of her head as she saw the big pressure bruise on Luci's bottom. It was time to move from the car to the inside of the FBC where I stumbled about awkwardly, Luci still connected to me via the umbilical cord. I attempted to get onto the bed, where I sat in a state of contemplation and shock from the speed in which I had just birthed. The midwives allowed me (us) to stay like that for about twenty minutes, letting us all get over the shock of our experience.

Luci was then freed and put under a heat lamp while I was brought a cup of tea and waited for the placenta to make its debut. Another twenty minutes passed and all was over — now it was time to relax and take it all in.

After all the reading I had done in the nine months, everything that I had been told seemed so irrelevant now. I know that I didn't have the 'normal' kind of birth but I did feel that perhaps too much emphasis is put on the educational part of labour and not enough emphasis is placed on the aftercare. Being a first-time mum I had not had exposure to many babies before and a little terror set in, knowing that I was now a parent. All of a sudden the responsibility of this tiny, helpless human is yours — don't get me wrong, it is wonderful, but scary at the same time.

I could not have asked for better support from the FBC — the midwives and the environment get you ready for normal life ahead. It was off home just before 6 p.m. and this time there were three of us. The experience was wonderful and I am ready to do it all again, but maybe not in the car!

10.

WATERBIRTHS

Anne and Mal's Beautiful Waterbirth

It was in the early hours of the morning when I woke up from a deep sleep having sworn, I had just heard the phone ring. You see I had been in a deep sleep dreaming that the woman I had been waiting on to go into labour, who was now 21 days over her estimated date of birth, was having her baby. Her baby was clearly happy inside; we all realised this as Anne went to have her little baby's heartbeat monitored daily, scan done and the placenta checked to make sure it was functioning beautifully, and it was. Anne (the Mum to be) was doing really well health-wise and all was going as it should. It was the home-birth midwife and myself who had to wait patiently, and encourage Anne and her husband Mal to do the same.

My dream was beautiful; it was dark outside and everywhere I looked I could see candles lit up around the house and

Anne birthing in my waterbirth tub which was filled with lovely hot water on this cold windy night. My heart pounded with excitement and then I was suddenly awoken with a jolt as I sat bolt upright in bed as I swore the phone had just rung. I sat there for a moment waiting for the phone to ring again. I looked at the clock, it was 1.30am. In my confusion I thought to myself they must have hung up as they felt it was just too early in the morning to call me. So, with that thought, I got out of bed, went to the toilet and made a hot chocolate drink. Then, deciding I was tired, I hopped back into bed where I must have fallen back to sleep. I knew full well if they needed me and had rung me previously, they would call again in the not-too-distant future.

Upon drifting back down to sleep it dawned on me, maybe the phone call was part of the dream I had been having. Again, I felt excited because when I dream about my clients' birthing, I know that it is about to happen very soon, in the immediate future. Not long into my sleep the phone did ring, for real this time and it was Anne explaining how at 1.30am in the morning she was awoken having a 'bloody show' and contractions. It was our strong connection that woke us both up experiencing a jolt at 1.30am? So often I am very in tuned and connected with the women that I doula for, experiencing these little 'unknown' and 'inexplicable' signs due to my heightened psychic abilities and intuition which come in very handy at times. So, when Anne's phone call came in the morning, I was not at all surprised and thanked my ability to connect and intuition for the prior warning.

As Anne and I spoke over the phone I could tell how relieved to know things were beginning and her body was moving into action. Anne had decided just the day before that she was going to be induced on the Friday having waited for 25 days to go into labour. Friday was the day she had decided to succumb to a medical induction. So as Anne described the period type sensations she was now experiencing, there was pure excitement in Anne's voice. Being that Anne was in early labour, she suggested that I go about my day and that she would call me when she needed me at a later time.

The morning passed quickly with me keeping my dentist appointment and managing to do a pregnancy massage for another client who was birthing that week also. Three times throughout the day I touched base with Anne and Mal via mobile phone and at 1.00pm they asked me to come on over as Anne was really needing some physical touch/massage as well as emotional support. When I arrived, I explained to Mal and the Midwife about my dream and wake-up call, and how Anne had had her first sensations then as well. We were all amazed and excited about what this implied and the sequence of events that had led to Anne being in full labour at that very moment in time.

With labour coming on I gave Anne some Homeopathic remedies to really get things moving along and like clockwork her contractions went into full swing putting her into great established labour, which is what we were all waiting for. With this rhythmical intensity change it was not long before Anne decided that she wanted to get into the tub and off the fitball which she had been sitting and rocking on for quite some time.

Like all women who enter the tub, the look of pure elation swept over her face as she slid on into the water. It was here that Anne laid down in the water in-between having contractions, and then sat up on her knees to have a contraction. She felt a certain amount of freedom in the tub to move about easily and really made the most of letting her mind and body go through surrendering to all the contractions as they came and went. After a period of time, Mal hopped into the water as well and applied the massage which I had taught him during one of my Labour preparation workshops.

We were a great team. Mal applied the great massage and physical support. I kept whispering positive affirmations and words of encouragement and Ruth, the homebirth Midwife, performed all the necessary medical checks from time to time to make sure both Mum and bub were fine. With all bases covered Anne was left to just get on with the job of labouring not having to worry about a thing.

As time passed by, Anne decided that she had had enough of the water and decided to hop out of the tub and use gravity for a bit to get the head further down into the pelvis. With this, she moved about the house rocking and leaning on Mal for support as the contractions came and went. After a while she leaned over the kitchen bench as it was a perfect height to lean on and over, and in-between doing this she sat on the fitball from time to time. Moving around from position to position really seemed to be helping Anne who was so strong and positive with an amazing ability to just close her eyes and go within to the beautiful calm place, a place where women can take themselves off to when they are in labour.

After an hour of moving about it was back into the tub for Anne where she laboured away beautifully. We filled the tub up a little higher at this point, so she was able to float if she wished, but mainly she wanted to sit upright and lean against the back wall looking out at all of us. Being that she was really calm and content, Mal took it upon himself to offer us the wonderful stew Anne had prepared earlier that day (with no recipe!) Anne took the opportunity to joke that she hoped it was all right as she didn't want to be left labouring on her own if we all got sick! It was a funny moment and nice break just for a moment for Anne who still had a great sense of humour amidst all of her intensity from the contractions. Even Anne braved her own cooking to have some fresh bread roll dipped in stew. We all felt wonderful having a full belly and feeling like the tank was full.

Anne laboured for another hour before she decided at about 6.30pm to have a VE (vaginal examination) in which Ruth, being very skilled, did whilst Anne stayed in the tub.

Anne was approximately 6-7 centimetres in dilation and Ruth explained that her cervix was so soft and stretchy it could easily go to ten with a little more pressure from the baby's head on the cervix. Anne once again decided to get out and use gravity again on her body and did so by sitting on the ball, walking around and leaning again on Mal during the contractions. This time it was my job to massage and keep assisting Anne in any way I knew possible. At this point we were all due some Sports drinks diluted with water and some chocolate and snakes. This worked a treat and everyone's energy picked up for a period of time as we continued to support Anne in our own special ways.

After a period of time Anne said to Ruth "I am just so tired I want to go to sleep".

Knowing how close Anne was to pushing her baby out and how she needed to be strong and really have some strength on board, Ruth suggested to Anne and Mal that they go and lay down on the bed to rest/cat nap in-between the contractions and work on focusing on breathing through the contractions. With that, Ruth assisted Anne and Mal to the bedroom and into bed where she left them to have some time out together.

When Ruth returned to the kitchen, where I was making us a cup of tea, Ruth said to me, the reason I got them to lay down is because it is going to do one of two things. It is going to slow Anne's contractions down a bit so she can get some rest before pushing the baby out, or she is going to come flying out of the bedroom very soon in transition and dive into the tub to birth the baby". Well Ruth was right about the latter comment. After about 10-15minutes, Anne started to make those deep primal noises that come from women when they are birthing their baby. These noises were echoing down the corridor. With that Ruth and I looked at each other and smiled; it had worked, and Anne was now on her way to pushing and birthing her baby.

Ruth and I turned to see Anne walking quickly down the corridor. Mal was in toe assisting Anne as she stripped off her dressing gown and flew past us before hopping into the tub with a spring in her step. It was here that she proceeded to push and birth her baby. While Ruth checked the baby's heartbeat, I picked up the cameras to film and Mal hopped into the water to support Anne and receive the baby from behind. It all happened so fast but at the same time was so calm and relaxed.

Not long after hopping in the tub Anne let out a huge primal noise and with that, pushed what Mal and I thought was the head out of her body. It was in fact her membranes full of amniotic fluid that looked like a huge balloon. Ruth tried to break them manually for what seemed like an eternity. It was truly amazing to see and acknowledge how tough to break they were, but eventually they did, leaving a smoky cloud of amniotic fluid in the tub. Ruth and I both knew that following that membrane balloon was the baby's head. With that we all watched in the mirror that was sitting on the floor of the tub as

Anne gently birthed her baby's head out of her body. It is always such an amazing and awe-inspiring event when you get to witness up close and personally.

Soon after, Anne gently birthed her baby into the beautiful warm waters of the tub. It was Mal who gently received their baby, along with Ruth who guided the baby through Anne's legs so she could receive the baby on her chest. It was here they both sat in wonderment and amazement for what had just happened. Emotions were running high, and we all cried in happiness and joy for what was and is the most remarkable birth journey of this beautiful baby from the womb into the world. After ten minutes or so Anne looked at her baby discovering that this baby in her arms was a girl and more tears of joy were shed by Anne and Mal.

After a period of time Anne got out of the tub to birth her placenta whilst sitting over a catch tray on the toilet while Mal and I held this beautiful little cherub close to our heart and chest to keep her warm. Not so long before this, Anne's baby had been still in utero, totally warm and snuggled up inside feeding off the placenta hearing all the muffled sounds of this life outside. And now here I stood holding onto this beautiful girl bright eyed and looking around curiously, so perfect and so small. It made me so proud of Anne and her ability as a woman to birth naturally and so peacefully and it made me so aware of how wonderful it is to be able to be a part of something so meaningful and real. It truly is an honour to be asked to be a part of the wonderful journey that women are on leading up to their labour, the labour itself, the birthing, then mothering, breastfeeding and beyond.

Katie's Birth Story

My little one (Harrison) was born on 09/12/15. My waters broke at 11:30pm one evening and I was determined to bring on contractions without induction so did some nipple stimulation then had a nice sleep/rest at home before getting up in the morning to be active and try to bring the baby down onto my cervix. I bounced on a fitball to music and the contractions started straight after.

I took myself off alone into a room and breathed through them, tried a TENS machine for a little while and a hot shower. At 3pm in the afternoon I told my husband we had to go in NOW as I was afraid of being stuck in rush hour traffic. I don't remember much of the car ride except telling my husband to put his foot down to get through amber traffic lights.

I was examined on arrival at the Family Birth Centre (well, it took about 15 minutes for me to get comfortable enough to let my midwife get a feel!) and asked not to be told what my dilation was. My midwife then rushed off to fill the bath and I later found out I was already 10cm! The moment I hopped into the water I changed completely; a sense of calm just came over me. I pushed for two hours but it didn't feel that long. I had two midwives, my student midwife and my husband in the room with me, but they were all so unobtrusive it really just felt like me and my husband. They were all fantastic.

I got through the pushing stage unscathed, just a tiny tear that didn't need stitches and I wouldn't have known it was there had they not told me- thanks to some of the things I learned in your class Gaby, and also the coaching of my midwife on the day. One of the midwives took photos of the birth, which I didn't ask for (my husband decided it would be good to have), but I'm so glad I have now. I remember chatting to the midwives after I pushed the head out "should I wait until the next contraction to push the shoulders out or push in between contractions?" Ha ha.

We were given lots of alone time for skin to skin. I had some trouble expelling the placenta. We waited 1.5 hours for it to come naturally but it wasn't budging and was starting to annoy me so I opted for the syntocinon in the end, which also took a while to work. I ended up having to have it tugged out of me! It was a big relief when it came out; I'd given Harrison (the baby) to my husband for skin to skin because having the placenta still inside me was really uncomfortable and distracting.

I wanted to come home, as planned, 4-6 hours post-birth. Unfortunately, I had to be admitted to hospital though due to a 19.5-hour gap between my waters breaking and Harrison being born. The hospital's policy is anything over 18 hours, without antibiotics, requires a 24-hour observation for the baby due to increased risk of infection. I hated being in hospital, I found there to be constant disturbances, so I got no sleep, and I was also upset at being separated from my husband (visiting hours are from 8am and I was admitted at 11pm). When the clock struck 6:55pm the next day (24 hours post-birth) and Harrison was given the all-clear to leave, we practically ran from the hospital!

I'm so happy to have experienced a non-medicalised water-birth and I feel a little sad for people who give birth on their back with an epidural! There are obviously times for medical intervention but when everything is low risk and normal, I just don't see why you would want to experience a natural birth without intervention! A few people have commented that they are "impressed" I gave birth without drugs, which implies it's what people 'expect' or view as the 'norm'. I went in with an open mind, knowing what I wanted, but not ruling anything out either. I did have a thought that I would try some gas and air however once in labour I totally forgot that drugs / gas even existed as options as I was just so in the zone and it all unfolded very naturally.

Cheers, Katie

Candice's Birth of Stella

Leading up to my estimated due date, I decided to see Gaby for a hypnobirthing session and because of this, I can now tell a story of a beautiful, positive and empowering natural water-birth experience.

At the early stage of my pregnancy, I read Gaby's book, A Labour of Love which really resonated with me. Gaby's name kept on coming up in conversation with various friends, so I knew it was a sign to see her.

During my session we worked together so I could get a strong understanding of the physiological process that my body was about to undertake, and we talked about the incredible connection between our mind and body during birth. I spent time writing my ideal birth plan and soon after Gaby hypno-tised me based on my labour and birth vision. Before seeing Gaby I thought I was having a boy but during my session with Gaby she sensed very feminine energy and we both acknowl-edged that I was holding onto male energy, from my last little angel, the baby who miscarried at nine weeks, but it was now time to let him go. On my way home from my hypnosis session the name Jade strongly came into my mind and at that point I had a sense that we may be having a little girl.

At the early stage of my pregnancy, I was fortunate enough to be accepted at the family birth centre and I had a beautiful midwife, Wendy and student midwife Sinead supporting me through my pregnancy. I felt confident and knew that my body was designed to have a positive pregnancy and birth experience.

My story started on Wednesday, 20th September 2017, I felt contractions commence late afternoon and I knew I had to be by the water, my calm and happy place. My husband Luke and I headed to the beach for a walk. It was a truly beautiful afternoon; we were in our bubble and no one around us knew that I was in the early stages of labour. We went to get some spicy Thai takeaway for dinner that evening, and Luke gave me the most relaxing massage with Clary Sage essential oil around my pressure points, as we were keen to get things moving! Around 9pm I tried to fall asleep as at this point the contractions were still bearable.

At 11pm I woke up with the presence of a lady standing over my bed, call it my imagination or whatever you like but I knew that was the spirit of my husband's grandmother who had passed away the night before. My dreams were so vivid, I also dreamed that my father's mother was handing me jasmine flowers, jasmine was her favourite flower. This Grandmother I had never met. On my birth plan, I wrote that when I go into labour, I wanted to invite the energy of my grandmothers and my Mother to come through to support me through this journey.

Once I was awake again, I decided to lay on our couch in the lounge, with an app and time my contractions as they were getting more intense. Around 1:30am I woke Luke up and we went to a room which had my yoga mat, fitball, calming and grounding essential oils ready to use and my crystals all set up. I remember how quiet and peaceful it was in the early hours of the morning. I started playing my hypnosis sound track that Gaby gave me and it automatically took me back to our session. I was sitting on my fitball, walking around and felt great comfortably swaying from side to side with my heat pack on my lower back. My husband was sitting calmly with me. I was trying hard to focus on surrendering to each contraction, I was trying to welcome and embrace them as this meant that I was getting closer to meeting our baby.

Around 5am, the contractions started to get more intense. I was in and out of the shower, using a tens machine and listening to the hypnosis soundtrack which really helped me keep my head in the game. Luke was giving me fluids, light snacks and massages. I was focusing on the power of my breath. My midwife was away on holiday, but we had a team of other very supportive midwives guiding my husband through the labour over the phone and advised us to come to the centre at 8am.

So we headed off and got stuck in the morning peak hour traffic and after an hour or so arrived at the centre and just wanted to get this baby out. After an internal examination the midwife said that I was not even 4cm dilated and they recommended that I go home so I could feel calm and continue to progress through my labour.

I felt like it was going to give up as I really thought I would be further along. Luke was so supportive and encouraging, and we left the centre knowing what we had to do. I continued to labour at home, looking back now that was the best thing that I did. At around 12pm I said to Luke that I wanted to go to the hospital and have an epidural due to the pain that I was experiencing.

Luke reminded me why I wanted to have a natural, drug free birth. He softly reminded me what I had always told him whilst pregnant, I wanted to be fully present in my birth experience, I wanted to be in whichever position my body required as I knew that freedom of movement would make my labour easier. I knew that by giving birth, drug free meant that there would be less chance of medical intervention, and I knew I wanted to create a calm environment for my baby to enter this world. I also had a strong sense that an epidural would interfere with my hormones and potentially slow my labour down. I knew that being in a drug free state, oxytocin the 'love hormone' would send endorphins to my brain which would work as a natural pain reliever and those hormones would continue assisting me during the pushing phase. I wanted to be able to feel the movement in my body and feel my baby coming down the birth canal, so I could ensure that I was able to push when my body needed me to do so. After this breakthrough, I went back to listening to the hypnosis for birth soundtrack and continued reminding myself of my 'why' and my head was back in the game.

At this point I couldn't talk through the pain, so the midwife advised us to head back to the centre. I remember being in the car for the second time thinking I wanted to escape this reality but soon enough we had arrived and this time I went straight into the birth suite. I asked the Midwife to fill up the bath, whilst that was taking place, I had this intense urge to start pushing. I was under the shower and kneeling on the floor over a chair. I was making extremely loud primal noises, so the midwife did an internal and I was already 8cm dilated. I walked over to the bath, across from my room and I felt this immense sense of calm as I got into the water, it felt as if my pain had gone away.

I had Gaby's voice in my head, and at that point I was able to transition into a state of pure calm and surrender from her listening to her voice. From that moment on I was quiet as making noise for me was too much effort. I felt most at ease breathing through the pushes, I knew that I was well on my way to pushing my baby out. After 50 minutes of pushing, I felt the head coming out of me and a moment later, our daughter emerged from the water and was placed on my chest. I was in a state of shock from the entire process and felt the adrenaline in my body.

Our perfect Stella Jade, a true miracle and a gift from above was born on September 21st, 2017, International Peace Day at 2:59pm, 7 days overdue. We have since found out after the birth that my husband's Grandmother (the lady who passed the night before Stella was born) her grandmother was called Stella.

I am so grateful to Gaby, the amazing team of midwives and my incredible husband for supporting me through the experience. After our final checks, we were cleared to go home from the centre at 9pm that evening. It was bliss being able to be back in our home and in our own bed with our daughter, who we felt like we had known forever. When we decide one day to have another baby, I hope to have the same pregnancy, labour and birth experience.

To all the amazing mums out there, whether you birthed naturally, with medical intervention, C- section, drug free or with pain relief, we are all warriors and have all brought our baby into the world the way it was meant to be.

Laïs's Waterbirth; at the Birth Centre

On Sunday morning, I was 41+5, bub and I was monitored in the hospital to see if all was fine. It was great timing seeing my midwife on the Friday before, at the end of the week, so as not to get pressured for an induction at 41+3, which they would have liked to have seen happen up in the main hospital. During the monitoring that Sunday morning some of my fears came up in discussing things with a midwife. I didn't feel comfortable getting a stretch and sweep from her as I felt this overwhelming pressure was on me to go into labour. It was during this appointment that my baby girl's heart rate dropped and they went into a bit of a panic, suggesting I be induced that night. Even though we discussed what happened during this appointment to have this happen, we all agreed nevertheless something had not been right, so I agreed that I would get induced that night, after speaking to some great obstetricians.

My partner and I enjoyed a good 'last' lunch before we drove home later that afternoon. I took about an hour nap around 3 pm and after that nap I could feel these cramps coming and going, which then felt like contractions. I knew what these felt like due to my other pregnancies in the first trimester that were lost. I knew all was good with bub, but I felt my body somehow 'didn't get it', or just didn't do the right thing at this stage and so I checked into my body. I had learned some amazing tools before this pregnancy doing body work that I decided to apply, and I ended up seeing that my cervix didn't want to let go and was literally holding on tight, doing its work very well, as required up till now! I could see that for years my deepest prayer had been for a baby to stay inside and my cervix to hold strong and not to let go and I was amazed to see how this was playing out now.

I checked in, cleared and created clarity in what was needed for my body to do now. At this very moment with this full-term baby that was probably ready and for me and her to have a natural birth. Bang! I felt my first proper contraction around

5.30 pm. I stayed quiet for an hour and then went to my husband sharing my wonderful news.

We did two birthing courses but we had the biggest fun googling about fake contractions "no" ..."no, don't have that"...."no", and then about real ones "yes"... "yes"... "YES". We called the hospital early that evening and they still wanted us to come in and check me. We went late that night when we felt ready, still in early labour. Once there we became not very popular. We had a doctor who still wanted to induce me with placing a balloon in my cervix, which I refused. He sat behind me with two students and kept talking to me during my contractions. I was leaning over the bed on a ball and I suddenly felt everything I had read about when the circumstances for birth are not right. I felt disrespected and stressed by all the questions at that moment.I needed to be left alone and I explained this to my husband.

Poor hubby's task to deal with this. He politely asked the doctor to continue the conversation in the corridor so I'd be at peace. The doctor said "no, she is my patient, I want to talk to her", and continued to ask me what I meant by having a natural birth and more questions like that. In my own language (Dutch) I said, "this doctor needs to leave now", so my husband explained to him this was not going well and asked if there was perhaps another doctor on the ward. The night then turned very quiet and I relaxed again...Later, while walking around in an almost deserted ward, around 05.00 my husband found me a bath which he filled himself strangely enough. Possibly the timing wasn't good for labour but I enjoyed it immensely after sitting on the ball all night doing purely my breathing exercise, 4 in 6 out.

At 6am it was really time to come out of the bath and an hour later the midwife checked my dilation which was 4 cm. We called Gabrielle our doula a bit later to let her know and she said she would come. After the shift change around 8am another midwife who actually read my birth plan started to arrange things for us since, as she said, I was doing everything myself anyway, was occupying a room in the hospital (they didn't like how I darkened it and used the spare bed as a towel rack) and I didn't want to be in the hospital if it was not necessary.

She surprised us by asking if we wanted to be transferred to the Birth Centre which was our original place to birth this baby! My husband almost started crying; Yes! We were going! We had to sign all medical release forms and off we went. My husband moved the car, Gabrielle who just arrived couldn't believe her ears, took my suitcase and the angelic midwife put me in a wheelchair and we were on our way to the Birth Centre. We all rushed in excitement, and I put on my ridiculous pink gown that of course hardly closed at the front giving everyone an eye full as I was pushed in the wheelchair in active labour.

At 9am, we raced through the hallways and tunnels of the hospital, and I remember passing the laundry guys and

Gabrielle quickly trying to get me decent by crossing my gown further. We were taken down a tunnel going downhill that connected this main hospital to the Birth Centre. The midwife yelled at Gabrielle running next to us "I don't know if I can hold the chair", while in front of me was just a fully grey concrete wall with only a door 90 degrees to the left, lucky for me Gaby grabbed the chair and took over. I felt like I was in a movie, it was so bizarre. The next thing I recall was the warmth and delight of the massive, amazing bath. I hadn't been to a room in the Birth Centre before and felt like I had been dropped straight into a beautiful environment.

There I laboured. I hung onto every little thing Gabrielle said, her encouragement and suggestions and felt I was only physically there in between her words. I had a wonderful midwife from the Birth Centre as well as Gaby and my supportive husband. It still took quite a few hours for my girl to arrive partly due to the waters having only partly broken in the bath, and because of my full bladder and my inability to do a wee. I had to get out of the bath a few times to try to pee with no result and for that reason I had a quick in and out catheter placed into my bladder to empty it. That was pure relief once that was done.

My membranes were also bulging full of amniotic fluid and were sitting in front of my baby's head. So they were broken to release that pressure. After that I went back in the warm supportive water and had to start pushing again. I was very tired after that interruption though. However, I did apparently have a time limit which was discussed quietly between Gabrielle and the Midwife. Gabrielle figured if I knew I was on a time limit it might help to push me a bit. It did; for sure I wasn't going to be wheeled back to the hospital or have anyone pull on my baby; so I pushed bub out!

I had a friend who had told me about having a short cord when she birthed her baby. When my girl shot out through the water in the bath she got pulled straight back to me like a bungee cord. When it stopped pulsating, my husband cut it and then I could feed her as it was hard to hold her up due to the short cord. The placenta hadn't come after an hour, so I got an injection and it came soon after that. I had no stitches, just a little internal tear that healed by itself perfectly.

Our precious girl, Laïs arrived at 2.53pm, seven minutes before my deadline. She weighed 3180 grams at almost 42 weeks. I'm so happy for her to come when she was ready, which was two weeks before I turned 41 years of age. I have truly beautiful memories of how Laïs chose to be born.

Bec's Story

When I found out I was pregnant, homebirth was the last thing from my mind.

I fretted about insurance and which was the best private hospital to attend for a month before deciding on an obstetrician and a hospital. It was only then that I realised my private health insurance wouldn't cover me for a private OB in a private hospital as I was two weeks out of the required time needed. My concerned partner Dion and I pondered what to do, until it was decided that we would budget to make sure we had the $10,000 needed to have our baby under the best health care, heaven forbid if something should go wrong.

At my first appointment with the OB, I waited over one hour in the waiting room. The friends who had referred me explained that this was normal as he was a very good OB who treated each patient like a special case. When it was finally my turn, I went in, sat down and proceeded to cry. I explained how although I was so happy to be pregnant, but how I was very fearful of giving birth after hearing so many awful stories and stated I wanted to have an elective caesarean if I could? However, I also had an excuse ready to tell my family should I need to have one, so they wouldn't know what a coward I was. I was petrified.

Over the next few months, I met with my OB a few more times; I also went to a baby expo. At the baby expo there was a stall for Chiropractic Care. I had heard how much Chiro could benefit children with colic, as well as pregnant women, so I decided to take up the complimentary offer and go myself, for research into my unborn child's health.

This was to be a life changing event.

The Chiropractor's wife and the clinic's manager, Cath, gave me some holistic magazines to read and I read up on how Chiropractic care could actually help reduce labour. I started regular adjustments and also began to borrow some positive birth books and magazines from the personal library. My negative birth thoughts were shrinking by the day and not long after I decided I didn't want an elective caesarean any more. My brain became a sponge; an inquisitive force to be reckoned with. I was exhausting Google, and I automatically switched my thought process about birth from negative to positive. I withdrew from private health care and registered with a local public hospital where I would be under the care of midwives. When I look back, I can honestly say it felt like I'd been thrown a lifeline.

On one of my Chiro visits, Cath told me she had organised a morning tea for all the pregnant ladies who came to Chiro practice as a client. She told me Gaby would be speaking. I had read 'A Labour of Love' borrowed from Cath and looked forward to the morning tea and meeting Gaby in person. Gaby spoke for two hours and at the end of the talk and having read her book, I had an epiphany, I wanted a homebirth! I now knew that the hospital was definitely not for me; I wasn't a special case, I was a normal healthy woman of 31. Both of my Grandmothers had their babies at home as did millions of women, and the benefits of a homebirth for both mother and child made for such a good case.

I voiced my thoughts to Cath. By now I was 34 weeks and I figured I couldn't change care at this stage, I also had no idea who to contact about homebirth. My trusty confidant Cath got me the information I needed. I emailed the Community Midwifery Association, and low and behold, they had a spot for me and I met all their guidelines. I withdrew from the hospital straight away, requested all my test results which they sent me promptly and withdrew from the hospital's antenatal classes I was enrolled in. The feeling of relief was amazing, like a tone of interference instantly removed from my life. I was taking charge.

My antenatal appointments with my midwife involved a hug and long chats over tea and cake at home. Dion and I, along with his mum Maria, enrolled in Gaby's birthing course. I'd always been told to do nothing but laze around when you're pregnant, but I finally started some light exercise each day. I was walking, using my fitball at home and would crawl around on my hands and knees each day for 20 minutes, no more lay-ing around with my feet up reclining on the couch! My new wealth of knowledge made me proactive to be as physical and healthy as I could possibly be.

Maria and my sister Emma were to be our support people. Emma read Gaby's book and wished she had had this knowledge when she'd birthed her two children. My support system was strong, and I was excited!

I'd decided on a waterbirth, and we had everything ready and set up to go. My EDD came and went, and my baby finally decided to come out at 42 weeks. I started contractions at 2:30am, because of all the knowledge I had gained from Gaby's book and couples' course, I knew I could handle this on my own and my support crew and midwives needed their sleep. I quietly went into the spare room and timed my contractions until 6:30am, breathing, surrendering and resting. I had tears of happiness already flowing, knowing that my baby would come to me soon.

At 7am I woke Dion and called my midwife, who asked how close the contractions were. At this stage they were ten minutes apart. My midwife needed to see another lady that morning, so she arrived around 10:30am to check on me. I was contracting beautifully, and she was very proud (all thanks to Gaby's couples childbirth education course). She gave me a kiss and left. She went to see her other girls and Dion called her once my contractions were two minutes apart.

The day progressed with me just lounging around, concentrating on one contraction after the other. Dion set up work from home and supported me when I needed him.

Emma, Maria and then my midwife arrived by 12:30pm. By this stage the intensity of the contractions meant all hands on deck. Dion began filling the birth pool and setting up the camera to record this momentous occasion. At 3:30pm it was time to get into the pool where the pain relief was instant! I was in and out of the pool during my labour and Dion hardly left my side; he was an absolute tower of strength.

Together with Maria and Emma, everyone took turns heating the pool, pouring water over my back and massaging me. I couldn't tolerate noise, so everyone was very quiet. I needed total concentration.

Finally, my baby boy came into the world at 8:50pm. The joy and happiness I felt was the most intense feeling. My Mum arrived while I was birthing the placenta. My mum and sister showered and dressed me afterwards while Dion held our baby. We were in the comfort of our own home with our five-minute old baby; it felt so natural, so right!

I wonder what my first experience of giving birth would have been like if I had stayed with obstetric care and not taken this path.

My little Ari is such a happy, placid and relaxed baby. I have had no problems with breastfeeding as most of my friends and family have had. My midwife came to see me every day for ten days after the birth, followed by every week for four weeks.

When Ari was four weeks old, I took him to my Chiro for his first check-up. We are now regulars and get our spines checked every few weeks. Ari has only needed a couple of minor adjustments.

My whole approach to life has changed because of Ari's birth. I no longer have blind faith in all I hear as I did before. I am a proud mother with a holistic approach in everything I do.

I will never forget Gaby's closing words from my very first meeting with her at the Chiro that day,

"If you don't know your options, you don't have any".

Thank you Gaby!

Matthew's Birth Story

I was woken at 0700hrs with an almighty contraction. I'd had a feeling the night before that it was just about time, so I was well prepared. I was planning a homebirth this time around as I'd had a previous hospital and Birth Centre birth. This time I preferred to stay at home in my own environment with my husband Brett, and two other children, Jarrod and Melanie.

I was planning a waterbirth, as I had done previously. I had the tub set up ready in the lounge room, where I could see out into the garden. I had all my special things arranged in the room – my picture of the 'Madonna', some fresh flowers, crystals, an oil burner with all my oils ready, a C.D. player and music (relaxation and belly dancing music), and a family photo. I had my flower and gem essences ready to take and my Aromatherapy massage blend all set to go.

At 0815hrs I rang my midwife, Kate, to let her know I was in labour. I hadn't had a show at this point and my membranes were still intact, but I felt like things were moving along quite quickly. I was contracting every 2-3 minutes. I also rang my parents, who were my support team. Mum had been my 'Doula' for the previous two births and Dad had been at the first but missed the second. They always proved to be a wonderful help with support for Brett and myself, and the other children.

Once I'd called everyone, the contractions seemed to slow down to 5-10 minutes apart. I decided to have a shower and eat some breakfast just in case it turned out to be a long day after all. Brett cooked up a big pot of porridge and we all sat down to eat. I managed to get through with only a couple of contractions and it felt like labour was fizzling out.

It was about 10 o'clock when I called my team to come back over. Dad had to be called back home from the golf course, and Kate had to drive across to the other side of town to pick up all her instruments. They had been dropped off for sterilising, following a birth the previous night.

There was a knock on the door. I answered it to find Mum and Dad expecting to see me in full on labour. I was feeling like a bit of a fake at this point. Once they were in and settled, I got a couple of whopper contractions which took me completely by surprise. But when they were finished, I felt bright and alert. It wasn't until Kate arrived at 10:45 that it really started happening! I had full on, sharp, bottom piercing contractions that I've ever experienced. It felt like I was sitting on a spear! Now I was desperate to go to the toilet (as a midwife, I know this is a sign of second stage – but I had to go!). I was sitting on the toilet when I felt the head looming down and all I could hear was Kate saying "get off the toilet Faye, you're having your baby".

It was lucky that Brett had taken charge of getting the tub ready for me because I had to perform a cross-legged manoeuvre across the room to get to it in between contractions. I climbed into it with great relief, just in time for the head to start emerging. I had the pleasure and the honour of guiding my sons' head out into the warm water. Matthew Joseph Read was born at 1118hrs (just 33 minutes after Kate's arrival), on Wednesday 5th July 1995.

The first thing Matthew saw was a sea of faces peering in at him from the edge of the tub. There was Mum and Dad, his brother Jarrod, sister Melanie, Gran and Grandad and Kate. He floated around for a while, taking it all in before settling into me for his first breastfeed while we snuggled together in the warm tub.

After about half an hour we decided to get out of the tub for the birth of the placenta, which came away nicely and all together. I cut the cord for Matthew, which seemed very symbolic. Later we showed the inquisitive kids what it was and how it worked. They were rather fascinated. We then wrapped Matthew up all nice and warm while I went off to have a shower.

The birth took place on a Wednesday, and as this is the day that my family usually gets together, we phoned my two sisters and invited them to come over and have 'family day' at our house. They both arrived soon after, loaded up with food and drinks for lunch. We all sat down together to celebrate the wonderful event with a mandatory glass of champagne. When I came down from my 'High', I decided to slip upstairs and sleep with my new baby. The others crept out quietly a little later on.

About a week later, we had a private little 'naming ceremony' in our backyard between those present on the birthday, and then we planted the placenta under a special rose bush that we had bought for the occasion. I had the most wonderful birth experience that I could ever have hoped for. I thank my wonderful family and midwife for all their fantastic support in creating this memorable experience.

Hayley's Story of Oceana

I met with Hayley just the week before she began labour after she flew down from the town of Tom Price in Western Australia's North East.

For a couple of weeks, we had been talking on the phone about me being her doula and using the services I provide. Just briefly we had touched on labour and what she wanted to happen on the imminent day or night going forward. It was from these conversations that I knew I would be working with a woman who had a really good vision and belief about herself and her body that it can and will give birth. Right from the get-go, I could hear in her voice and words that she used that she had been preparing mentally for her labour. In hindsight this was a good thing really as we had very little time to do much together preparation wise, just managing to meet for a three-hour session before Hayley went into labour the following week.

It was a Saturday morning, and a text came through saying, 'Please call. Confusing circumstances occurring'. When I rang, Hayley told me she had been having period pains which had been building from about 4am in the morning. It was now 8am in the morning when I called back. Next, I had to try to work out – was this the 'real deal' or just a 'warm up?' I asked the formidable questions, "Have you been doing any poos?" She replied that she had been doing number twos all morning!

"Any bloody show or mucus?" She replied, "No". "Have your membranes broken yet?" To which she said "No".

All I had to go on was that she was stirring up and maybe it was a warm up episode. One thing I knew that would tell us for sure was getting Hayley to go and lie down in bed and see if she could get some more sleep or not. I explained to her that if the sensations kept going and became even stronger and more regular then she was definitely in labour. If it just went away, it was a warm up episode, and she could get some more sleep.

Two hours later Hayley rang to say she tried to lay down and get some sleep, however after about an hour it started to get so strong, she could no longer lie down and had to get up out of bed. We also spoke of her partner Ben and whether or not he should get on a plane in Paraburdoo where he was working, as the only plane on that day was about to leave in an hour. I said "YES, just get him on the plane because I do think you are having your baby today". My intuition was red hot on this day as I could really sense Hayley was powering along, even though she was still in disbelief and shock that she had even begun labouring. This was mainly because Hayley still had three weeks to go to her estimated due date and had come to Perth early to meet with me to gather a little more education as well as to exercise in the pool in preparation for the labour. Well, that went out the window!

I arrived at Hayley's in-law's house, where she was staying, at 1 pm that afternoon. Hayley had done a brilliant job of warming up her body and getting it ready to go into established labour. When I arrived, she was in the lounge on her hands and knees working beautifully through the contractions. Soon after she was clearly in established labour as she went from wanting to talk to needing to be very quiet and just breathing through each contraction.

I made her go to the toilet to empty her bladder which is so important in labour and while she was there, she told me she had lots of pressure down in her bottom, particularly at the end of the contraction! She was finding it harder and harder to get off the toilet as well. I asked her if she needed to push at all and she responded with "I just feel like I need to keep pooing!!!"

Not long after this Ben flew in the door and ran to change his dirty clothes as he literally just raced in his car to get onto the plane with only minutes to spare. He was covered in the red dirt of our outback and looked a mess, but luckily made it just in the nick of time.

I thought 'OK, time we get going' as she really is powering along beautifully. I rang the Birth Centre, left my number and they rang me back promptly. On the other end of the phone was Judy, a wonderful midwife I had known for many years. I was delighted that we would be seeing her soon, as I knew Hayley wanted to labour and birth in the tub they had at the Birth Centre. Due to the new law enabling women to legally waterbirth in hospitals in Western Australia, Judy and I were very excited. For years Judy had been campaigning for this to happen, and finally here we were with a willing woman and a very experienced and trained midwife. Everything was as it was supposed to be for sure.

Before we set off in the car I asked Hayley to put some baby nappies in her undies and put a heap of towels on the floor of my car just in case her membranes broke in my car. I didn't want the amniotic fluid going all over the upholstery as it really does stink and is so hard to get rid of the smell. As I drove Hayley and Ben to the Birth Centre, we had a brief chat about waterbirth which excited all of us. I told Hayley that the midwife she was about to have was trained and experienced and was already running the bath for her as we spoke.

All the way to the Birth Centre Hayley laboured away in her calm and serene way in that beautiful labour space. I felt so happy as it was a warm winter's day, the sun was shining, and I was about to attend a waterbirth. I really love my job!

When we arrived, we were greeted by Judy who did a few necessary medical checks on Hayley and the baby and then it was off to the bathroom where the tub was full and ready to go. The time was about 4.30 pm and Hayley got into the tub and looked like she was in heaven. She floated, relaxed and knelt forward leaning on the side, and then squatted and moved about bringing her baby down through her birth canal.

When Hayley hit transition, which seemed to last about half an hour, she said the familia, "fuck" and "when is this baby coming?" She also started to make the low groaning noises and verbalise what she was feeling; all very normal and reassuring to Judy and I who could see and hear what was going on for Hayley. It was great to witness as this, to me, is what birth in its pure essence looks like. This was truly an innate birth experience. In between this state she was calm, relaxed and even smiled at me, cracking the odd joke which made me respond with "you must be ok as you still have your sense of humour!" She just smiled at me.

As she got closer to birthing, I went and asked Ben, Hayley's partner, and his mother if they wanted to come into the bathroom. The bathroom was full in the end but wonderful having all those people quietly witness the waterbirth of Oceana.

Hayley pushed for about half an hour and finally bub's head emerged with the membranes completely intact like a water balloon. We could not quite see her little head, but we knew she was in there. On the next push her head and body gushed out of Hayley, in a dramatic entrance, she flung open her arms and legs and broke her own membranes. It was the most incredible thing to see. Oceana was then placed onto Hayley's chest where she confirmed with Ben that this was in fact a little girl as they began their mother/father/daughter journey together. It was so beautiful.

After a short period of time, we all assisted Hayley to get out of the tub and ten minutes later she birthed her placenta having a physiological third stage. Ben cut the cord and to-gether they chatted and bonded with their beautiful daughter.

I felt so honoured and elated to be able to witness this amazing birth experience. From the waters of the womb to the waters of the world this beautiful baby girl Oceana was born. In the most peaceful, loving way.

Dianne's Birth of Arlee

Monday 29th March 10.36pm. For over a week Dianne had been in what I call the 'warm up' to labour. This is where you have really strong Braxton Hicks and period pain that comes and goes each and every day and sometimes through the night. All of this activity is necessary in order to ripen the cer-vix, by thinning it out in preparation for opening with the di-lation once labour begins. So, it is all positive. However, it is very tiring especially when it goes on for days as it had done in Dianne's case.

On the Monday 29th March the same 'warm up' activity continued, only this time Dianne called me as she felt some-thing was different. She had noticed a bit of a 'show', not the cabaret type but the 'mucus show' type, which told me things were on the go for sure. I did my usual questioning over the phone such as "so have you had the need to do a big poo yet, anything at all…diarrhoea, lots of poos?" She replied that she had needed to go to the toilet a fair bit but nothing would come out. I assumed because there was so much pressure down low from the baby's head descending that it was preventing her from going. "Yahoo" I thought, the baby must have engaged now which I was relieved about as I knew Dianne was beginning to get a little frustrated and fed up with all this little stuff going on. She wanted the big contractions to start as she was so positive and excited about meeting this baby, she had been growing inside of her.

The first time I met Dianne I could tell she had this inner strength about her. Even though she came across as being very soft, feminine and the most honest and sincere person I had ever met, she was no push over. In fact, I was thinking to myself you really don't want to mess with this woman as she is really strong and determined and to a greater degree stubborn. I knew she would be applying and asserting herself with all these traits when she was in labour. Upon meeting her I had this inner knowing that she would labour her baby out very well and would not give in at any cost if things were no matter how hard labour became. Besides, she was working on having a beautiful waterbirth and really wanted to prove to herself she could do this. She employed me as her doula to make sure all the conditions were in her favour for creating her dream birth.

Before I hung the phone up from our discussion, around 11.00am in the morning, I finished by saying "Dianne, you sound as if you are probably in true labour warm up so just chill out, try to take a nap to get some rest and call me if you need me at any time. I will touch base in a couple of hours."

The day went on and with our next conversation Dianne still talked through her sensations. She said they "Were a little more than a period sensation" as they had a little peak to them, but nothing she couldn't handle, so she just pottered around the house moving from place to place. Her husband Chad did a brilliant job of massaging her whenever a sensation came, and together they stayed quietly in their home. Over the phone Dianne did mention to me that at the end of the sensation she had this deep pushing feeling in her bottom that stayed for a while then disappeared, but always came back on the next contraction. I said '" you probably just need to poo, go and see if you can because you might actually feel better if you do". This non – pooing had started to get Dianne a little pooed off, literally. She kept trying but it just would not happen! Often the opposite can happen when you do go into labour and you can't stop pooing. This is nature's way I reckon to clean you out before you push your baby out. But this did not apply in Dianne's case at all.

Dianne was happy to just carry on, outlining that she felt great and did not feel she wanted me with her yet. Besides she had an appointment with her Doctor that evening at 6 pm which she wanted to attend to have a stretch and sweep of her cervix to get things moving along.

Dianne had been patiently waiting for this appointment and her vaginal examination with a stretch and a sweep, hoping it would instigate true labour! As the Doctor proceeded with the vaginal examination, the look on his face changed and apparently was 'priceless' Dianne later told me "you should have seen the look on his face; he was so surprised and shocked, just like we were ". You see, Dianne was eight centimetres dilated and was still thinking she was in 'warm up labour' with a long way to go.

Still in disbelief she called me to tell me the news. I was so happy for her and we had a bit of a laugh about it, followed by a discussion about meeting at the hospital. I asked her "by the way, how are you still able to laugh and talk through the contractions?" In all honesty, I could not believe Dianne was actually in established labour as she was so calm and blissed out and still able to hold complete conversations!

As I drove to the hospital I was thinking about Dianne and her pain threshold. It must be a case of either Dianne has an incredible pain threshold or just maybe Dianne is one of these amazing women that just labours and births with very little peak sensation at all. I was trying to analyse and figure it out, but I thought without seeing Dianne in person I could not tell which of these scenarios it could be.

As I entered the labour room at the hospital I arrived to be greeted by a very excited and happy Chad and Dianne, both who were chatty and ready to fill me in on the Doctor's appointment scene. We all laughed and talked away as I began to get some homoeopathic remedies ready to give Dianne to get this show on the road. You see, labour at this point had almost stopped, which Dianne was almost relieved about, so she could actually get her head around and prepare for giving birth in the not-too-distant future.

I asked Dianne again "how is it that you are eight centimetres dilated and have got here to this place in such a calm peaceful way?" She said at first she didn't know then said "I just felt like it had to be more than this. I just kept expecting it was going to be so much harder than it really is; I had this expectation of labour and this was just not it. All day I have waited for something more to happen and it didn't". (I also had this expectation that my contractions had to get closer than 10 minutes apart)

I witnessed Dianne begin to relax just a little and chill out as we got her sitting on the fitball and leaning forward on the bed. I gave her some big hits of calming remedy as well as made her drink lots of water to rehydrate in preparation for the pushing stage, which was looming just around the corner.

After about an hour of re-focusing her attention back on labouring, Dianne was again having contractions 2-4 minutes apart, some which looked like they barely touched her, others she had to stand up for due to the pressure in her bottom. It was at this point I decided it was time for the bath to be run in readiness for Dianne's waterbirth. Dianne had been dreaming and focusing upon having a waterbirth since our first meeting, and I was so excited for her that her dream was about to become a reality.

Dianne entered the tub at 9pm stating "oh my god that feels so good. How good does the water feel?"

I knew the feeling having had three water births myself, I just smiled at Dianne.

Dianne continued to labour away beautifully, and we welcomed the new midwife into our labour room with welcome arms as she was very experienced with waterbirth and was so excited to be able to assist Dianne and honour her birth plan. With that, Dianne began to make some deep primal birthing noises as she began to push her baby out of her body. This was the only time she said "this fucking hurts", then proceeded to apologise to everyone for swearing. Chad and I gave a little chuckle as we had not heard Dianne say anything like this before this moment. I figured she must be in transition now as this was very un-characteristic of Dianne to swear and talk like this.

A short time after this I looked at Dianne who looked so beautiful and relaxed in between the pushing as she was reclined back in the tub, arms outstretched, one leg over the side of the tub and one leg in the water stretched straight out, head back and eyes closed just floating. I could tell she was now completely in her body and just allowing the sensations to pass through her as she worked her baby down and out of her body. I reminded Dianne to just trust in her body as it knew what to do, so she just needed to allow it to get on with the job of opening and she just needed to surrender.

Chad and I attended to Dianne's needs by giving her cold-water drinks, putting ice water towels on her neck and forehead, and I washed her face down with an icy flannel. Women love ice and cold water when they are pushing as they get extremely hot, especially when labouring in water and Dianne was no exception.

At 10.36pm beautiful Arlee entered this world so calmly and peacefully. She was gently placed on Dianne's chest skin to skin, all soft and slippery when she arrived out of Dianne's body and into the water with two final pushes. It was a quiet and peaceful birth apart from the midwives who were present all buzzing around doing all the medical things necessary when birthing in a hospital and me taking lots of photos.

A short time later when the dust had settled and time had been given to Mum and bubs, who were still bonding in the tub, Chad cut the cord that had stopped pulsating. We assisted Dianne to get out of the tub and sit on the birthing stool while she fed Arlee to assist with the physiological third stage to birth her placenta.

The drawing down of the colostrum while breastfeeding a newborn baby can assist with the birthing of the placenta as oxytocin is released which can assist in the expulsion of the placenta. So with this in mind we suggested Dianne try this and it seemed to work beautifully as the placenta arrived 40 minutes after the birth of Arlee.

After Dianne fed Arlee on both breasts, it was time for her to get comfortable on the bed and eat some much-needed food and have a hot chocolate drink. This is something I always try to give women when they have just given birth as the combination of the hot liquid and the sugar from the chocolate always helps women to feel better and more present straightaway. It seems to somehow ground them by elevating their blood sugar levels and helping to bring down the birth adrenalin, something women are usually very high on after a normal vaginal birth.

I was in awe of Dianne and so proud of her for reminding me how labour can be for some women; even though she was probably in denial and disbelief for the most part! She created this birth, no doubt about it. She owned it and worked towards creating this with her strength and determination, and most importantly, inner belief in herself. I was so blessed to have been witness to this beautiful experience. Thank you, Dianne and Chad.

I hope this story inspires women to really stay positive and not set their expectations of just how the 'intensity/pain' of labour is going to be. You cannot go into labour thinking you are going to expect a certain level. I cannot stress this enough. The first rule of labour is; make no assumptions at all about the intensity you think you are going to experience. The second rule is, you have to just trust and believe in your body that it can just get on with the job of opening and birthing.

Rebecca and Trent's Water Birth Story

When I fell pregnant with my first baby I knew I wanted to have a homebirth. I had done a lot of research prior to conception and I knew that an intervention free birth was the best for me and my baby, and that homebirth was the most likely way of achieving this. I was also very keen on having a waterbirth and there was very little chance of this happening in a hospital. Besides, being a nurse I knew I really didn't want to have anything to do with hospitals; I wasn't sick, I was just pregnant!

My husband and I chose to enlist the services of an independent midwife as we felt that gave us the best possible standard of care. When I met Abbey, I knew she was the right one for us. I loved the fact that she was relatively young, as were we, and seeing as everyone else I had come across was a lot older she was a great fit for us. She had such a beautiful presence about her and truly supported us in the decisions we made. She would come to our home regularly, weekly towards the end, and I loved the time we spent together during our appointments.

My pregnancy continued on smoothly and I found myself enjoying it greatly. I had a real affinity with water and loved going to my aqua classes and finding the opportunity to swim whenever possible. I also attended yoga towards the end and kept up other gentle forms of exercise. Mentally I really tried to remain pragmatic about the whole process, I didn't let it become bigger than it was and tried to live my life just as I would normally. Particularly towards the end I really made sure I didn't focus on 'being due' or become fixated on the pregnancy finishing. In fact, it was quite the opposite, I was really enjoying having my baby belly and didn't want it to end, even with the increasing aches and pains and that shocking Perth summer!

My 'estimated due date' came and went without me even realising and I continued to have the attitude that my baby would come when she was ready. I was very much preparing myself to go 42 weeks or over, although there seemed to be something about the 28th/29th of Feb. I just put it down to the fact that it was a leap year so that was why I was fixated on it. I didn't feel too much pressure to birth, and when people did try to make a fuss over it I shut them down pretty quickly. I did find the phone calls to 'see if I had birthed yet' irritating and I know for next time I will add three weeks onto my 'due date' to avoid that happening again. The only true pressure I felt was from my MIL who had timed her visit home from overseas to end on the 3rd of March, which was only eight days past my due date. I really didn't hold much hope that I would birth before then and felt quite disappointed that she would miss out on meeting her first grandchild. But I did have to remember that she was a capable adult who had made that decision and she therefore had to live with the consequences. Again, I came back to the fact that my baby would come when she was ready, nothing I could do could change that, so there was no point worrying.

On Thursday 28th (40+4) I did feel a little strange, but I didn't allow myself to think about it too much. I noticed a bit of mucous discharge, but it wasn't what I had heard the plug looked like, so I didn't get too excited. That evening I took myself off to aqua classes and during the relaxation part Gaby worked on my pressure points for about 30 minutes. She was very excited because I was quite twitchy and narky, but I didn't notice. I returned home for dinner and then all of a sudden something came over me. You see I had wanted to do up a sign pretty much saying 'Homebirth in progress, go away and do not disturb'. I had been meaning to do this for weeks and in fact we had joked that when I finally did my sign I would go into labour. Well, all of a sudden, I HAD to do my sign! So, it was 10pm and I was on the computer. Trent was telling me to come to bed but I just couldn't, I was fixated. I got it finished and felt much better! Then we had a bit of 'couple time', not with the intention of bringing anything on but because we both really felt like it! As I was falling asleep at midnight, I just knew it was going to happen, I would be in labour soon. I didn't realise it would be quite so soon however...

I was having this really strange dream about my waters breaking...next thing I know I woke up very quickly and could feel a bit of wetness between my legs. I put my hand down and realised it was quite watery, so up I jumped and ran into the ensuite. GUSH...there goes my waters! I didn't get any in the bed either, which I was very impressed with. So it was 1am on the 29th and my waters had most definitely broken, they were nice and clear and pinkish too, which I found reassuring. My next concern was what on earth do you do to stem the flow? I needed an 'Amniotic Fluid Management System' and I needed it now! I ended up with a newborn nappy followed by a towel stuffed into undies and then I carried another towel with me to sit on. I did try to get some more sleep, but it was pointless, so I got up. I couldn't decide whether to tell Trent or not; part of me said to let him sleep because I knew once he woke, he would be too excited, but the other part wanted desperately to tell him we would be having our baby soon!

At about 2am I decided to spill the beans, so I climbed into bed and whispered the news in his ear. I had to whisper a couple of times before he woke up of course. He was pretty excited, and that was the end of the sleep. So we were both up, him pottering around getting things tidy, and me sitting on the computer and finishing up baby related things. I was starting to get a bit crampy but nothing that resembled contractions. At around 4am Trent decided to go back to bed, I tried but couldn't get comfy, so I came out and sat on my fitball. I noticed I was starting to get regular cramping, with a bit of tightening as well, which was pleasing but I didn't pay too much attention to it. It was at about 5am that I noticed a definite pattern to the tightening, and they were getting a bit stronger. I timed them for a little while and they were coming every 4 minutes on the dot, lasting a minute exactly. I thought that was pretty cool, but then decided to stop timing them and just let it be. I was getting very tired by this point, so I moved into the lounge leaning over my ball and tried to sleep alongside the tightening. I stayed like this for quite a few hours, with my beautiful birth music playing (a special version of Pachelbel's Canon that we had listened to during aqua classes). It was very relaxing, and although I didn't sleep, I certainly rested. The journey had started!

At around 7am Trent woke up and we decided to let our midwife and our birth support person know what was going on. We decided that Abbey would come over at 9am to check me out and administer the first dose of intramuscular antibiotics that I had chosen to treat Strep B. I told my close friend who was going to support us during the birth that I didn't need her yet and would probably get her to come over later that day. I continued to contract away at regular intervals, of course I was starting to feel they were painful but in hindsight that early labour is nothing in comparison to what comes later! I did try to remind myself of that fact. I had seen so many women get carried away and believe early labour was really painful. Of course, when it does get serious, they've got nowhere to go. To combat the sensations, I stayed over my ball and breathed deeply to get through.

Looking back now I realise that they weren't really painful, more like 'intense'. When Abbey arrived my labour stalled, which was a classic indicator that I was in early labour, and the fact that whilst the contractions were regular there was no need to get too excited. Once she had done her thing, she sat with me while Trent popped out to the shops and picked up last minute supplies. I would have gone with him if not for the leaking fluid. Interestingly I did not have one contraction in the entire time he was gone. When he got back Abbey headed home with the instruction to call her when we wanted her back. Pretty much as soon as she headed off, I got back into a nice regular rhythm of contractions and that was where I stayed for the next few hours.

At about midday they started ramping up a bit; I really had to breathe through the sensations and began starting to vocalise. I felt really comfortable doing what I was doing, either sitting on the fitball or leaning over it, sometimes with Trent holding my hands. It was around this time that we decided to call our support person Jayde and asked her to come over. When she arrived my contractions once again stalled, which frustrated me. I really just wanted my space with my husband; I wasn't in the mood for others. I tried to be very quiet and focused, to get back into a nice rhythm, which eventually happened. Once I got back into it I was very pleased to have Jayde there; it was nice to have another woman who knew what I was going through. Both of them supported me through my contractions as they started getting more and more intense. In the meantime, Trent started baking lactation cookies; I think it gave him something productive to do!

It was around this point that I headed into established labour and my memory starts getting hazy from all those wonderful hormones. I was really vocalising through contractions at this stage, as well as stomping my feet as it seemed to help. I tried out many different positions, mainly utilising my birth ball. My favourite turned out to be sitting on my ball and leaning over the back of the couch while someone massaged my back, and I stomped my feet. I had one particular contraction on my way to the toilet that got everyone's attention and Trent decided to call our midwife and ask her to come around. I was still protesting saying I didn't need her. She arrived at about 4pm. They sneaked her in to avoid things slowing down; even still I really had to focus on not thinking about her arrival; I couldn't even look at her.

Not much later my thoughts started turning to my beautiful birth pool. In my mind it was a sort of reward to be able to get into it but I wanted to wait until I really needed it, and I was concerned about getting in too early. I decided, much to everyone's amusement, that I would get in at 6pm! From that point on at every contraction I would ask what the time was. Finally, my target rolled around, and I jumped in there so quickly. It was so warm and soft and I instantly relaxed. I could let my heavy pregnant body float and I felt so cocooned and protected. The contractions on the other hand got mighty intense in the water; I would even say they were more painful. But I was happy with this because I felt like I was getting somewhere. Increased pain meant increased productiveness. Being in the water meant that I could truly relax in between contractions and recharge before the next one, something I couldn't properly do on land. I was supported by my fabulous team; Trent sitting close by and massaging my head, Jayde pouring water on my back, and Abby sitting on the mattress doing what all good midwives should do, nothing!

As the sun started to go down and we headed into the night I continued to labour away in the pool. I verbalised with every contraction, low and deep groans. I banged my hands on the side of the pool or squeezed Trent's hand. In between sensations I would rest and relax every muscle in my body. I had my music going (the same song I had been listening to from the start) and candles burning, it really was a beautiful calm space.

I would occasionally get out to make a trip down to the toilet where strangely, even though I was in my own home with people I knew and trusted, I felt like that was my 'time out'. What a sight I must have been, a heavily pregnant woman in labour trudging down to the back of the house hastily covered in whatever towels her support people could throw on her. I would moan and cry and have full blown contractions in the toilet, before quickly trudging back to the pool to get back into the beautiful water.

Sometime in the early evening I started vomiting. It wasn't too much of a problem; in fact, it was quite a relief to clear myself out. It did however make me convinced that I was getting close to fully dilated. And herein lies the problem; I just couldn't get out of my 'nurse' headspace. I constantly analysed everything that was happening and drew assumptions from the signs I was getting from my body. I remember wondering exactly what I should be thinking during a contraction, because my brain was so switched on; internally of course, externally I had really gone within by this point.

For some strange reason I started trying to push not long after this, at around 10pm. I felt ever so slightly pushy, but I'm not exactly sure what I was trying to do at this point, I think maybe I wanted to get things going. I tried unsuccessfully to push for a while, and probably did nothing but tire myself out. My contractions definitely slowed down, and any pushy urge disappeared.

Abbey knew that this wasn't 'it'; she could easily see that my pushes were ineffective and forced. This was clearly different from the full-blown pushing urge you get later on down the track, but of course I didn't know this. She suggested a change of scene, so I got out of the pool and Trent and I tried to have a lie down. That was just pure agony; everything seemed so much harder to handle lying down. I started shaking uncontrollably, a whole body shake that I couldn't stop if I wanted to. Trent tried to hold me tight, but I was too agitated. It was at this point that I started to doubt myself. Could I do this? It was going on too long. The pain was too much. I felt like I was losing control. I briefly contemplated heading to the hospital, it was only when I realised that on arrival at the hospital, I was still going to have to push out a baby that I gave up on that idea. At that point I just wanted someone to take it all away. Of course, in retrospect I believe this was when I headed into transition.

I went to Abbey and sought her solace. I remember saying I couldn't do it anymore, yet she reassured me I could. I wondered if I should ask for a VE to find out how far along I was, and as it turned out, she was wondering that too but neither of us verbalised it. For this I am very grateful.

Around 11pm I got back into the pool and this was when things started getting serious! My contractions returned strong and regular, I started vomiting again and the intensity of the contractions was like nothing I had experienced to this point. I did everything and anything to get through them. I wriggled around the birth pool, attempted to keep my breathing under control and tried to keep my birth noises low and deep. I felt like I was hanging on for dear life. As we went on, the intensity shifted to my bottom and the urge to poo started to become very strong. I was very nervous about doing a poo in front of everyone and again Abbey assured me that it would be ok. I did trot down to the toilet on a few occasions to see if I could do the 'poo' but of course it resulted in nothing but some horrendous contractions and me hankering for my lovely pool.

Around 1am I began feeling very 'grunty' at the peak of contractions and all of a sudden, my body took over and I found myself pushing my baby out towards this world. I started to push outside the pool, leaning over and then progressing down towards the floor until I was on my hands and knees. Trent supported me and I went with what my body was doing. I wouldn't say I pushed with all my might, I would say my body pushed with all it's might, I really wasn't doing anything. I stayed there for a little while but was aware of the fact that I wanted to give birth in the pool, so I got back in. I continued pushing, all the while supporting my perineum with one hand. At first, I could feel her head inside my vagina, then I could feel it coming further and further down. After about an hour of pushing I could feel beautiful soft hair floating in the water, which I proudly announced to everyone present. They all found this to be a hilarious moment given the fact that I hadn't spoken for a couple of hours, and then all of a sudden I loudly exclaimed "she's got hair!" Fifteen minutes later her head was on show with contractions, and it was another twenty minutes, and her head was out.

I could feel her just there and waited patiently for the next contraction. Suddenly, I gave a final push and before me I saw a little baby sitting on the bottom of the pool. Immediately I scooped her up and brought her to my chest. She was so beautiful! Smaller than I imagined she would be, covered thick in vernix, and she had a full head of hair. She didn't breathe immediately but we weren't too concerned because she was still getting oxygen from the umbilical cord. Trent and I kissed her, blew air on her face, rubbed her back and spoke to her. All these things were instinctive. In the end Abbey did give her just a touch of suction and we all gave her a good rubbing up. After what seemed like forever, she took a big deep breath and pinked up immediately. Then she let out a big, lush cry and opened her eyes to greet her parents. That was about it in terms of crying. From that point on she just lay on my chest and took in her new surroundings. She was very alert and bright eyed. We stayed in the pool for about ten minutes and then I got out to birth the placenta. After that, all three of us snuggled up together in bed, our freshly born daughter and her parents. Just the three of us. Perfect.

Abbey continued to visit us in the days following her birth, and for many weeks afterwards. We are forever in debt to her for her fantastic level of care, support and love.

So that is the story of my first child's birth, a home waterbirth, boringly normal and beautifully exhilarating all at the same time.

The Birth of Hudson (12th April 2012)

I woke at 6am on the morning of 12th April with a dull cramp in my belly. I caught my husband Phill as he left for work to say that I think something may be happening today, and that I would call him later with an update. My last labour had stopped and started a few times, so I didn't feel an urgency about this. As I was up early I thought that I'd get a head start to the day and get into the morning jobs of unstacking the dish-washer and putting on a load of Phill's work clothes to wash.

Once my daughter Lucy (19 months) woke, as it was such a beautiful day, we went for a morning walk. As we walked around the streets of Hilton, I began to notice that the dull cramps had increased and become waves of contractions. When we arrived home, I ate some breakfast and got changed, as I thought that this baby was well under way. Despite this thought, I still imagined that I would have a good while to 'kill' before I was seriously in labour, so I decided not to let Phill know at this stage.

That morning we had a 2nd birthday to go to in Hilton, but I still had a few errands to run, picking up bits and pieces before the baby came. So I decided to drop by Big W on the way to the party. At Big W, I definitely knew that things were happening, and fast! Even though the party started at 10am, I thought we could drop in a bit earlier to help with some things for the party, with the intention of only staying a short while and racing home to set up for the homebirth.

The decision to have a homebirth came about over time. Once finding out I was pregnant for the second time, we decided that we wanted to give birth at the Family Birthing Centre attached to King Edward Hospital. I was also interested in being a part of the Community Midwifery Program but was pretty sure that we didn't want a homebirth. We visited the Birthing Centre and liked the look of it, so decided to apply for the CMP with the venue being the FBC. Throughout the CMP appointments, I was becoming quite comfortable with my midwife. She was so encouraging and informative and took the time to discuss any concerns with me. The point came in my pregnancy where I had to decide whether I was going to lock in with the FBC or opt for a homebirth.

My midwife asked me whether I would consider a homebirth and what my fears or reservations might be. It was great to have an open, unbiased discussion with my midwife who was happy to support me in whatever choice I made. I took about a month to consider all the possibilities and reservations that I had and decided that I was actually more at peace with a homebirth than with the thought of having to transfer to the FBC to get set up and feel comfortable there. However, Phill was still quite unsure. He was able to chat with a few people and read some testimonies and we prayed together. Once we had decided on a homebirth, I was feeling really at peace and excited about the possibility of it.

On arriving early to the party, much to the host's surprise, she put me in charge of cutting up fruit for a platter. I had been told that pineapple can bring on labour, and as I was cutting up some, I thought I would try out this theory. Having a job kept my mind off the labour and on the task. I was able to hide away in the kitchen and wiggle my hips when needed.

As the other guests arrived I tried to hold conversations with them while staying chilled and calm. For the most part I went unnoticed apart from the host who followed me into the kitchen to check on me. She thought I should go home, but I responded saying "it's ok, they're only about 15 minutes apart." But no, she said my contractions were really 10 minutes apart and I should leave. As I was starting to leave the cake appeared, and Lucy had her heart set on it. To take her now would have caused a drama I was in no state to handle. We stayed for the cake, but by the time I left I really needed to be home.

Once home at 11:15am it was all action stations! I put Lucy in bed for her nap, called Phill to tell him to come home (NOW!) and then called the midwife. Unfortunately, my midwife was on her day off (she hadn't had one for two weeks, so she really needed to be off!) so the back-up was grocery shopping in Midland (40 minutes away!). I thought I should get the washing on the line before the baby came, so I was hanging out Phill's work clothes while on the phone to her. I tried to tell her that I was in established labour but she wasn't getting it. She was asking me if this was my first pregnancy and how close my contractions were. I tried to tell her, but she found me too calm to really heed my urgency.

On hanging up I called my student midwife to come ASAP and tried to get my friend to come to collect Lucy when she woke. Unfortunately, she was on a train into the city to get her hair done, so she suggested calling her husband who was the first to arrive (11:40ish) and I asked him to set up the birth pool while I gathered all my labour bits and pieces (drink, food, oils, TENS etc.). He got busy setting up the pool 'OUTSIDE' and began to fill it with water. Once my contraction had passed, I called him to move it inside to fill up from the kitchen tap. It was at that time that Phill arrived (12ish) and I asked him to put on my TENS machine that I had been hanging out for. Phill scrambled around to find the tap connector as he had put it in a 'safe' place. While they did that I was labouring away in the bedroom with my student midwife supporting me.

The midwife still hadn't come, and we called her again to try and explain the urgency of her arrival. At 12:30, the pool was being filled and it was time for Lucy to leave. Phill woke her up and packed a bag, and our friend took her back to their place for the afternoon.

Around 12:45, the midwife arrived, just as my waters broke. She raced in to set up her baby kit and then came straight in to see me. She asked me to quickly move to the pool as my baby was about to be born. I jumped in the pool while the water was still filling up, the music was on and things were becoming calm and controlled. Then, the phone rang! I was ready to scream at it, when there was a knock on the door and another midwife, and her student walked in. I was definitely in transition at that stage, as I remember feeling frustrated at the casual nature of everyone's greetings, and just wanted peace and quiet.

At 1:05 I had the urge to push. After three big pushes, a few cries for help and less than 10 minutes, my beautiful baby, Hudson William was born at 1:12pm. Birthing him into the water seemed to slow things down. As I was leaning over the edge of the pool to push, he came out behind me, and I had to turn around to lift him up. Phill said it felt like an eternity before Hudson arrived on my chest. On picking him up and leaning back, it was the biggest relief and so amazing to look into the eyes of my sweet boy. It was the most beautiful way to give birth – in water and in my own home.

The labour of Hudson happened so fast that I don't think I would have even made it to the hospital or Birthing Centre in time anyway. Knowing that I didn't have to leave my home, gave me comfort to continue labouring and certainly brought about a smooth labour journey where I felt relaxed and calm.

11.

ALL SORTS OF BIRTHS

Sarah's Powerful Birth

Sarah came to me with such a positive and strong attitude, and an amazingly positive outlook on life. What struck me most about Sarah was her beautiful smile. Sarah just always smiled. I realised sometime after we met what her inner radiance and glow was about. Against the odds she had conceived and was going to become a mother, finally. What I also found interesting was Sarah's determination to avoid a C-section due to her age and not have a 'happy cervix' according to her Ob. We often laughed about the fact that he was pushing her so hard to agree, however she stood her ground and worked on creating a 'happy cervix' that would dilate and open beautifully, and it did. Here is her story.

Tilly (against all odds!!!)

I truly believed that I was not meant to have children. I had reached this belief after ten years of interventions because of my 'unexplained infertility'. Interventions and treatments over the years had included having an ovarian cyst removed and treatment for endometriosis, intrauterine insemination followed by two failed attempts at IVF with ICSI in Singapore. For anyone who has been through this you will understand the devastating effect it can have on your self-esteem and looking back, I think I experienced some episodes of depression as a result.

Three years ago after moving to Perth I fell pregnant out of the blue. However at thirteen weeks I discovered the baby had Down syndrome and was struggling to survive so I had a termination. That was the end as far as I was concerned, and I completely gave up on becoming pregnant.

I visited a homoeopath to try and improve my sleep and general state of well-being as I felt run down and very stressed. She treated the source of my symptoms using iridology to diagnose that my body was highly acidic, and I was treated over a period of eighteen months before I again fell pregnant out of the blue; finding out I was pregnant on our fifteen-year wedding anniversary. This time the twelve- and nineteen-week scans showed that all was as it should be and we were over the moon; yet we still did not quite believe that this could finally be happening for us.

My obstetrician was very honest about his bias towards C sections, especially for women of my age (39 turning 40) who were far less "elastic" than younger women, and therefore more likely to have complications and to tear when giving birth. It was only when I started antenatal swim classes and took part in the four-week pregnancy and childbirth education journey that I began to question this and to think that it was entirely possible for me to give birth vaginally. Each time I visited him it was the same pressure to have a C section. I developed gestational diabetes and there was a concern that I might have a big baby (another possible reason for a C section) but my scan at 35 weeks revealed the baby was only slightly above average. By this time, I was confident that I would aim to have a natural birth and only have a C section if necessary, for medical reasons. As my estimated date approached again, my obstetrician with his usual pessimistic outlook told me that the head was high and my cervix was "unfavourable" meaning nowhere near being ripe for birth, and I was unlikely to go into spontaneous labour.

At five days past my estimated date and after Gaby pushed my trigger points during our relaxation at aqua class, drinking lots of raspberry leaf tea and having homoeopathic drops to ripen my cervix, my labour started spontaneously at midnight. The contractions were about twenty minutes apart and this continued for the next twelve hours at which stage we went to hospital. I was sent home as I was not in established labour, but eight hours later my contractions were ten minutes apart, so we returned to the hospital where a vaginal exam revealed

633

my cervix was fully effaced and one centimetre dilated. We were admitted to a birthing suite and left to labour away where I encountered the first of two supportive and encouraging midwives who would help me through this experience.

My contractions moved to five minutes apart then back to ten minutes, which was a bit frustrating. Six hours later I was only two centimetres apart and utterly exhausted, as was my husband, who had been incredibly supportive throughout providing heat packs and back massage on every contraction. At this stage the midwife recommended some pethidine pain relief so I could get some rest before my obstetrician arrived at seven am. When he did arrive, pessimistic as ever, he said this was a bad situation as the head was in an unfavourable position and I was only two centimetres dilated. He then broke my water and I burst into tears when cleaning myself up in the toilet. I was almost at the stage of saying go ahead and do the C section but something in me decided to keep going.

I was given Syntocinon to strengthen the contractions and hopefully turn my baby's head into position. I also had an epidural at this stage as I thought a C section was on the horizon and I was truly exhausted. The syntocinon had a dramatic effect and just three hours later I had reached ten centimetres dilation and the midwife said it was time to push. She called my obstetrician who arrived just fifteen minutes before my baby girl was born after pushing for just forty minutes (her head had turned into position beautifully by itself!). I had a minor tear which required a few stitches but nothing major and my placenta arrived without me even noticing. The feeling of utter joy after waiting for so long as she was placed on my chest was indescribable and I truly felt that she was an absolute miracle!! I couldn't believe how perfect she looked, and her long fingers were amazing to behold.

I think I surprised my obstetrician and I really hope that he won't be so quick to recommend C sections to women of my age in the future.

Waterbirth Using Hypnosis

I attended a private hypnotherapy session with you Gaby in late February of 2010 and wanted to share with you how my birth went using your techniques I learnt during my hypnotherapy session.

My labour was such a positive and healthy experience. I laboured for four hours at home from 7am (just like I'd hoped!) with Brett, and then I went to Kaleeya, where after the internal examination they said I was 5 centimetres dilated (halfway there - yes! :)

I requested the bath straight away just as you suggested, hopped in where I laboured for three more hours. Throughout my session with you, you suggested I should use water as it was an amazing natural intensity relief option and that maybe I could have a waterbirth, which I didn't really consider until you said it.

Funnily enough, once I was in that bath I didn't want to get out; the midwives asked me to and I refused! So, they went and found a qualified waterbirth midwife who helped me birth my beautiful baby boy Boden.

I used your techniques throughout my labour, and I believe they were the key to my success. I am so proud and overjoyed to talk about my labour with friends, and always tell people how helpful the use of hypnotherapy was for me. In my Mother's group and even within my group of friends I am the only one who had an all-natural birth, let alone waterbirth! I thank you for that.

Being a mother is so much more than I thought it was going to be and I'm loving it more every day. I can't wait to birth my second baby- which I hope will be a positive experience once again. Alannah

I Loved My Labour and Placenta Peacetime

I am just watching a documentary on Perth and thought of you. I thought you would like to know that my son Taj Gordon was born on the 13 August, weighing 9-pound 12 oz.

I was starting to think I would never have a baby; I was fifteen days over EDD and the doctor wanted to induce me at thirteen days over because he was off on the weekend. I agreed to be monitored every day but there was no way I was agreeing to have an induction. I had been experiencing highly stressful situations which I think Taj didn't feel safe to come out into. So, on Saturday night I sent my daughter Kihara off with my Mum and spent some quality time with Laith, my husband.

I began feeling the contractions of my SPONTANEOUS START TO LABOUR that night. I slept on and off that night and woke up in the morning very excited to finally be able see my baby and take on the challenge I had been preparing for.

The contractions increased quickly, and before I knew it, were only a minute or so apart. At 9am I called my midwives and headed off to the hospital. After a very slow walk into the birthing room, I found myself sitting on the loo leaning on Laith rolling with motions. I could feel my baby pushing his way into life, but the back pain was excruciating. I crawled into the bath and my waters burst soon after. I was so surprised by this feeling that I thought my baby's head had shot off with the pressure. Crazy thought I know! Once I realised what happened I was excited again to feel the true feelings of natural labour.

Now I needed to push, and I sounded like a primal animal. After some time of pushing, I needed a new position, so out of the bath and on all fours I went. I still couldn't bring him down. I then tried on my side, the birth stool, and squatting. I desperately want to see my baby now. I let the doctor talk to me and decided to get help with suction. On arriving in the delivery suite, we were left alone for one more try, and I threw myself on the floor for one last heave ho. I couldn't do it. I was so close. So up onto the bed I climbed and in a flash the suction cap was on the baby's head, and a few moments later he squeezed out with the cord around his neck and all. I had my beautiful blue almost 10-pound baby on my chest.

After another three hours and a catheter was put in (as my bladder was full) my placenta came out. To the disgust of the doctor, it was STILL ATTACHED to my baby, where it remained until day four.

Taj enjoyed his PEACE TIME, with his placenta. He had a large hematoma on the whole right-hand side of his head, which I felt really bad about. I am sorry to have had that intervention on him. However, I made a conscious informed decision and had full control over our birth. I am VERY happy and proud of our effort.

Taj is now ten weeks old and is a very peaceful person. Last night he slept through to the morning! I am disappointed not to have had a waterbirth, however I am satisfied that I did my very best in labour. I am very satisfied to have experienced a natural start and to feel the water burst was exhilarating. I am also so pleased that we followed through on a lotus.

You have been such an inspiration on my journey along with my angelic midwives. Thank you for being a part of this significant time in my life.

I later gave your book and advice to my sister who had a baby last week. She also found your work more informative than any other birthing class her hospital or midwives offered. Melissa had a beautiful experience giving birth with a completely submerged face and all. Her baby Willow was born out of her with a smile on her face. Amazing. I am so proud of her.

Thanks again. My whole family is going really well. Laith and I are connecting with each other and our children on a deeper level of understanding and love.

I am happy and wish you my happiness too! Love Kylie

Friday, 20 October, 2006

Siena's Birth Story

To my darling Siena, I thought you might enjoy knowing how you came into the world and what a truly special day it was for your Daddy and I.

Well, your estimated due date was the 8th January. In the weeks after that I tried everything to help you arrive. I was doing lots of walking, swimming and cleaning; lots of activity is supposed to help. I even washed the car (in my bikini no less; poor neighbours!). On the 21st January I went for acupuncture and I also saw the obstetrician. She told me you were very close.

At 2am on the 22nd January I felt some pains in my tummy. I got out of bed and realised that this was the beginning of your arrival. I was pacing up and down the kitchen and my breathing was heavy. I started writing down the time of each contraction.

Daddy woke up and came out to the kitchen. He thought my loud breathing was Mercedes (our pussycat) coughing up a fur ball. He soon realised what was going on. So we rang the birthing suite and they said we should wait till the contractions were three in ten minutes. I was also extremely glad as I had the desperate urge to go to the toilet before we left.

So off we went to Subiaco and arrived at the birthing suite. They took us to our room, and I kept pacing and breathing with each contraction. I asked Daddy to text Grandma and it was not long before Grandma was there too; around 5am. The midwife (Marion) was already coaching mummy and asking me where I was feeling the pain. "In the back" was my answer. This apparently was because you had your spine against mine instead of your spine facing my belly.

Marion suggested I go in the shower, which I did. The shower was very soothing. But after a few hours in the shower, I was getting very tired and by this stage had also lost my dinner. Daddy was massaging my lower back with every contraction. I was going from the shower to the bed to lie down in between the contractions. Then we put a beanbag in the bathroom so I could rest in there instead of walking back to the bedroom. I always felt like I had to stand for the contractions.

I wanted to push but Marion kept telling me not to because you were the wrong way around and if I pushed now, I would make the birth a lot longer. So, Marion suggested we go into the bath to calm things down and to help me to avoid pushing.

Daddy and Grandma were kept very busy the whole time massaging my back and holding the hand-held shower head with hot water on my back for pain relief.

After a little while in the bath Marion suggested we had a few options. We could go to the hospital and they would give me an epidural, which would stop me having the urge to push. Or we could try to wait for two more contractions and then Marion would have a look and feel to find out what was going on with dilation doing a vaginal examination (VE).

We chose the second option. When Marion was doing the exam, I told her I could feel another contraction about to start and this time she asked me to push. Marion pushed at the same time (and got the cervix in a better position). With the next contraction I felt you turn inside me. I sighed "it's turned, it's turned". Remember we didn't know if you were a baby boy or girl at that point, so that's why you were an "it"!

"Great!' said Marion, 'NOW you can push!"

Within a couple of contractions Marion said she could see your head. She got me to kneel down, and she said that if I used my hand I would be able to feel and guide your head. I looked down and could see this perfect crown of dark hair. Marion kept telling me, "Breathe, Rebecca, nice and easy, we don't want to tear." So I kept breathing but not pushing too hard, and before long your head was out (and don't forget, under water!).

"What do I do now?" I asked Marion. Marion was so calm so I knew everything was going just as it should. "Just wait for the next contraction and push a little bit more".

With the next contraction you were out. Marion caught you in the water and put you in my arms. The cord was around your neck, so Marion got that out of the way. Daddy said to me, "we have a little girl!". It was 11am.

I kept looking at you; I could not believe how beautiful you were. You were perfect in every way. Your skin was rosy, and your lips were red. You weren't squashed or scratched, just a doll! I kept you at my breast. I will never forget the feeling of first having your skin against mine. Daddy was already on the phone to Aunty Ange in Melbourne while I was still in the bath! I think perhaps he forgot that we weren't done yet!

After about half an hour Marion cut the umbilical cord. I passed you to Daddy. There was certainly no need to wash you; you were perfectly clean and perfectly baked! Marion then gave me a small chair to sit on in the bath to birth the placenta which just took a couple of extra pushes. We examined the placenta together to make sure it was all intact and it was. Good job!

We weren't planning on a waterbirth, but we are so grateful that was what eventuated. We think it has got something to do with the fact that you gravitate so strongly to the water and that from your very first bath it looked like you were in another dimension entirely!

And that, my darling Siena, is the story of your beautiful birth!

Birth of a Boy!

Shaun and I were so happy when we found out we were going to be parents. Nine months seemed so far away, and we couldn't wait to meet our baby.

We really wanted to have a waterbirth. For us it seemed the most natural and relaxed way to birth, for both mother and baby, so when we went for our first appointment at the hospital, we discussed it with our midwife only to find out that waterbirths were not allowed at hospitals. The only way to have a waterbirth was to have it at home, and not knowing anything about homebirth, we didn't bother about pursuing that avenue and settled with having our baby at the hospital.

I started going to Gaby's aqua natal classes from about eighteen weeks and also did her four-week pregnancy and child-birth education journey and her antenatal class for support peo-ple, with Shaun. Not only did we learn about pregnancy and birthing, but we made friends and Gaby told us about the com-munity midwifery program. Unfortunately, there was no room on the program for us. So once again, disappointed, we settled with the notion that we were going to have our baby at the hospital.

It wasn't until I was thirty weeks that Gaby, knowing how badly I wanted a waterbirth, suggested I call her midwife Mary and ask her if she would be a midwife for us so we could have the waterbirth we wanted. After having all of our questions answered about home birth, and Mary agreeing to take us on, we finally were going to get our water birth.

At 2am on Wednesday morning I had a bloody show and by 6am I was in pre-labour having period-like pains. I called Mary to let her know but she was coming for a scheduled visit at 11am anyway. My contractions increased throughout the day and by five o'clock I got Shaun to fill up the birthing pool. As soon as I got into the pool, I became instantly relaxed, and the intensity of the contractions eased. Mary arrived at eight pm, after going home that morning after her scheduled ap-pointment to leave me to get on with the job of labouring. I laboured away with Shaun who massaged my lower back and gave me food and drink regularly. Mary gave me some Bach flower rescue remedy and encouraging words occasionally.

I was coping really well in the pool and with the breathing technique Gaby taught me, so I felt confident and relaxed. Mary constantly monitored the baby's heartbeat and at 4am she became concerned about the baby's irregular heartbeat and discussed a transfer to the hospital to monitor the baby. I fully trusted Mary's advice and was totally fine with the decision; I only wanted my baby to be safe.

Shaun drove me to the hospital with Mary right behind. Being out of the pool I started to really feel the intensity of my contractions. When we got to our labour room, I was asked to lie on my back to have the monitors put on my belly. I found this incredibly hard to handle and would stand up for each contraction, leaning on Shaun until they passed. After being on the monitor for a while, the midwives were happy that the baby was fine and we moved to the birthing suite where I went straight into the bath.

I laboured for a while in the bath but with being prodded, poked and made to lie on my back beforehand, it really made me lose my concentration and I couldn't get back into my breathing rhythm. I was exhausted and wasn't coping, so I asked for an epidural. Shaun was fully supportive of my decision, giving us both a chance to rest. After the epidural had worn off and I was fully dilated and ready to push, I refused to go onto my back and opted to be on all fours; Shaun was with me holding my hands. I started birthing my baby. I wanted to stop, unsure I could do it, but with reassuring words from Mary and Shaun I gained the confident boost I needed, and I pushed my baby's head out. After having a little rest, I birthed the rest of my baby. Someone immediately passed my baby between my legs and into my arms, and with Shaun right beside me, we said hello to our baby for the first time. Tears of pure happiness flowed, and it wasn't until someone asked what sex the baby was that we thought to look. We had a gorgeous baby boy!!

It wasn't until after that I was told about the concerns the midwives had for our baby. His heartbeat had slowed as the cord was around his neck, but I wasn't made aware of it at the time. All I knew was that my instincts were telling me to get my baby out, so I did.

Our baby boy is three weeks old now and he is happy and healthy, and breastfeeding well. I thank Gaby and Mary, for their support and world of knowledge. My advice to first time mums…….. Be informed, knowledge is power, know your rights and have the birth you want. Enjoy the experience as it is the most amazing thing you'll ever do!!

Liz's Story

When I met Liz she was '100 miles an hour'. I could totally relate to her because she was a physical education/dance teacher, as I had been for many years; English, as I am, and '100 miles an hour' as I am sometimes too! However, my initial impression was "could this wonderful woman ever slow down enough to actually surrender and give birth in a calm and relaxed way?"

I was honoured when she asked me to be her doula. I had thought to myself that I could really assist her and help her to let go and relax in labour, as well as help her to let her body just get on with the job of labouring.

I was very excited when Liz decided to come and have a hypnosis session with me as this would really clear the pathway to a more calm and relaxed experience. I figure women have absolutely nothing to lose by trying everything they can in creating the experience they want to have, and Liz did just that. After her labour she told me how she had gone through her entire labour as she had seen it under hypnosis, down to when and how she thought she would birth. I just laughed and said something like "see you can't underestimate the power of the mind and the subconscious. I keep telling you all this but you just don't believe me. Do you believe me now?" Liz replied "oh Yeah, I sure do" and we both smiled and laughed.

When I woke up on Monday 26th May I awoke to a text message at 7.28am that read "morning Gaby X - bloody show 5am. Intensities are pretty frequent..... I'm at home. Can you call me when u have got kids sorted 4 school etc". Now anyone who knows me will tell you that just about every day of my life

I receive text messages about someone going into labour, or from someone who has just given birth. It is all part of this journey and course I am on. Fortunately my clients are so considerate in that they understand that I see to my own children first, before seeing them, which is so lovely and why I have been able to do this work for so long.

At this point in time I rang Liz to do what I call 'check in'. It is where I talk to a woman in labour and see how she responds to me and to see if she wants me to go to the home where she is warming up in labour. Often women in the early stages of labour are quite happy to just stay at home with their partner and potter about the house, getting themselves prepared for the labour ahead both mentally and physically on their own. Liz was no exception and said that she was doing fine however, was surprised with the intensity that was coming on so early into her warm up stage. With this comment I suggested she get into the shower and try to use water to distract her from thinking about the intensity and to assist her to relax and let go.

At approximately 9.30am I received another call from Simon stating that Liz was working extremely hard and that she was not getting much of a rest in between. I could actually hear her in the background making some noise on her contractions and I knew she was doing some great work, and 'Yes' this was the 'real deal' and not just a pretend run! I stayed on the phone for a while and asked to speak to Liz where I reminded her of her breathing. I then spoke to Simon, realising that I had in front of me a forty minute drive down south, and then we all needed to come back up north again to the hospital. With the amount of noise Liz was making I really did not think Liz would actually make it up to the hospital if she did not leave home now!

I calmly stated to Simon that I felt it would be in his and Liz's best interest to head up to the hospital, swinging via my house on the way, as I did not think we had eighty minutes give or take to spare on my travel and their travel back up. Thankfully Simon agreed and let Liz know what I thought, and luckily she agreed to get on the road. As requested by me they rang when on the road to let me know they had left home and that all was fine.

I was in my car waiting in the driveway and they followed me to the hospital in a slow and relaxed manner. Very different to the way in which Simon drove, getting a speeding camera flash on the way up from the South!! Oh well, it is all in the name of birth and justified, I think!

Upon arrival we had the most beautiful midwife who was an absolute angel. She knew of me and my work, so that was a lovely surprise to say the least. Liz was totally honoured and respected by this midwife who was so positive and supportive of Liz and Simon and myself. This always makes for a great birth journey together.

When we finally got into the labour room Liz was powering ahead 'full steam'. I was so amazed and impressed by her inner focus and calm. I had to admit it was the first time I had seen Liz speechless as she was literally unable to talk through the contractions as they were coming on every two minutes and lasting for 40 to 50 seconds. All she could do was breathe and surrender, and she was doing this so well.

After a period of time, Liz had a VE which indicated she was seven centimetres dilated with her membranes intact and bulging. I was so proud and happy that she was this far along. I also realised that this was the journey of labour she had seen under hypnosis in her 'mind's eye' playing out before the both of us. This made me feel very excited and happy for I knew how this journey played out and prayed that this was how it was going to end.

Liz decided to go on her hands and knees in the shower after her internal as unfortunately the bathtub was already occupied. It was here that Simon, who was holding the handheld shower head on Liz's back, exclaimed "something just went pop and came out of Liz's body." I had a look and could not see anything, so I felt for the head. All of a sudden Liz had this enormous urge to 'POO' and 'PUSH' and we all knew what that meant!

After a few more contractions in the shower we, Simon and I, assisted Liz back to the bed where initially she felt cold and then all of a sudden intensely hot and wanted to strip off. This

650

is so common when women begin to go through transition and begin to push their baby out.

At this point Liz was up on the bed on her hands and knees leaning over the top of the bed, which was now nearly upright on a 90°angle and meant she could be upright and lean forward on pillows. This worked so well for Liz as she began to push and breathe as she moved through transition.

Simon and I fed Liz lots of water and sweet drinks on a regular basis. Liz also had the hot heat bags on her back and cold icy flannels over her neck and face. Women, during this stage, love freezing cold flannels to help cool them down.

After a period of time it was decided that another VE was required just to make sure full dilatation had been reached and to check which position the baby was in. It was also hospital policy to put the continuous foetal monitors on the labouring women if the baby does a poo inside the mother. There was evidence of this in the fluid that Liz was oozing out of her body. Fortunately, the baby's heartbeat was perfect throughout this stage of labour and came into the world so calm and peaceful.

Liz began pushing at approximately 1.45pm in the afternoon and pushed for about one hour and fifteen minutes, which is quite a short amount of time for a first-time woman to give birth and given the baby's presentation in the pelvis. You see, Liz birthed her baby in a very unique position in that her baby's face was not presenting up or down but sideways.

She was looking at Liz's hip bone in a totally lateral position. This is something I had never seen before which totally amazed me and surprised the midwife!

To push a baby out in this position takes so much strength and power. I have to say all of Liz's dance strength and fitness came to the party. Simon and I assisted Liz in many positions including: standing up then squatting down on the floor and standing back up again, repeatedly, then she squatted on the bed, before she tried kneeling in the knight's position alternating one leg up then the other, over and over. Then we tried Liz in a semi-reclined position with her feet up on our hips pushing. Finally, after about an hour, the head began to stay on the perineum and not slide back in.

I thought to myself in all honesty, with this amount of pushing "how is it that Liz had not pushed out her baby yet?" I began to question, as did the midwife, and then even Liz said she felt beaten and that this part had got the better of her. She was bright red in the face and pouring with sweat. As soon as she had taken a drink, out it poured in sweat. I just stood and prayed this baby was going to come out right here and right now as this was what Liz deserved given all the work she had done. Her pelvic floor pushing was awesome, so strong and directed; she was doing everything absolutely right, no doubts about that.

No sooner had I said this to myself the baby made an appearance looking towards Liz's leg, and both the midwife and I glanced at one another and said "that's why". It was truly a moving moment and one I will not forget in a hurry. The baby had the biggest cone head and swelling on her head where she had been applying pressure on the cervix; it was like she was wearing a little cap on the top of her head.

As soon as the head popped out, the body followed beautifully, and Liz finally received her baby at 2.58pm in the afternoon. Their baby girl, Isobel, made her way into this world weighing 7 pounds 11 oz and was so chunky and healthy looking. She proceeded to breastfeed almost straight away.

Liz's placenta came away with no Syntocinon drug to assist its expulsion and her blood loss was next to nothing. Liz was truly amazing and after it was all over, I was in awe of her ability and strength, and we spoke about the whole day and how it had gone according to her hypnosis plan. Like lots of women after a great natural birth experience they are high on hormones and feel so invincible, proud and empowered, and so she should have been, it was an incredible effort.

I feel so blessed to have been present for this wonderful birth and learning journey. Thank you from the bottom of my heart.

Liz's story in her words, of Isabelle Frances Randall born Monday 26th May, 2008.

I found out about Gaby's Aqua-fitness classes through her website, which I looked at whilst reading her book 'A Labour of Love- a guide to natural childbirth without fear'. I knew from the word go that I wanted her input; as I found her to be so warm, friendly and knowledgeable. As a graduate of dance and having taught dance and Physical Education in Secondary Schools around the world, I felt a connection with Gaby, on several levels as Gaby has the same background.

The first Aqua-fitness class that I attended made me really excited about my pregnancy and about giving birth. (I was 19 weeks pregnant at the time.) Up until that point I had been worrying about EVERYTHING to do with this pregnancy and birth! I was busy working full time (teaching Dance at a high school) but from then on, the preparation for birth was on my agenda. Simon (my husband) and I went to Gaby's support person's workshop, which was excellent. Simon really felt that he understood the process of birth much more clearly.

A week later I began the four-week pregnancy and childbirth education journey alongside a really excellent group of women. These four sessions were exactly as Gaby indicated ..... 'A Journey'. I gained lots of knowledge about the actual mechanics of childbirth, which was really useful and thorough, not like any antenatal class or information that the hospital offers.

I gained awareness of myself, which enabled me to mentally prepare for birth and motherhood. We discussed, in detail, all of our options and choices, before, during and after giving birth. Up until this point I was unaware that I even had choices! We also watched some amazing and beautiful births. By the end of my 'journey' I felt like a powerful woman who could set out to do something and successfully DO IT! Gaby created such a positive and empowering belief system, that from then on, I was on a mission to create the beautiful, natural birth that I desired for me and my baby.

It was at this point that I asked Gaby if she would be my doula, she said she would love to. I immediately felt calm and relaxed because she was now fully on board. Throughout the remainder of my pregnancy, I kept in close contact with Gaby, doing her classes and getting positive input whenever I felt I was lacking a little! I finished work at the end of week 37, which in retrospect was a little late, in terms of mentally preparing I mean. I felt that I had a lot to do in my final two weeks, if in fact I even had two weeks! From then on I concentrated on creating a wonderful birth.

I was already doing a yoga class on a daily basis via a (DVD) as well as Gaby's hypnosis scripts every third day or so. So now I decided to do the hypnosis scripts daily and really try and relax. At this point I knew I needed Gaby's help, I tend to think too much, and I needed her to talk to me calmly when I was winding myself up. I booked a one-on-one hypnosis session;

which for me was the clincher .... that is, from that moment on, my body was ready to give birth. I experienced the whole birth process so powerfully in that session, it meant that for the next three days (which was when I gave birth) I was so focused, so mentally ready that my body just did what it needed to do. Here's how it all unfolded...

I woke up at 5am on Monday 26th May, 2008 and needed a wee; this was nothing unusual seeing as I was almost forty weeks pregnant! As I was walking to the loo I thought "oh no, I have just wet myself!" Again, this was not totally unusual with the pressure on my bladder! The big 'splodge' in my undies though was blood! At that moment I felt a mixture of excitement and nerves. I was thinking "this is it, I am going to have a baby today!" I intended to grab new undies and an enormous pad, from my half-packed hospital bag, without waking my husband but he was already awake. We talked and hugged for a while when I got back into bed and then I said we ought to get a bit more sleep if we could because it could be a full-on day! We had gone to bed quite early on Sunday evening and I had slept really well, so another hour would just make it even better.

By 6.30am I was awake and aware of waves of period-like back ache. I stayed in bed until 7am, which was when Simon was getting in the shower and ready for work. We discussed what we should do and decided that I would text Gaby, then just potter about, finish packing the bag, have breakfast and take a shower. Simon went into work to tell them that he would not be staying and then he had been instructed, by me, to buy some slippers because I didn't have any to take to the hospital.

As Simon went off to work, I sent a text to Gaby and put Pachabel in D minor on... this track was the one that we relaxed to at the end of Gaby's class on a Thursday evening in the Hydro pool, and always made me feel instantly relaxed. I was just making toast and a cup of tea when Gaby rang, we chatted about the intensities, and about what to do over the next few hours. I did feel unable to be still and I was a bit worried that if I was only in the early stages of warming up that I would not be able to cope when it was REALLY happening! Nevertheless, I said I would call in a few hours to let her know how I was. I then swayed and hummed away to myself whilst eating breakfast. I could not sit down!

The next hour or so were a bit of a blur, I was trying to stay in my logical 'here and now' brain, but my body wanted to leave it and get on with birthing this baby! I managed to finish packing my bag and get in the shower. I had only just got out of the shower when Simon got back home. It was 9.20am and I was really pleased to see him. I think from that point on I left my 'here and now' brain .... I really did not want to speak or communicate. I was in another place; everything was fuzzy, I was concentrating so hard on each intensity and saying the following to myself, 'relax', and 'my body is opening up to allow this baby out' and 'I can do this!'

Simon spoke to Gaby and between them they decided what to do. This was good because I needed someone else to take charge of the mundane decisions about being at the hospital or at home for longer! I was to get in the shower while Simon packed the car, then he would help me to dress ..... which was really funny because the intensities were happening every couple of minutes or less and I had to kneel down to get through them! Poor Simon, he had this grunting, non-speaking wife to try and dress! I remember he asked me what pants I wanted to put on and the question was too much for my brain ..... I just grabbed a pair that I had worn briefly the night before. Questions are not a good idea for a labouring woman, I remember Gaby saying that and it is so true!

Simon slowly helped me to the car where he had pulled the passenger front seat right forward to enable me to kneel on the floor in the back. With my head stuffed into the pillows and blankets on the back seat, we made our way to Gaby's. I was totally oblivious of where we were, and I was not worried now because I knew I was in good hands. Looking back, I bet I was a real sight to be seen. I have a fuzzy memory of us stopping at some traffic lights as another intensity hit; I was groaning loudly and rocking with my head stuffed into a pillow on the back seat. We were right next to a lorry and I could fleetingly see the driver looking at me, I wondered what he thought was going on!

When we got to the hospital, I took ages to emerge from the car, my contractions were really full on and I knew I could not handle one standing upright! I eventually, with the encouragement of Gaby and Simon, made my way into the hospital and up the stairs. I stopped halfway up to honour a contraction, Gaby was talking to me through my breathing as people were walking past! We were led to Birth Suite two and introduced to our midwife who was really lovely; she had read my birth plan and was really excited to meet Gaby! They chatted while attending to me, although I was so focused on each contraction that it was only later that I could fully appreciate how wonderful they had both been.

The midwife asked me if I would like to have an internal examination to establish what was happening, I agreed, and we were all pleasantly told that I was seven centimetres dilated. I laboured away on my hands and knees on the bed, with my arms holding onto the back of the bed; this was a good place to be and all the while Simon, Gaby and the midwife looked after me. I drank a lot as Simon or Gaby were constantly offering me water and juice. After a half hour or so both the midwife and Gaby suggested I get in the shower. For a while I couldn't move or register what they had said, but I nodded to Simon that I was in agreement. Simon and Gaby then escorted me to the shower. Once there I was very comfortable leaning over a fitball and kneeling on a foam mat whilst Simon showered me with hot water on the base of my spine. My contractions at this point were really intense and at one stage I thought I had bitten a hole in the fitball!

Then all of a sudden, when I felt that my body could not 'open' anymore, at least without splitting in two! I felt a release of pressure and a gush as my membranes exploded! Simon, who was concentrating on rubbing my back and keeping the water hot said "something just happened!" Gaby and the midwife came over to investigate and of course all of the membrane had gone down the drain! With my next piggy backing contraction, I really felt hot and that I needed to push. It really does feel like you need a poo! You can't describe it; you have to experience it to understand it. The brilliant thing is that your body knows exactly what to do and it just gets on and does it, if you let it! I spent a bit more time in the shower then was helped out and onto my hands and knees on the bed. I was cold then hot, then the more I pushed the hotter I got! Gaby and Simon were offering me water between contractions, which I readily accepted, and Gaby had got loads of cold flannels which she kept applying to my forehead and the back of my neck.

I had another VE at this stage, which was quite painful, mainly because I had to lie on my back. When a baby's head is almost ready to be born this is the last position you want to be in! Interestingly, my contractions stopped for about fifteen minutes after the internal examination. (I think my body reacted to being interfered with and shut down for a while) the midwife took a while because she could not establish whether the baby was facing up or down (Anterior or Posterior presentation). As we discovered when Isabelle finally appeared, she was in neither of these positions, but instead she was facing sideways (transverse presentation), looking at my hip bone! This is apparently quite unusual, both Gaby and the midwife had not seen a baby birthed like this before. The baby had done a poo which meant that I needed a monitor attached to me. This was a bit of a hassle, although at the time I had no idea what was going on and I was just concentrating on pushing!

Isabelle's heartbeat was fabulous even through really intense pushes. After a while I can remember sensing that things were not quite as they should be and that I had been pushing for so long to no avail. At this point I said to Gaby "I can't do this! I can't believe that I have gotten this far and now I'm really doubting my ability to birth this baby". Mentally this was make or break time for me and Gaby's words saved the day, she said that most women pushed for longer than this and I could do this. Then she said "get angry! Use the power that is inside you, get angry and push this baby out!" That was it for me! I had to find some power to finish this job and it had to come from me! I then proceeded to rant and swear! I wound myself up and felt really angry; I actually felt more powerful and I concentrated hard through each contraction. Gaby suggested different positions for pushing. I stood up, squatted, went on my

661

hands and knees, did the knight's position, squatted again and so on. Another thing which really helped at this point was watching myself push with a mirror. I know it sounds strange but there you are being told to push, and you are pushing with all of your strength, but you're not sure where the push is being concentrated unless you see it! Once I had seen at what angle I needed to push, I was away.

Finally, after what seemed like hours, the baby's head stopped playing peek-a-boo! With each contraction Isabelle was now edging her way out of my body. For the final pushes I was semi-reclined on the bed pushing with my legs wide open, wedged against Gaby's and the midwife's hip bone, the leverage was really important, and it worked really well. I can remember saying to the midwife "tell me how big a push I should do." I was thinking of my perineum and trying to prevent it from tearing.

The midwife was excellent and once Isabelle's head was out, she told me to do little pushes with the next contraction and out she came. Covered in goosies and plonked straight on my chest was my baby daughter! Wow how amazing! I did it and I was so pleased that I had done it with no intervention at all. I birthed exactly as I had wished, naturally and in a really honoured environment. Both Gaby and the midwife were elated! They could not believe that my pelvic floor muscles had been so strong and able to push my baby out facing sideways, first her head then her body! I was just so glad I had found the strength to do just that. The placenta was born thirty minutes after the baby, with no syntocinon drug to assist its expulsion.

I am truly in debt to Gaby for Isabelle's awesome birth; without her input I really believe it could have ended with major intervention. With Isabelle's transverse presentation a doctor would have definitely advised some intervention. Without Gaby's constant, even relentless positive words, I'm not sure I would have kept going. Plus, her interaction with the midwife was invaluable, because at one point she (the midwife) thought that I had been pushing for long enough, but Gaby convinced her to give me more time, which was all I needed. Consequently, I had a fabulous birthing experience, and Isabelle Frances was born at 2.54pm, weighing a healthy 7 pound 11 and she came into the world calmly, and breastfed soon after. Simon and I were really emotional at this point and Gaby took lots of pictures of the happy and rather overwhelmed new Mum and Dad with their gorgeous baby girl.

Simon and I are both really glad that Gaby was a part of our very special birthing experience. We are both convinced that had she not been a part of it, things may not have turned out quite so beautifully. Thanks Gaby x

12

TWIN AND TRIPLET
BIRTH STORIES

Olivia's Triplet Birth Story

Olivia and Mick came to me some months before the birth of their triplets to find out about my doula services and what I could offer them. I could tell from talking to Olivia that she was very well educated about natural birth and was very clear on just what she wanted to create for the births of her babies. What also struck me about this strong intelligent woman was her awareness about her body. Being a Chiropractor I knew that she was in really great shape physically, particularly skeletally due to having weekly adjustments. She had also been attending my pregnancy specific aquatic classes to keep fit as well as walking and listening to my hypnosis for birth scripts to prepare herself mentally.

At 36 weeks of pregnancy Olivia looked dynamic and was carrying the three babies with grace and ease. Olivia never once looked like she was having a hard time and never once looked like she was carrying three babies inside her body. Her belly swell looked just a little bigger than an average woman carrying a second or third baby and was not excessively big at all. She was and is a true inspiration to all the other women who attended my aquatic classes and to other multiple pregnancy women she came into contact with as well. I want to attribute her body's fabulous condition and ability to labour and birth beautifully to Olivia managing a good balance between her Chiropractic care, positive mental preparation and her physical fitness and health. Her story follows.

On 15th June 2007, just before midnight, three very special babies were born into this world. Clancy, Will and Tom were born weighing in together at just over 16 pounds. What makes this a remarkable story is that they were conceived naturally by Olivia Gleeson and Mick Ryan, with one egg splitting, making Clancy and Will identical and Tom non identical. Even more amazing is that they were born vaginally with Olivia using deep relaxation and breathing techniques, and no pain relief on board at all, until the very last minutes of birth, with Tom needing just a bit of help to come into the birth canal. You see, Clancy and Will had pushed him up into the higher section of the uterus and he needed to be assisted down into the pelvis to be born. I think they were all jostling at one point to be born first, as just days prior to Olivia's induction, they were all head down and working at pole position!

So, the day's events went along with Olivia and Mick arriving at the hospital in the early hours of the morning for an induction. Being that Olivia was now 36 weeks pregnant with very little room left and her cervix fully effaced and three centimetres dilated, it was time to get things going. With that she had her membranes broken and the Syntocinon drip put in as well as an epidural, however no drugs were put through the line as this was just a precautionary measure just in case one of the triplets needed to be born immediately via C-section. As it turned out, it was necessary at the very and was used as it was needed.

In the morning, Olivia and Mick had a vast array of medical people come into their labour room and all was very busy and buzzing leaving Olivia feeling a little overwhelmed. However this also reassured her that she had plenty of people around to support her. The realisation of this being the case however changed when everyone, apart from the midwife and Mick, finally departed to leave Olivia to get on with labouring and opening up her body to birth these three babies. This is where I came into the picture at 4pm, as Olivia and Mick's birth support (doula). Initially I was not even sure how exactly I was going to support Olivia. There she was attached to three foetal monitors and one monitor to record her contractions strength and regularity, a drip in the back of her hand and an epidural in her back with plastic film covering almost all of her back.

It was not long before I realised that Olivia just needed some verbal reassurance that she was opening up and labouring beautifully and doing an amazing job. I touched her through her shoulders to keep them down and 'let go' of any tension during contractions and used oral homoeopathic remedies to get her labour moving along and contractions more regular and stronger. I also gave her, from time to time, an oral calming remedy. Olivia had been listening to my 'Hypnosis for Labour' script just prior to me walking into the room and seemed to acknowledge and respond to my voice as I spoke to her softly. As she sat there upright and slightly moving through her pelvis on the fitball, she laboured away beautifully, surrendering to the necessary sensations when the contractions came on and passed by.

In between the contractions Olivia smiled and kept her great sense of humour, drank water and sweet drinks, ate a little food when she felt like it, and remained very calm. On three occasions we disconnected all the machines so Olivia could walk to the toilet having a break from sitting on the ball and empty her bladder and labour for a while on the loo. Meanwhile, I just kept thinking to myself "wow! What a woman!" Here she is demonstrating her strength, in a strong determined way as she laboured actively in the calmest and most peaceful manner, not fazed by anything, despite everything that was going on with blood pressure checks, temperature checks and all the machines attached to her and beeping.

It was around 9pm when Olivia's Obstetrician, Dr Craig came back to check on Olivia's progress and dilation. Just prior to this I had asked Olivia to visualise how dilated she was, and like always, women are usually always spot on with how open they are. The doctor's examination confirmed what Olivia had visualised which was nine centimetres dilated, with just one centimetre to go. With this news we all grew very excited. Dr Craig suggested that Olivia may take one hour to do this or ten minutes, whatever time it took was ideal as this would give him a little more time to prepare the theatre as this was where the triplets were to come into the world in case an emergency arose.

It was not long before Olivia's urge to push became evident, as with each contraction that came on, she felt more and more pressure down. With that we calmly headed up to the birthing theatre so that Olivia and Mick could meet their boys. When we arrived, Mick and I were taken to the Male and Female change rooms to put on the attractive theatre attire; navy blue pants, a top and a very attractive shower cap to keep the elusive hair from dropping out in the theatre room and shoe covers that looked like shower caps for your feet! Upon walking in Mick and I were reunited in a little room just outside the theatre where we got to talk about the births of the babies. Having been in this theatre and birthing situation with other women having one baby, I knew what to expect and tried to reassure and let Mick know what was going on to the best of my knowledge. It was here also that we were met with a private photographer employed by the hospital to capture these births on film. It was all so exciting!

Upon entering the room, we came face to face with a vast array of medical people. In total there would have been eighteen people in the theatre, all who had a job to do and a role to play. And of course, most importantly, Olivia was there in a semi-reclined position and working at pushing Clancy out of her body. It was here that as Olivia's doula I washed her face down with an icy sponge flannelette and talked her through her pushing as I supported her back and shoulders as she pushed. Such was the force and intensity of Olivia's dynamic effort, she had the unfortunate timing of a blood nose through the first five minutes of pushing, so my next job was to mop up the blood from her nose and pinch her nose to try to stop the flow of blood.

Clancy, like all the babies, was looking up to the sky in a posterior position and was proving a little squashed in the pelvis. Dr Craig suggested a little assistance was needed with some suction on his head, and as Olivia pushed, he applied just a little pressure to his head and out he came looking beautiful and perfect. He was placed immediately on Olivia's chest and it was here that we all touched him, rubbed him and Olivia got to see him face to face and skin to skin while Mick had some photos taken and kissed Olivia. The Paediatricians that were on standby then took Clancy over to the baby warmer where it was recommended, after a period of time, that he go downstairs to the nursery as he needed some assistance and monitoring of his breathing.

Next born was Will, who was guided down by Dr Craig into the birth canal with forceps where Olivia then pushed Will out. This seemed to take very little time as he just seemed to appear so quickly. He was really upset by having to come out and he let everyone know this as he lay on Olivia's chest crying. This actually was a good sign as he cleared his lungs and all of the fluid in his mouth by crying. He was very alert and settled down very quickly after his initial arrival. He was then taken over to the baby warmer for observation as well. After a while he was wrapped and swaddled and seemed very happy and content to wait for his brother to be born.

The epidural drug was administered before baby number three, Tom, was born as he needed some assistance and suction. Tom was positioned up the top of the uterus in a transverse position (sideways) and was going to need to be assisted down and into the birth canal. To make this bearable for Olivia it was better for her to have some pain relief on board during this time. So, we waited for about five minutes for the block to kick in, which gave Olivia a little time out in which to rest, relax and let her body go. It was not long before the next contraction came, and Olivia worked with Dr Craig to bring Tom down. It was in fact in the blink of an eye that he slipped out of

Olivia's body, probably because his brothers had opened the door and paved the way for him to be born so easily. He too was placed on Olivia's chest. This is when I felt the full enormity of what had just happened hit everyone, including myself, and I felt the need to shed a tear or two!

Tom, being slightly smaller than Clancy and Will, needed immediate medical assistance and monitoring and headed straight down to the nursery. Meanwhile, the placentas were born as well as the membranes and remaining cords. The cords on the babies were cut properly by a very proud Dad. Will was looking for a feed and went straight on the breast, as did Clancy when he was reunited an hour later with Olivia. Tom however, remained in the nursery for the following days being fed expressed colostrum until day three when he finally had a breast-feed from Olivia.

After a few stitches were given in the perineum, Olivia was taken to the recovery room where she continued to feed Will, who once he got the hang of breastfeeding, did not want to come off.

Finally, we arrived back in the labour room where Olivia was observed and monitored as she had post labour shakes and went very cold followed by feeling incredibly hot with a temperature. This, I assured Olivia, could be a response to the labour hormones as well as having the epidural in. Olivia was hungry and thirsty upon arriving back at the room, and we attempted to feed her as much drink and food as possible while she continued to breastfeed.

Mick and I went down to get Clancy as he was given all clear to be reunited with his brother and Mum. He looked so big compared to some of the babies down in the nursery where he was, and particularly big next to his brother Tom, who was just gorgeous and perfect. One of the neonatal nurses assisted us to bring Clancy back to the room where Olivia breastfed Clancy for the first time. In the meantime, Olivia's work practice partner, fellow Chiropractor Ali, came into the hospital at 1am to adjust the babies. Immediately upon adjustment the babies calmed right down and seemed very placid, relaxed and aware of what was going on. Olivia too had an adjustment and felt much better for it.

It was really difficult to leave the hospital that morning as I was so full of adrenalin, excitement and elation to have been able to be a part of something so special. I will always be indebted to Olivia and Mick for this experience. Thank you both from the bottom of my heart for allowing me to be involved in this truly amazing experience and being able to welcome your three beautiful boys into this world.

Gen's Birth Story of Natural Vaginal Twins

When I met Gen she basically had made the assumption that she was going to have to have a C-section because she was having twins. She really knew very little about her options and was just being led along by everyone who was seeing her. This is totally common with many women as they just don't know they have choices at all, and Gen was no exception.

Over the weeks that followed our first meeting at the pregnancy aqua classes I ran, I began to whisper into Gen's ear and worked at planting the seeds of possibilities! Hence Gen decided to register for my women's four-week pregnancy and birth education journey and make an appointment to see an Obstetrician that I recommended, that I had worked with as a doula previously to assist triplets to be born vaginally, only eight months before. Gen was definitely open to the idea of having the twins naturally, and was intrigued about what she didn't know and set about educating herself.

I can tell you now that the woman I met some four months before was a completely different woman I witnessed giving birth. Gen had taken everything on board in such a positive and meaningful way, and never once looked back. Each and every day she grew heavier and more tired, but she still managed to be very matter of fact and direct about what she wanted.

Gen really looked after herself, exercising regularly and having chiropractic care as well. She really did a great job of rising above all the potential dramas and kept on smiling, which helped.

I was so happy to be asked to be Gen and Stu's doula. Here is their story.

At 37 and a half weeks Dr Craig wanted Gen to have gone into labour. So Gen did everything she could, drank a glass of wine, had sex, ate hot curry, ate a whole pineapple and took homeopathic remedies and had acupressure point stimulation by me, as well as acupuncture by a specialist; but still no true labour. However, she did experience good period cramping as a result and during the warmup. She definitely stirred the pot and got things moving gently, so it was not in vain!

So on the evening of Tuesday 20th May, Gen went into hospital to be induced with a foley's catheter. When a foley's catheter is inserted through the cervix it is gently pulled through a closed cervix forcing it to open with the balloon on the end that is four centimetres in diameter. Well after about half an hour it just fell out of Gen's body! So much for that I thought! This was fantastic news because it meant Gen's cervix was soft and stretchy. Gen had definitely ripened herself up for labour to begin. Next they put some prostaglandin gel into her cervix and let her sleep the night through.

Come Wednesday morning Gen was feeling ready, strong and excited in her usual style and said "come on, bring it on!" as she was ready to have the babies. It was mid-morning when they broke Gen's membranes and the contractions began, induced by the Syntocinon drip that was being fed into a vein in her hand. Initially it was turned down very low so Gen could get used to the contractions, and slowly, over the course of the day, they were increased, which was the best approach.

By 6pm that night Gen was really beginning to work hard, and they called me into the hospital. Upon walking into the room, I was greeted by Gen's beautiful smile and Stu who looked happy and relaxed. Stu was doing a wonderful job of supporting Gen, massaging her and supporting her physically and mentally all day. They worked together as a team and I could see a strong loving bond between them which was beautiful. All was going to plan, and Gen was given the opportunity, when she wanted to have a shower for twenty minutes or more, to give her a break from being connected to a machine with cords. They did this at this hospital as they wanted to monitor the babies closely to make sure they were handling the drug induced labour.

At about 11pm Gen had another internal, using some gas this time, as she seemed to be very uncomfortable. However, she was elated to find out she was seven centimetres dilated. We were all so happy as we knew that Gen was doing amazingly well, breathing beautifully on the contractions, standing up next to the bed, sitting on the fitball, using heat bags across her lower back and receiving a massage. For a woman being driven to contract via the drug Syntocinon she was doing so well demonstrating her strength and determination. I was so proud of her and just knew she could do this.

At seven centimetres it was decided that Gen would have an epidural put into her back - just in case the second twin needed assistance out. Gen had decided beforehand and was quite adamant that she did not want any drugs and made this very clear. Gen agreed on having the epidural in her spine but for no medication to be put through the tube in her spine which they complied to her request. Gen pushed on working and breathing beautifully through the contractions.

At about 12.30am Gen could feel so much pressure down below and was beginning to feel incredibly tired. She opted for a very low dose of anaesthetic to go through the epidural, just to take the edge off. This worked incredibly well as Gen basically got to full dilation very soon after this and began the pushing stage. Gen initially was on the bed on her hands and knees and pushed with great effort and intensity. I became very excited as I could see the baby's head after about half an hour.

As the head descended down the birth canal Craig asked Gen to turn over and Gen pushed with one foot on my hip and one foot on Stu's hip. I then gave some instructions to Gen as to how to push on a contraction to make the most of it, in which she listened and took on board. It was hard going for Gen, but she got there in the end and birthed a beautiful baby boy first at 2.32am.

Stu and Gen had no idea of what the sexes of their babies were so when Gen received baby number one, they cuddled and checked him/her over to discover this baby was a boy and named him Harry. It was so wonderful to meet this little person finally. Before long though, Gen began to feel the contractions brewing up a storm. She stated in her very matter of fact way to the paediatrician "ok, come and take him as I have to push the other one out now!" And with that the cord was cut by Stu and I went with the baby to the baby warmer to make sure he was all OK. Harry weighed 6 pounds and looked healthy and strong. He was perfect and beautiful; however, he was breathing a little fast and making some noise. Later that night he ended up going to the nursery to be watched over as he had swallowed some amniotic fluid and needed antibiotics.

Next came baby number two. Gen felt the need to push, assisted by Craig, and out slid this beautiful little bubs in three pushes. Gen then received this baby on her chest to discover she was a little girl, and named her Rose. She weighed 5 pounds and was a little light weight!

Finally, they were born after a long day and night. Thankfully the placentas came away easily and Gen could get herself into Mothering mode. Gen had a bad case of the shakes, which can be quite normal after such a long labour and a side effect of having an epidural and from the adrenaline produced naturally for the pushing stage.

To help overcome this we fed Gen hot chocolate drinks and pâté on bread as she was starving after all that labouring and pushing! We covered her in a warm blanket that had been in the warmer and gave her homeopathics to counteract the shakes. I know this may sound strange, but I also laid my body over hers as the heat and weight from my body forced Gen to relax and let go. This was a technique I had learned years ago from a midwife. I talked to her, getting her to imagine every muscle relaxing, and slowly it began to stop. It all did the trick, and not long after, it all just disappeared altogether.

Not long after Gen was feeding Rose who took to the breast immediately. I figured she was making up for her brother's absence and trying to get a head start on the boobie feeding and colostrum.

I am so honoured and proud to have been present for this wonderful experience; I will always hold this dear to me. Thank you Gen and Stu for allowing me to share in your special journey, bringing these two special little people into the world.

13

BIRTHS THROUGH
A DOULA'S EYES

I thought that it might be appropriate to write about three very different births that I attended in one year to give a little insight as to what it is we Doulas actually do! It is often hard to explain exactly what we do because for each and every birth we attend is different and the support we offer is so varied, unique and autonomous. The fourth story in this chapter has been shared by a colleague and one that I am sure you find very interesting.

Birth One

This client came to me as a referral from a midwife who thought that having a doula in her chosen hospital might work better than having an independent midwife who would have to negate her authority to satisfy hospital policy with regard to the birth. And so this is where I came into the picture.

Jane decided after much consideration that I would be the person to support her during her labour and birth at her chosen hospital. What I would like to stress here is that a doula doesn't just commit to attending the labour and birth. A substantial amount of work is done in meetings prior to the actual birth itself. In fact, this is where all of the necessary groundwork is done, over cups of tea. The more cups of tea the better the education, communication, rapport and trust!

With the cups of tea in mind Jane and I met once or twice a week to connect and get to know each other; most importantly to discuss the type of birth Jane really desired. Jane was one of those women who had read everything she could get her hands on and was full of information about all types of topics to do with pregnancy, labour and birth. What I felt we needed to do was weed through all the rubbish she had read on this and get down into the more important issues at hand. I always begin by asking a woman "what type of birth do you really want to have?" From there we begin our journey to hopefully arrive at a place prior to birth where my client feels mentally, physically and emotionally ready for her baby's birthday.

I would just like to mention here that women often do over-read to the point that they get overwhelmed with information that they then cannot define for themselves what they really want or or define what is important to them when preparing for their own birth.

After many hours of pre-birth preparation, educational sessions and discussions, finally the phone call came to let me know that Jane's waters had broken and slight niggles were occurring in her uterus. However, there was nothing to panic about, and I reassured her to relax and just let go and allow her body to find its own pace and timing. After a day and night had passed I decided to venture over to Jane's house where I found her doing some Yoga with an instructor to bring on the labour. A few hours later, I thought it might be a good idea to have some lunch and then go for a little walk. We did all of the above and still the contractions kept at bay, neither increasing nor decreasing in sensation. Jane was still very content and happy to remain at home and did not want to proceed to the hospital.

In fact, 28 hours had passed and still no change. I decided at this point to phone my own midwife and mentor Mary to discuss our possible options, and after our long conversation, I decided to phone Jane's Obstetrician and explain where Jane was at and what she felt we should do. I was very pleased when she suggested that we stay a little longer to see if things changed. However, she did say within the next two hours I would like to see Jane in the hospital so that she could have the necessary medical and standard checks of both baby and mum, given that her membranes had been gone for some time now. Giving antibiotics to reduce the risk of infection was part of this care.

With the threat of me suggesting we go to the hospital, as her Obstetrician had suggested, some rather big contractions started to occur. It was then That Jane decided that it was a good idea to have the baby's heartbeat monitored, and Jane's blood pressure taken to make sure all was fine. So we headed into the hospital with arms loaded full with gear as we headed for the natural birthing suite which we discovered was available on this night, much to Jane's delight. The Obstetrician came in after a short period of time doing all the standard checks and was quite happy to let Jane continue on as she had planned and requested. In the meantime, I massaged, spoke quietly in a positive reaffirming way, gave water, juice and food on a requested basis and suggested various positions as she progressed along in her labour.

As a result of being aware and informed about the various labouring positions, Jane laboured in the bath, on the floor, on the bed, in the shower, on the fitball and walking the corridors. However, her labour did not progress at all, and by 7am in the morning, after a full night of activity she was exhausted and wanted an epidural.

Jane's epidural was granted, and to try to get the contractions going, the syntocinon was put up in a drip as well. This stayed in for a period of time but unfortunately, a very short time after the epidural went into her body, Jane's baby went into foetal distress and Jane underwent an emergency caesarean-section.

Occasionally, time is against a woman and when the membranes have been gone for such a long time and a woman does not go into labour with strong dynamic contractions it is almost inevitable that she is going to need some form of intervention, unless of course she can relieve herself of any stress, anxiety and fear she may be presenting. As a Doula this can be very challenging, however I do believe that all the preparation and education prior to the birth makes women feel stronger, more empowered and positive, and confident not only to birth but in becoming a mother. This helps women enormously to deal with birth outcomes that were not what they had even considered to be an option.

Having said all of that, one thing I do notice with the women I work with is that when a woman is adamant, she does not want to have this or that, and she focuses on that thing telling me how much she does not want it, she almost always ends up with that exact outcome and thing happening to her!

It is the law of attraction at its best. I call this the self fulfilling prophecy- attracting to themselves the very thing they don't want! Women should be focusing on what they do want to have happen; this is far more beneficial and productive in bringing what they do want as an outcome to them as their reward.

Jane had a beautiful baby girl who was just adorable, so the outcome was a positive one despite the actual way the baby came out of her body being not what Jane would have liked at all (which she told me often). The bringing into the world of a gorgeous little baby is the most important thing here and this birth was a great example about the law of attraction and thought processes, and how they really can dominate what goes on despite a woman's best intentions.

This story also demonstrates how much time and effort is given to women pre-birth and during the labour. A doula not only provides hands-on support, she is a coach, mentor, advocate, negotiator and educator giving tirelessly of her time and energy.

Birth Two

Robin and I had been friends for years and shared mutual female friends. Robin had also previously been to my aqua antenatal classes throughout her second pregnancy, so you could say a lot of the ground work had been done between us and I knew where I stood and what would be required of me when the time came.

Robin and I had lots of cups of tea and chatted over the phone on a regular basis right up until the seventh day over her estimated due date. Robin was at this point very heavy, very tired and very big, and had had enough. However, she knew that she really wanted a quick, to-the-point birth with no messing about. She decided the following day to be induced as she was really worried about the size of the baby, as the other two had been big and it looked like this one was 'just as big'.

The time was 7.30pm in the evening when we spoke about the induction that would take place in the morning and what her options were, as well as what she would like to have happen. So I hung up knowing that I would be at a birth the following day. At 8.00pm the phone rang and it was Robin on the other end, in full labour. At first I thought she was pulling my leg, however I soon realised very quickly after two contractions in the space of four minutes that this was the real deal and she was well on her way to getting into established labour right at that moment in time.

As soon as I put down the phone I ran to my car and was on the way to Robin's house and arrived five minutes later to find Robin and her partner in the car, reversing out of the drive. I just flagged them on and followed in my car. When we got to the hospital Robin continued to labour beautifully, not missing a beat and working totally with her body, surrendering and breathing her way through her contractions. She was so focused and centred within; she was in that place where women go to when they are in true established labour.

As Robin's doula I spoke quietly suggesting affirmations, I massaged her lower back and ran the shower nozzle on her lower back when a contraction came on, alternating to running the water over her belly when the contraction was off. We soon found our rhythm, which worked so beautifully and seemed to help Robin cope with the intensity. I assisted to give rescue remedy on a regular basis and fed Robin liquids through a straw when I got the chance. It was Robin and I working together calmly and quietly with her partner in the background, which he was happy with. We agreed during the pushing stage he would be at the head end of Robin, encouraging her and supporting her, while I would be receiving bubs down the other end!

Before long Robin had hit transition in which she changed from her calm, quiet demeanour to being direct and outspoken, putting her hands on her hips and stating "oh, when is this baby coming out?" Robin then removed herself from the shower and headed for the labour room once again. I followed behind trying to get a towel over her butt naked body, as she walked down and across a public corridor with not a care in the world. (Which of course was totally acceptable during this stage of labour) I call this stage of labour the anything goes stage in labour - as anything can happen and it does! Once she was back in the labour room she lowered herself onto a mattress on the floor leaning over a beanbag and began pushing with absolutely no noise at all. She was as quiet as a mouse, but working really hard on each and every contraction.

After about twenty minutes of pushing she decided to get her body in a more upright position and moved where she was leaning over the bed, still on her knees on the floor. It was here that she pushed her very big, nearly 10 pound baby out with the assistance of myself, the midwife and the obstetrician looking over our shoulders, guiding the both of us where necessary. It was a wonderful experience and one that I feel very honoured to have been a part of. This was actually my very first experience of having received a baby totally and was absolutely amazing. Robin had given birth to a baby boy in less than three hours of labour from first contraction to pushing the baby out with no tearing of the perineum! "Wow, what a woman!"

Robin taught me so much about the inner strength women possess and how women can birth in a calm, natural and empowered way when they are left to do so. She also taught me that the perineum really can stretch WIDE open as it was designed to do!

Robin's ideas about having a Doula.

I chose to have a doula because I wanted a more positive birth experience than what I had had during my previous labour/birth.

With my second baby I had my husband, friend and an uncommunicative midwife in a hospital. Hence, I had no direction in my labour and the birth became frustrating and painful, leaving me with bad injuries (perineum tears) that took a long time to recover from. I felt traumatised after that birth and really did not want to go through that again.

The lesson I learnt from the second birth is that women like myself really need a professional birth support person, who is connected to me and able to assist with the spiritual and emotional aspects of birth.

From my experience I felt a doula can and does provide this support. Doulas are guides for birthing, in which the act of birthing is a very spiritual experience. As well as the spiritual support a doula also looks after your physical and mental state and uses her intuition to assist and guide accordingly. Birth after all does put you in a very vulnerable position and I feel a doula is able to protect your interests in a way that your labour progresses and in which direction it goes.

So my third baby was the biggest at 10lb4oz and I am here to tell you that there is such a thing as a positive 'beautiful birth' and little Noa is living proof that a doula can and does make a huge difference. So, thank you Gaby for assisting with my third birth experience which was amazing.

Birth Three

Sam was a friend of a friend who had actually heard about Robin's birth (above). She knew I had assisted Robin to have a three hour labour/birth and how she didn't tear birthing a

10lb 4oz baby. This really intrigued Sam and she rang me to make an appointment over a cup of tea! It was at our first meeting that I felt very connected and comfortable as we had many similarities in our lives.

Sam came along to my aqua antenatal classes as well as childbirth education classes where our friendship developed very quickly over a short space of time. It was in fact, only six weeks from the time we met to the time Sam gave birth, and in that time she had a complete shift in her understanding and concept about birth and birthing.

How this shift came about was firstly, Sam decided to block out the entire negative outside influences that she felt both exposed and vulnerable to, from family and her girlfriends, most of whom had had babies born by caesareans. Next she decided to start to listen to positive birthing stories and seek out alternative childbirth education and read books with positive informed content that assisted her to feel empowered about her imminent labour and birth. As a result she soon realised that she could birth naturally if she wanted to make that decision and put her trust in her body. Over the next couple of weeks she did a lot of mental preparation with me through meditation, visualisation and relaxation, as well as physical preparation through aqua and fitball classes.

After six weeks of mental and physical preparation, Sam went into labour naturally on her estimated due date at about four in the morning. At 7am she rang me to let me know 'today was the day'. Like all the births that I attend, I always go over to see a client in the early stages of labour to 'check in' with them and see where they are at mentally. It is a visit to connect on many levels and see what language they are using and observe what physically is going on, and to see if she is surrendering and letting go. I usually stay for half an hour or so, then I leave if I sense the woman needs more time and space, so as not to bring on what I call "Performance Anxiety". This is where a woman in labour feels like she is being watched and observed.

Sam was contracting really well from 7.30am when I arrived till when I left at 8am. I went home to leave her to get on with her labour in the peace and quiet of her home. At 11.00am Sam called to say her contractions had stopped and I suggested that she get some rest, and possibly have a sleep. I suggested this so she could reserve her energy for when contractions started up again. I also said that nature had been really kind and enabled her to have a really great warm up and to experience first-hand how contractions feel. On that note she took off to attend her pre-booked reflexology session to help her relax, rest and perhaps get things going.

At 2.00pm a call came from Sam's partner that they wanted me to come back over, so I jumped in my car straight away. I arrived to find Sam labouring in her lounge room on the floor. Not long after she sat on the couch next to John to give and receive a hug and kiss from John. I walked out to give them some alone time together. Within a minute Sam made a strange noise out loud and I ran back in as Sam's membranes had broken all over the couch. With that I helped her up and said go straight to the shower. She waddled down the corridor leaving amniotic fluid every step she took. It was literally pouring out of her and was all over the house and instantly her contractions came on really strong. I have never seen a woman lose such a great amount of amniotic fluid before, it literally was like a never ending bucket of liquid! I gave everyone a hit of Rescue Remedy to calm everyone down, me included, then I proceeded to mop up and clean up the couch while Sam was in the shower leaking more and more fluid!

After the shower where Sam stayed till no more amniotic fluid came out, she returned to the lounge room wearing a nappy just in case and continued to laboured on the floor, fitball, lounge and her bed, to well into the evening. Towards 10pm she felt she needed to travel to the hospital. On this particular night Perth was experiencing one of the worst storms in twenty years, lights were out all over the place due to severe lightning, thunder and torrential rain, not to forget major flooding on the roads! They say that women often give birth in strong stormy weather, when the barometric pressure drops. Well on this night, Sam was true to form.

John and I experienced one of the best lightening shows we have ever experienced, not to mention having to drive the car through flooded streets and along the freeway where the Swan River water was crashing over the car in huge waves with the

693

wind making it impossible to drive any faster than 20kms per hour. It was absolutely insane! All the while Sam was oblivious to the whole thing, and just continued to labour away in the car burying her face deep into her pillow.

Upon arrival it was suggested that Sam go into the hot tub and labour, and she did so for the next four hours. After the birth she said she wished she could have stayed in the tub longer than half an hour. With that I looked at her and said "Sam, you were in the tub for four hours". She couldn't believe it. Birth hormones affect time in a distorted way, so much so that what may seem like one hour for a labour woman can actually be two or three hours. This is an awesome fact about labour that women are so often not aware of. After four hours in the tub Sam started to feel the urge to push and felt like she needed to get out of the water and get gravity working for her. As her Doula I ran around to the room and prepared it with a mattress on the floor, with a big bean bag and pillows on top for her to lean over if she wanted. I dimmed the lights down and put the music on. I also found her dressing gown and socks for her feet, as I knew she would feel cold in the room after being in the hot water for such a long time. Then the power went out. I opened the curtains as the room was pitch black, to let in the light from outside. For the next hour and a half we could hear all the alarms in the hospital going off and got to witness the most incredible lightning show from the storm that was hitting Perth at this time. For the next couple of hours I continually gave Sam rescue remedy and spoke some positive words of encouragement and affirmations as I massaged her back with essential oils.

On the floor is where Sam stayed for the next three hours, panting and avoiding the urge to push; waiting for an anterior lip to move so she could push her baby out smoothly. (An Anterior lip is a swelling of the tissue around the neck of the cervix, which should never be pushed against no matter how strong the urge is as it can cause damage to the tissue.) As a doula, during those last three hours I continually supported both physically, mentally and emotionally assisting Sam to stay positive and strong and not lose sight of the fact that she would be meeting her baby soon and to try not to push. Not pushing when you have the urge to push is incredibly hard to do. Finally, with another internal examination, the midwife managed to flick the tissue out of the way and Sam was at last able to push freely which was such a relief.

Sam had the most amazing stamina and strength as she pushed out a very big first baby who weighed 9pounds 9oz. I was so honoured to have been a part of this fantastic experience and in awe of Sam's body and its ability to birth. Sam softly and gently worked with each contraction by pushing her baby down and out, little by little, with no pain relief, as she at this point had understood what it meant to just 'go within' and 'surrender' to the intensity of labour and work with it, not against it. She couldn't wait to tell all her friends about her amazing labour experience. I thought she should, as she really succeeded in giving birth naturally through sheer belief in herself and her body and through absolute determination and stamina.

I learnt so much from attending Sam and John's birth. Firstly, I learnt that in six weeks women can go from wanting to have a caesarean to believing they can naturally birth in an empowered and informed way. What they need to do is find a doula willing to install that belief through discussions, educational material, and positive childbirth education and information.

Secondly, I realised that women can keep on labouring, like running in an endurance event provided they have the right support around them, are given ample food/nutrients to keep them going, lots of water and sweet drinks and receive lots of natural intensity/pain relieving methods so that they keep on going.

Sam's thoughts about having a Doula.

Our Doula:

- Helped make the whole experience a pleasurable one by giving us support and encouragement and positive affirmations.

- Was the person we chose to attend the birth to explain the technical and medical jargon in the hospital so we understood what was going on.

- Assisted us to stay at home as long as possible before heading off to hospital which allowed us to relax and do this without any stress.

- Offered us alternatives to chemical pain relief, eg: massage, hot tub, breathing and relaxation techniques etc. (This was one of the reasons why I had a doula - because having a natural childbirth was important to me).

- I truly believe having a doula attend our birth allowed me to relax and therefore focus on breathing through the contractions and let go and surrender. As a result I didn't feel 'pain' and I didn't once feel as though I needed pain relief/treatment.

- John and I felt being able to focus just on the birth and not worry about other issues was the key to having a positive birth experience in a hospital setting and Gaby enabled us to do that.

John's points about having a Doula.

- Having an experienced person with us in the room offered Sam and I to work as a three-way team.

- Having a doula meant it turned two people who didn't know what they were doing into an effective three-way support network who trusted what was going on.

- A doula, to us, was an additive to the experience rather than an alternative to what is offered in the hospital today.

As you can see from these three birth stories the role of a Doula varies considerably depending on the length of the birth and how easy or hard the birth is at the time. I often find that it is hard to define what it is that I do as a doula, however I understand that it is a lot more than just attending a birth and supporting a couple during the labour and birth.

When people ask me why I choose to assist women during childbirth I always reply, because I love birth and I feel passionate about women being able to experience a positive birth. Seeing women give birth in an empowered and positive way, observing the look on their faces when they hold their baby in their arms for the first time is the most rewarding and uplifting experience that a support person can have. Birth is so special and unique and seeing that little head appear from deep within the body is an absolute honour and privilege to be a part of. I am very grateful that I am able to be of service to women who want and need support during the most important event in their and of course their baby's life.

Witnessing the Power of Birth

In some ways, my decision to become a doula was prompted by a desire not to feel like I was missing out anymore.

I've known for a long time my body would never allow me to birth a baby of my own and yet, as a massage therapist, I have played a very intimate role in many pregnancies. So often, when I gently knead and stroke these beautiful pregnant bodies, I feel the heat and energy from life-swollen bellies, or the kick and sweep of a baby inside, responding to my touch.

Then, after months together, my clients go away and have their babies. I don't resent them or feel jealous that they can experience something I can't, but so often I am left feeling as though I am standing outside the door, missing out on something really special.

In 2006, I started studying via correspondence to be a doula. My teacher told me all I needed was a pair of hands and a heart. I knew I was cut out for exactly this kind of work as it fitted in with my own philosophies as a massage therapist and teacher: that to be a good therapist, you need to open your heart and be fully present for every client.

I knew I could take these skills into a birthing space and offer a client emotional support by focusing completely on her. Many of the expectant mothers I have worked with over the years told me they felt like everyone focused on the baby and the pregnancy, and that they were lost in the whole experience.

What a doula can do is focus on the woman without being emotionally attached. The time they are together is her time to connect and be intimate with somebody.

699

One of the requirements of my course is that I attend three births but, three months into my study, I hadn't yet approached any of my clients about supporting at a birth.

Just three days before her estimated due date, a woman I had massaged regularly for nine years, asked me to be at her baby's birth. Rebecca had organised a homebirth with a midwife and a support person who fell through.

I was so excited that I didn't sleep properly for three days, waking up about thirty times a night, thinking the phone was ringing when it wasn't.

Finally, her midwife called me at 3am on a Saturday. As I hadn't been expecting to be the support at this birth, I hadn't been able to clear my schedule, so I was due to run a course that day starting at 9am. I knew I couldn't even think about that; my priority was Rebecca.

Rebecca had been labouring for twenty hours, the midwife told me, and the baby's father Max was exhausted as was Rebecca and in need of extra support.

All my nervous energy from the past three days dissipated and I felt calm and present as soon as I walked into the birthing space. The room was hot and intense. Incense was burning, filling the space with the scent of something ritual. Rebecca was lying on a bean bag, moaning, while Max and the midwife were by her side looking tired but in control.

I walked in and said, "Max, you need to go and have a sleep" and I suggested the midwife lie down on the couch nearby.

The thing that struck me was how unnecessary words were. Rebecca and I didn't speak; she was grumpy and exhausted in pain. I knew I needed to be an anchor and just hold the space, so I immediately started applying hot towels to her sacrum.

The room was well set up with a birthing pool at one end, and a Mexican sling and futon at the other. There was music and a heater to keep the towels hot ... which I was glad about as Rebecca let out a primal growl every time the towels got cold.

I continued hot towelling for a couple of hours while she moved into different positions until it became obvious that she needed to have something to eat and a rest. The midwife told Rebecca she needed to talk to her baby and let her know that mum needed to have a sleep.

Rebecca did a brief meditation, asking the baby to quieten down, which she did for about half an hour. It was amazing to see the communication between a mother and her unborn child ...I thought to myself, this was some of the special stuff I had been missing out on.

After her rest, Rebecca got up and asked to be taken to the birthing pool, which was where she stayed until she was ready to push. I could see her urge to push was strong, but she was scared and kept closing her legs together. As much as she wanted to, she didn't seem to be able to bring herself to open up to the intense sensation that was sweeping through her body, that I could only imagine.

During our massage sessions, Rebecca and I had talked about how there were times when we needed the warrior woman to emerge to face difficult situations. I leaned into her and whispered in her ear "it's time for the warrior woman, Rebecca" and asked her to take some deep breaths with me.

At that moment, I saw in her eyes what I can only describe as fire kicking in. We moved her into the Mexican sling so she could be in a supported squat and, with the midwife's guidance, Rebecca started to push.

I stood behind Rebecca to catch her if she slipped but I really wanted to see what was happening with the baby so I put my head around to see what I could see.

Max waved me around and I saw the baby crown. It really was the most incredible thing, and Rebecca let out this warrior-woman cry, and the baby's head came out and, with another cry, she birthed her baby's body.

She was a little girl.

Rebecca dropped onto the futon, and I stepped back, laughing and crying. I was in this total state of bliss and my whole body was shaking. The crying really kicked in, but I thought, 'this isn't the time and the place to be crying like this; this is about Rebecca and the baby'.

I gathered myself and I remember standing there just looking at Rebecca who, not that long ago, was overwhelmed, exhausted and whispering in my ear "I can see why women take pain killers". Here she was now with rosy cheeks, smiling and it was as though the previous twenty four hours' effort had never existed.

What surprised me most about the birth was how powerful Rebecca was. When she gave birth, I saw how powerful women are. That's a power that, as a man, I will never know. As a doula though, I will be blessed to witness that power, time and time again.

Baby Kate was born at about 8.40am. At nine o'clock I remembered I was supposed to be teaching a course and when I got to the venue, I leaped out of the car and the people waiting for me just stared as I was so high on birth energy. The whole day I was in a state of bliss, so 'oxytocinised' up and on cloud nine!

Andrew Barnes Man-doula

14

QUICK
FAST LABOURS

Louise's Birth Story

I woke up at 4:30am on my estimated due date (9/11/16) to contractions that were very mild. I stayed in bed until 6am and then got up to use the toilet. As I was going to sit on the toilet, my waters broke. I called the hospital and they asked me to come in for a check-up. We got there at 9am and the midwife checked that it was indeed my waters that were leaking and that I was having contractions. As they were still over ten minutes apart, they sent me home and asked me to return at 11:30pm to get things started if they hadn't done so naturally. I went home and paced the house as sitting during contractions was too painful. I started recording my contractions from 12-2:30pm and they were going from 4-5 minutes apart, down to 3-4, or sometimes even 2 minutes apart. I called the hospital and they said to come in when I can no longer handle the pain anymore.

Half an hour later at 3pm we decided to head in to beat the traffic and I was starting to struggle. I got to the hospital in a fair bit of pain, contracting in the car was hard. The midwife did an examination and found I was already 8cm dilated and they quickly moved me into a room ready for the birth. I got very emotional at this stage as I realised, I was too far along for any kind of pain relief and the contractions were taking over my whole body. It was very overwhelming. A hug from my husband got me back on track. The midwives got me into the shower, and I never left.

At the start I was leaning over a chair but moved into the corner on a padded mat under the shower head, holding onto the bars on the wall as I contracted. I started to get the urge to push so let my body do its thing, I could hear the noises I was making but it felt surreal and bizarre to hear those noises coming from me. I sounded like a wild mad woman, but it was what I needed to do. The midwife left me be and only interrupted me to check the baby's heartbeat with the doppler. I had no idea how far along I was but I could feel that it wouldn't be long until my baby was here. They moved me to the toilet as kneeling wasn't working and I was wasting my energy. I pushed into the toilet as I contracted and stood in between, sitting or lying down was still just too unbearable.

My husband had the shower head on me the whole time until she was ready to come out. They had me stand up at the end and lean against the wall as I birthed. A few pushes and she was out, and they caught her and handed her up to me. She was born at 5:52pm weighing 3.34kg.

After the birth of the placenta and breastfeeding the baby, I was up and walking around not long after which was a great feeling. I had some second degree tearing which didn't cause too many issues. I feel I had a really positive birth (although I was sure I wasn't going to get through it at the time) and am so amazed at what I have achieved and what the female body can do. I am so grateful for the empowering birth I was able to experience.

Louise Townsend

Eleanor's Birth Story

On the 1st November 2015, the night before I gave birth, I started feeling cramping sensations similar to when I get my period every month. It was a little bit uncomfortable, but fine so I went to bed and slept the night through. I was thirty eight weeks and four days pregnant. My husband left for work around 7am. I got out of bed at around 7:30am and started having contractions; by 8am, the contractions were five minutes apart.

I called the hospital and the midwife advised me to take some Panadol and lie down and see what happens. I took the Panadol, but there was no way I could lie down. By 9am, contractions were about a minute and a half apart. I felt like I constantly wanted to bear down and was moving between pacing around and rushing into the toilet to sit down. By this stage there was also a little blood, known as the 'bloody show'.

I called the hospital and they said I should come in. I called my husband to come and get me. I think he had heard stories about how labour takes a really long time, so he didn't hurry over. Consequently, he made sure he finished up what he was doing at work first. When he got home, he fed the dog and took his time. We then headed to Armadale hospital, which was about fifteen minutes away.

When we got to the ward, I needed to rush off to the toilet to push down while we were waiting. We were ushered into an exam room about 10:20am. The midwife, who was the same midwife that had conducted our antenatal classes, recognised us. She looked at me and said "are you pushing?" It had not occurred to me until that moment that I was actually pushing and had transitioned already. I said "yes I am".

I then removed my underwear, and she checked my cervix and said "you're fully dilated, the baby is coming down now". I was then put into a wheelchair quickly and raced off to a birthing suite. When we got there the midwife asked if I wanted to get in the shower, stand or get on the bed. I thought a shower sounded good. She said "this baby is about to be born now, so wherever you want to be, that's where this baby is going to be born". I was really surprised at how fast this was all happening.

I opted to stay holding onto the bed railing, standing. There was a rush to get paper on the floor and nurses around me. I ended up naked, and I was pushing, but I was still a bit reserved. The nurse said "come on Nashell, you need to get angry". So I just had to let go. I started to grunt.

I decided to move on to the bed, so we moved everything so that I was on my hands and knees on the bed. During all of these moves the nurses kept saying "the membranes are bulging and are just not breaking". They asked my husband if he could see this too.

Finally the baby's head was through. The midwife asked me to stop pushing, but I could not, and the shoulders and the rest of the baby came through in a rush, with a stinging feeling.

Eleanor was born in the 'Caul' with the membranes intact until after she was born. She landed on the bed, breaking them herself. She was born at 11:02am.

I turned over and lay down on my back and she was put on my chest, where she stayed for the next hour while I was stitched up from a second-degree tear. Eleanor was perfect, weighing 3.46kgs.

My experience was very fast yet very positive. Only three and a half hours in duration! I got dressed and walked the baby to the maternity ward and felt high on birth hormones. I stayed one night, leaving the hospital with our beautiful baby the next day.

Sandra's Experience of a Fast Labour

I was pregnant with my second baby and was three days past my estimated date. Everything in this pregnancy had been going along so well and I was actually enjoying this pregnancy, as it was so easy, and I was not uncomfortable at all.

It was a shock when I was woken up in the middle of the night when my membranes broke all over our bed sheets and I had three huge contractions one after the other and had the urge to bear down like nothing I have ever experienced before. To say it was intense was an understatement! My first labour had been pretty intense and quick, but it was not like this.

My husband jumped up and put the bedside light on to discover that the amniotic fluid was all over our bed sheets and was lime green in colour. It actually looked like car radiator coolant! It was bizarre to say the least. There I was in the throes of needing to bear down with this intense pressure in my bottom. I tried so hard to resist it but I couldn't stop at all, so I decided to give a push with this intensity to see what would happen as it just felt so right to do so at the time. In fact, when

I did push it didn't hurt at all, until I felt a burn and a stinging sensation and out shot our baby in one go landing on the bed, thank goodness!

Robert James came into the world in one BIG whoosh at 12.33pm much to the astonishment and amazement of my husband and I who just sat in this BIG pool of green amniotic fluid, poo from me and the baby and some blood!

Our beautiful baby boy was perfect and fine, pink slippery and divine and cried, bless him. I was not surprised that he was crying as one minute he was all warm in a big sack of amniotic fluid, calm and relaxed inside of me and next minute he was shot out landing on the cold bed in the cold of the bedroom, in a big puddle dripping wet. It must have been a shock for him. I scooped him up onto my chest to try to keep him warm while my husband ran to get some towels from the bathroom.

Everything happened so fast. Eventually I said to my husband I think you better call an ambulance now and the hospital to let them know what has just happened. We were all fine but in shock for days. Once we recovered, we just laughed and laughed, what else could we do as it was kind of funny.

A Fast Positive Accidental Homebirth

On the 10th of September at 11.00 o'clock in the morning I began to experience contractions at last. The reason I was so relieved was because I was now one week and one day past my estimated date my baby was due and due to my age had been given a really hard time about going over my 40-week mark. You see at the age of 44 the Family Birth centre wanted me to birth in the main hospital and I initially was very angry and upset about this and had to jump through lots of hoops to convince them that I am a very healthy, fit woman who has been a professional dancer all her life and had experienced a beautiful natural waterbirth before, so new what I was doing! Eventually they gave me permission to go two weeks past my estimated date with no need or pressure for an induction.

So here I was at home beginning my labour spontaneously in the middle of the day. At 12.27pm we called Gaby our doula to give her the heads up that this labour was starting but we didn't need her just yet. Not long after, my husband packed our daughter's bag at about 2 pm, called Gaby to say he was dropping our daughter off to our friend's house to leave me to labour. Gaby said she would be around very soon. I was happy at home walking around a little sitting on my fitball. When my husband arrived back home, he played the crystal bowl for me so I could really get into the zone.

Not long after this I visualised my cervix opening to ten centimetres and the baby moving down into the birth canal and within seconds of imagining this my baby dropped down and I had the biggest amount of pressure in my bottom. I thought to myself 'WOW' this visualisation thing really works! So, 'your thoughts really do create your reality!'

With this feeling of pressure, I began to feel very hot and like I could not breathe and in walked Gaby and came straight up to me and gave me a big hug from behind. After my contraction Gaby asked me what I was feeling, and I responded by saying just so much pressure in my bottom.

On the next contraction Gaby asked me to stand up to see if it relieved the pressure at all. It didn't at all. It was then that I said "I have to push". With that Gaby said "I am going to take your pants down now and see what is happening down there, is that OK?" I replied, "Yes".

As Gaby took my pants down another contraction came and I began to push spontaneously and poo as well which fell out of me and went all over the pants as Gaby took them down! I didn't know this until later on. So here I was leaning over our reading nook built into the wall, when Gaby suggested I climb on up and go on my hands and knees as I was about to have the baby.

When my husband heard this picked up the phone and called the birth centre. They suggested we call an ambulance and he hung up. Gaby then asked us "do you want to call an ambulance or are you happy for us to do this here and now or, do you want to get in your own car and travel now to the birth

713

centre?" My husband replied "we want it to just be us, but we can call them if we need to right?" I said, "Yes absolutely".

With that the birth centre called to say they had rung an ambulance which my husband told them to cancel as we were fine on our own.

I then began to push with the bearing down sensation as I could no longer resist the urge. It was so powerful and strong. Gaby was amazing and started to order my husband around asking for him to bring hot water for my perineum, towels to catch the baby in and wrap the baby up in, ice and face clothes. While he ran off and did this, she took some photos, and encouraged me as to what to do at the same time in a calm and composed manner.

As the baby came onto my perineum, I could feel Gaby applying lots of oil and the hot towels which felt amazing. As the baby started to be born Gaby spoke to me and kept me focused on what to do and how to nudge my baby out gently.

The room was very quiet apart from a little bit of music in the background which was just perfect. As the baby slowly appeared, Gaby told me our baby had membranes intact over her face, but they had also partially broken and were hanging down like a deflated balloon filled with water down one end which when I put my hand down to feel, felt very weird.

I slowly pushed and stretched and birthed my baby's head as guided by Gaby. Gaby had told me the baby had done a fresh baby poo but there was nothing to worry about and asked my husband to start taking some photos. My husband was relieved about having a job to do as it reassured him everything was going along normally, as he was looking at our baby's head thinking that doesn't look good because she had green amniotic fluid all over her face as well as the membranes which did look weird. The green baby poo looked like slime and it was hard to see her face. Once her body came out on the next contraction and she broke free from her membranes she cried and pinked up pretty quickly and took her first breath. Gaby just held her face down to drain all the fluid out of her mouth before I turned around to receive her on my chest skin to skin.

At 3.38pm our beautiful baby girl arrived.

There I stayed with this beautiful baby girl on my chest while Gaby and my husband looked on laughing and smiling at what had just happened. I was so happy and after a while started to share and re-tell what had just happened. I was in shock a little due to the speed at which she came. Everything was so relaxing being at home and in this moment it all felt very surreal what had just happened. A great remedy for a quick labour is to eat and drink and with that Gaby and my husband began to feed me some food which helped as I started to shake from all the adrenaline I had on board. Gaby asked if my husband could find a clean shoelace in which to tie off the umbilical cord as she didn't have any cord clips in her doula bag. He came back with a brand new clean one which Gaby tied in two places and he cut between the two with some sharp scissors. Finally, I could bring the baby onto my chest skin to skin as the cord was very short.

After a while our beautiful little girl began to breastfeed beautifully.

After half an hour Gaby suggested that I go to the toilet to do a big pee to see if the placenta would release itself from within me naturally. As I sat on the toilet I held onto the umbilical cord and within a second it had popped out of me and into the toilet. I screamed out to Gaby who was running to go and get a bowl for the placenta. Too late it landed in the loo.

I decided to take a shower at this time while my husband did the skin on skin. Gaby assisted me, dried me and helped me get dressed. After feeding my beautiful girl, we got into the car and headed to the hospital. Because my beautiful girl had done a green fresh baby poo in the amniotic fluid, she was required to stay in hospital overnight for observation over the next 24hours. I also needed a few stitches inside as well but not on my perineum which I was pleased about.

Upon arriving at the hospital we had a beautiful midwife greet us in the birthing suite we were taken to. She congratulated me for doing an amazing job at accidentally birthing at home and congratulated Gaby and my husband for assisting me as well. When she went to do the baby checks she laughed as she saw the shoelace around the cord and said well done, now that is creative! We all had a laugh at the beautiful bow Gaby had tied with the shoelace around the umbilical cord.

All in all, I could not have been happier with this amazing three and a half hour labour journey. As it turned out my Birth centre midwife was away and they were full so I couldn't have birthed there anyway. In hindsight everything turned out as it was meant to and I could not have been happier with my fast, natural, accidental, birth at home.

What a brilliant way to experience labour.

15

ANYTHING IS POSSIBLE

Trust and Believe in You

Over the many years that I have been attending births and working with pregnant women, I have heard of some extraordinary birth experiences, such as a baby being born off the coast of Western Australia, at Monkey Mia with the dolphins swimming around. The planning that it took to execute this birth was huge as the timing had to be just right to have a professional midwife in attendance. Monkey Mia is a 12 hour drive from Perth up the coast to this remote and beautiful place. The 'midwife' that agreed to be present wanted to arrive not too many days before or arrive late and miss the birth altogether, so it was very tricky to coordinate. Thankfully it was perfect and divine timing and it all worked out well. On the day of the labour everyone was ready including the dolphins who were already 'hanging around' sensing the imminent birth of the baby and when the time was right the labouring woman got into the water and gave birth with the dolphins all in attendance. It was a warm sunny day, and the water temperature was just right. What an incredible experience this must have been for both Mum and bubs and the dolphins as well as the midwife to witness.

Many years ago, a similar story occurred in 1993 in the Red Sea when a couple from England went to birth with some friendly dolphins off the coast in the beautiful warm water. A documentary was made about their journey and is still available today. They had arrived some four weeks before their baby was due to get to know the dolphins as they swam with them every day. On the day the labour started the mum entered the warm almost hot water of the Red Sea with midwife in tow and gave birth with a pod of dolphins in attendance all looking curiously on to see what was happening. I feel this story takes water birthing to a complete other level.

After the birth they returned to their native country and proceeded to teach their beautiful baby girl to swim and returned back to the same place with the dolphins in the Red Sea. The idea now was to film their beautiful little girl swimming underwater with the dolphins. What they had not counted on was one big female dolphin coming right up close and looking straight into their little girl's eyes as she swam happily along. The photos of this experience hang proudly in my studio and I feel so blessed to have heard this story firsthand from Estelle Myers, my mentor and teacher who was truly a pioneer in waterbirth and swimming and interacting with wild dolphins for many years. Sadly, she passed away a few years ago but the memory of what she achieved as an advocate for natural water birth will never be forgotten. Her legacy will always be her film 'Oceana', the promise of tomorrow. A film about waterbirth, Igor Charkovsky, the founder of baby swim, dolphin and whale interactions around the world and many other topics.

I know of a birth that happened in a Tipi in the south of Western Australia in a place called Cosy Corner between Denmark and Albany where a woman called in all her female friends to assist as she laboured around the fire built in the middle of the Tipi. What an amazing and primal natural experience this would have been.

I know of a beautiful baby called Amidases who was born in the natural bush setting of Byron Bay with just his sister present. This freebirth via water was free of any constrictions and restraints placed upon by the medical fraternity and was the most amazing powerful and empowered experience of birth for this mother and her son.

Lastly, I want to share with you that I met a midwife in one of WA highest interventional establishments and she was so excited to meet me as a doula with one of my clients as I was advocating for a natural birth on this day. She was excited due to the fact that this was going to be the first natural birth she had seen in three months since working at this hospital. She then went on to tell me how she had just spent a year in Ghana, in Africa and how the women there walk some twenty kilometres in labour with a basket with their belongings on their heads, to give birth in a small one roomed brick shelter they called the hospital to give birth in. Interestingly, when they arrive, they just lay down on a plank of wood outside that is raised off the ground by bricks and labour silently. The midwives have to watch them as to when they start to stir a little as this is a sign that the baby is coming. They then give birth silently. They spend a few hours or a day to rest and recover before walking back into the wilderness and back to their village. When I heard this story, I was in awe and thought 'WOW' we really have something to learn from these strong amazing women!

I know of stories from an African tribe that walk-in labour to 'the birth tree', with all their specially chosen women, and they hold onto a strong branch and swing their body literally whilst hanging as she works through a contraction. When the baby is ready to be born, she has the women around her lift her legs up into the air to assist the baby out as the baby is received by a few women assisting. How powerful and amazing would that be.

I find it interesting that 'we have forgotten' that women have been birthing through ions of time with no interventions and no assistance at all. Women actually know how to give birth as we are so strong and powerful, but we have just forgotten that we are!

Love your way,

Gabrielle

Something to consider, Today I will make a difference

Today I will make a difference. I will begin by controlling my thoughts.

♥

I am a product of my thoughts.
Because my thoughts create my reality!
So today I will choose to have happy and positive thoughts.
Therefore, I will feel happy and hopeful.

♥

I refuse to feel down about my pregnant body or my circumstances.
I will not let petty inconveniences such as doctor's appointments, routine check-ups, tests or scans annoy me.
I will avoid negativism - especially that associated with birth and birth stories.
Optimism will be my companion and feeling empowered will be my hallmark.

♥

Today I will make a difference in the way I think about my pregnancy and birth.

♥

I will be grateful for the twenty-four hours that are before me. Time is a precious commodity, and I will celebrate each day being pregnant.
I refuse to allow what little time I have to be contaminated by complaining, self-pity, anxiety, or boredom.
I will face this day with the joy of a child and the courage of the strong woman that I am.
I will drink each minute as though it is my last. When tomorrow comes, today will be gone forever. While it is here, I will use it for loving myself and those around me.

♥

Today I will make a difference and I will honour my body and mind and rest if I need to and not feel guilty.

♥

I will not let past birth experiences or stories haunt me.
Even though I may have experienced a not so positive birth journey previously I refuse to allow any negative thoughts associated with the past haunt my thoughts.

❤

Victoriously. I know I can do things differently. The loudest voice in my head is:-

I am strong and I believe in who I am and what I am capable of.

I trust in my body and its ability to birth.

It's OK to feel this way and I will not allow others to make me think otherwise.

❤

Today I will make a difference.

❤

I will spend time with those I love.

Five quality minutes with the people who are going to support me in labour.

Today I will spend at least five minutes with the significant people in my world.

Five quality minutes of talking, hugging, thanking or listening.

Five undiluted minutes, with my mate, children, and friends and support people.

❤

Today I will make a difference because of the positive way in which I am thinking and feeling.

www.ingramcontent.com/pod-product-compliance
Lightning Source LLC
Chambersburg PA
CBHW071726270326
41928CB00013B/2578